Atlas of
Surgical Anatomy
FOR GENERAL SURGEONS

Atlas of Surgical Anatomy
FOR GENERAL SURGEONS

Stephen W. Gray, Ph.D.

Professor of Anatomy
Emory University School of Medicine
Scientific Staff
Emory University Hospital
Consultant to the Medical Staff for Congenital Anomalies
The Piedmont Hospital
Atlanta, Georgia

John E. Skandalakis, M.D., Ph.D., F.A.C.S.

Chris Carlos Professor of Surgical Anatomy and Technique
Assistant Professor of Surgery
Emory University School of Medicine
Senior Attending Surgeon
The Piedmont Hospital
Atlanta, Georgia

David A. McClusky, M.S., M.D.

Former Chief Resident of General Surgery
The Piedmont Hospital
Atlanta, Georgia

Illustrations by John E. McClusky, M.F.A., A.M.I.

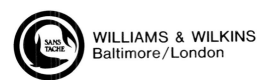

WILLIAMS & WILKINS
Baltimore/London

Editor: Toni M. Tracy
Associate Editor: Jonathan W. Pine, Jr.
Copy Editors: Rosemary Wolfe and Karen King
Design: Joanne Janowiak
Illustration Planning: Wayne Hubbel
Production: Carol L. Eckhart

Copyright © 1985
Williams & Wilkins
428 East Preston Street
Baltimore, MD 21202, U.S.A.

Library of Congress Cataloging in Publication Data

Gray, Stephen Wood, 191 -
    Atlas of surgical anatomy for general surgeons.

    Includes index.
    1. Anatomy, Surgical and topographical. I. Skandalakis, John Elias. II. McClusky,
David A. III. McClusky, John E., (1914-)   . IV. Title.
QM531.G73 1984   611   83–16883
ISBN 0-683-03733-1

Printed in Hong Kong

Dedication

To Thalia and Michael Carlos
In appreciation of their interest and support of
Surgical Anatomy and Technique

"Reach what you can, my child"

"Reach what you cannot"

Nikos Kazantzakis

(from *Report to Greco*, translated from
Greek by P.A. Bien, published by
Simon and Schuster, 1965)

Bernard of Chartres was wont to say that we are as
dwarfs mounted on the shoulders of giants, so that we
can see more and farther than they; yet not by virtue of
the keenness of our eyesight nor through the tallness of
our stature, but because we are raised and born aloft
upon that gigantic mass.

John of Salisbury

Metalogicon iii.4.

Preface

The purpose of this book is to present to the general surgeon the working anatomy of those areas of the human body which are within his special discipline.

The book is essentially the anatomy of the procedures of the general surgeon. We have occasionally introduced remarks on technique to emphasize the complications to be avoided, but this is not a book of surgical technique. There are many atlases of surgical technique, but there are few that emphasize the correct and practical anatomy upon which the techniques are based.

We have given special attention to the anatomical entities which may be injured in the operating room. We hope our drawings and diagrams will remind the surgeon of the pitfalls and risks, ranging from inconvenient to catastrophic, associated with each procedure.

General surgery is changing: for all practical purposes the diaphragm, not very justly, has been taken over by the thoracic surgeon. The general surgeon still claims the veins of the lower extremity, but this too may change.

Some of the sections are long; some are very short. This may reflect our own special interest based on our previous studies in the laboratory or experience in the operating room. In other cases, it reflects the relative complexity of the anatomy rather than the importance of the procedure.

The anatomy illustrated here is not only for the general surgeon but for the resident and young anatomist. It will explain to the last two the reasons why all anatomical details are not equally important to the surgeon, and why, with the introduction of new procedures, some anatomical details, previously described only in fine print, become of the greatest importance. One such example is the segmental anatomy of the spleen which permits partial splenectomy.

Another reason for this book is the decline in the teaching of gross anatomy which has become the stepchild of the basic medical sciences. The topography of the "surgical" anatomical entities is almost unknown to the medical student of today. The true anatomist is not a "sophisticated mortician" as some would have it, but a man or woman who advances the knowledge of the student and thus improves the quality of surgery being practiced on the patient. The true anatomist continues to study the body for clinical and surgical applications demanded by new and improved procedures.

Each of the drawings in this book was conceived as a primitive, classroom blackboard sketch and was born, often after a hard delivery, by Mr. John McClusky as an accurate and artistic illustration. We also acknowledge the influence of the great legacy of anatomical drawing beginning with Vesalius' *Fabrica* and including Anderson's *Grant's Atlas of Anatomy*, Hollinshead's *Anatomy for Surgeons*, Nyhus and Condon's *Hernia*, Pernkopf's *Atlas of Anatomy*, Warwick and Williams' *Gray's Anatomy*, and Netter's *The Ciba Collection of Medical Illustrations*. We may have seen farther because we were standing on the shoulders of these giants.

The illustrations and their legends have been graciously examined and corrected by Dr. Eugene Colborn and Dr. Norbert Jones of the Medical College of Georgia. Ms. Kathleen Manning kept track of the hundreds of illustrations through all stages of their development.

Contents

Atlas of
Surgical Anatomy
FOR GENERAL SURGEONS

PLATE 1-1
Development of the Neck

Only by the end of the first trimester can the neck be distinguished as a constriction between the cranial and thoracic regions. At first, the pharynx and its system of branchial arches and clefts dominate the postcranial region. By the seventh week the site of the neck is indicated by the branchial arches above and the relatively huge pericardium below.

At the end of the third month the growth of the pharynx has slowed, the branchial clefts are no longer visible, and the postpharyngeal foregut (esophagus) is elongating. This elongation carries the head away from the pericardial bulge. Subsequent elevation of the head and the appearance of the sternocleidomastoid and trapezius muscles will establish the form of the adult human neck.

A. The human embryo at 4 weeks of development. The branchial arches are numbered with Roman numerals I to IV.

B. By the seventh week the site of the neck is indicated between the branchial arches above and the pericardium below.

C. The neck approaches its adult form by the end of the third month. The numbered areas indicate the probable contribution of the branchial arches to the anterior and lateral surfaces of the neck.

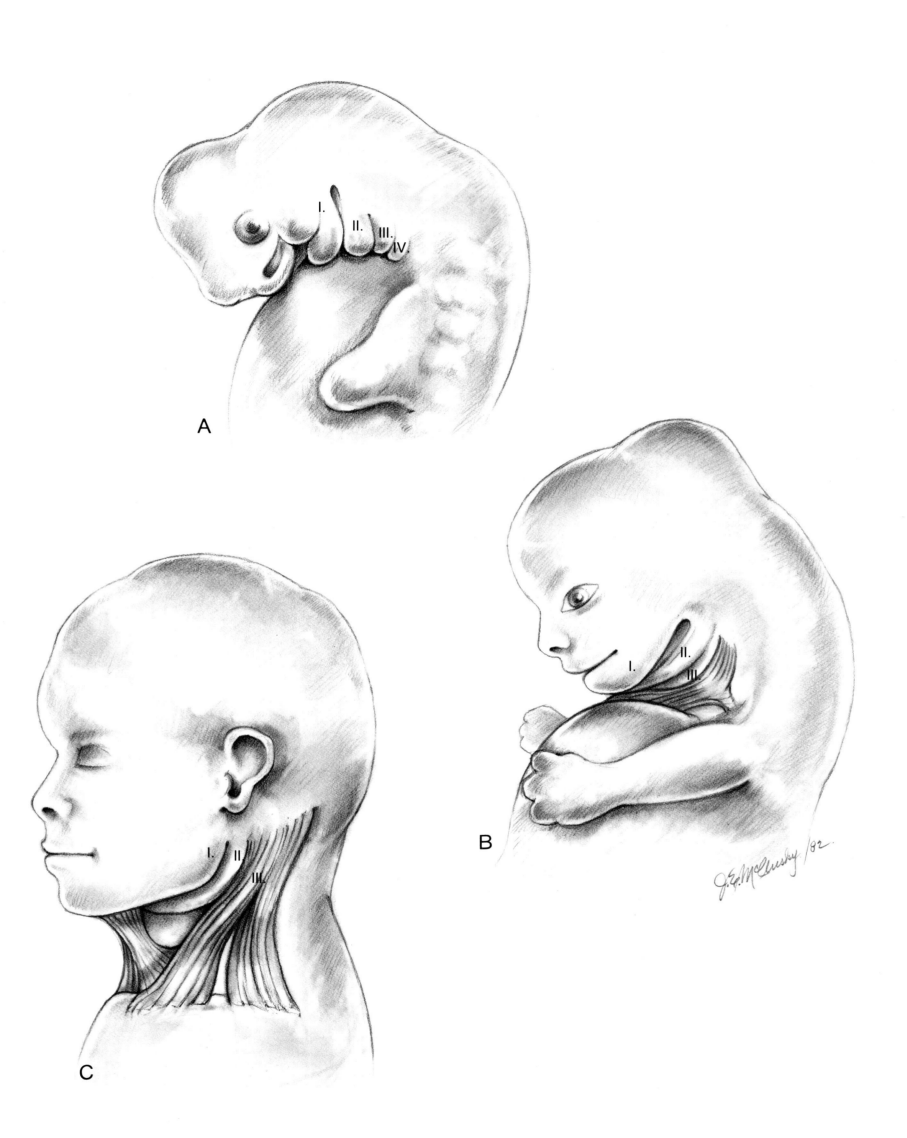

PLATE 1-2
Development of the Foregut: Thyroid, Parathyroid and Thymus

A. Ventral view of the embryonic foregut in the fourth week. Four branchial pouches and the thyroid primordium are present in the pharynx. The trachea, esophagus and stomach are elongating. The pancreatic and hepatic diverticula mark the caudal limit of the foregut.

B. Ventral view of the embryonic foregut and its derivatives at the end of the sixth week. Thyroid, parathyroid and thymus glands have appeared, and all branchial pouches but the first are disappearing. The dorsal portion of the first pouch will persist as the auditory (Eustachian) tube.

C. and D. The superior parathyroid glands and the thymus bodies are descending behind the thyroid gland.

Inset shows the usual position of the adult parathyroid glands. Notice that parathyroid III has become the inferior parathyroid gland having descended past parathyroid IV. The entire thymus is now below the thyroid gland.

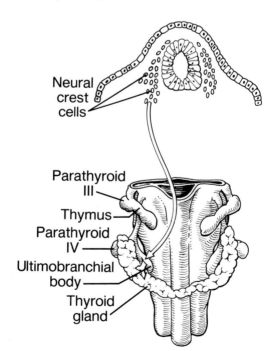

Migration of cells of the neural crest to the ultimobranchial body and subsequently to the thyroid gland. These are calcitonin producing cells (C cells). Medullary carcinoma of the thyroid is concentrated in the middle one third of the gland and may be due to the presence of more C cells in this area.

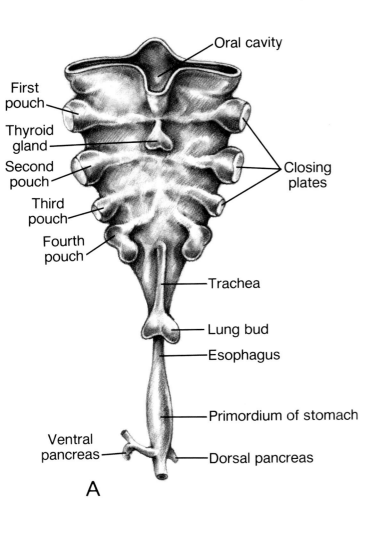

First pouch

Thyroid gland

Second pouch

Third pouch

Fourth pouch

Oral cavity

Closing plates

Trachea

Lung bud

Esophagus

Primordium of stomach

Ventral pancreas

Dorsal pancreas

A

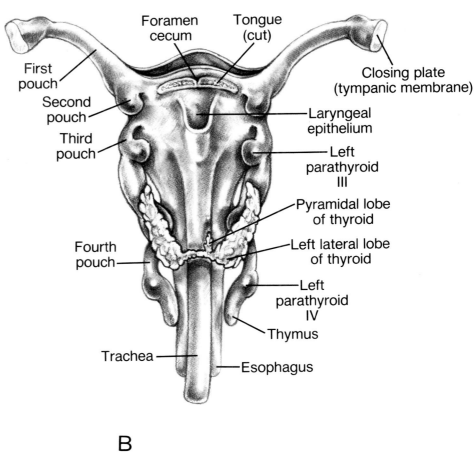

Foramen cecum

Tongue (cut)

First pouch

Second pouch

Third pouch

Fourth pouch

Trachea

Closing plate (tympanic membrane)

Laryngeal epithelium

Left parathyroid III

Pyramidal lobe of thyroid

Left lateral lobe of thyroid

Left parathyroid IV

Thymus

Esophagus

B

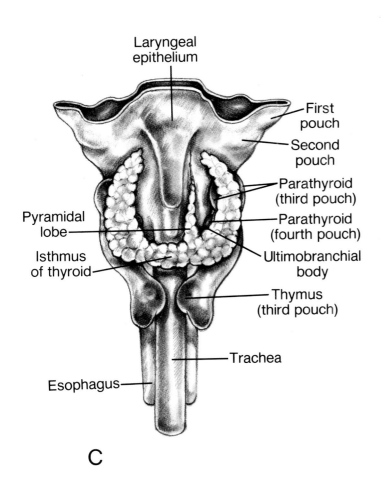

Laryngeal epithelium

First pouch

Second pouch

Parathyroid (third pouch)

Parathyroid (fourth pouch)

Pyramidal lobe

Isthmus of thyroid

Ultimobranchial body

Thymus (third pouch)

Trachea

Esophagus

C

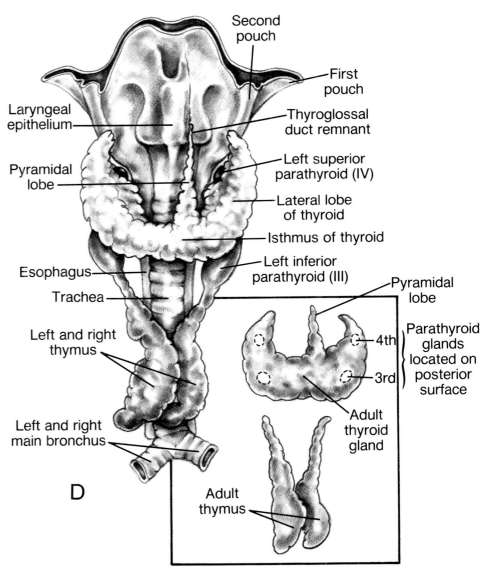

Second pouch

First pouch

Laryngeal epithelium

Thyroglossal duct remnant

Left superior parathyroid (IV)

Pyramidal lobe

Lateral lobe of thyroid

Isthmus of thyroid

Left inferior parathyroid (III)

Esophagus

Trachea

Left and right thymus

Left and right main bronchus

Pyramidal lobe

Parathyroid glands located on posterior surface

4th

3rd

Adult thyroid gland

Adult thymus

D

PLATE 1-3
Derivatives of the Branchial Arches, Clefts and Pouches

PLATE 1-3
Derivatives of the Branchial Arches, Clefts and Pouches

The Pharynx and Its Derivatives

	Arteries and Nerves	Dorsal	Ventral	Floor
I	ARCH Maxillary and mandibular branches of stapedial artery Nerve V$_3$	Incus Tragus and crus of pinna	Meckel's cartilage Malleus	Body of tongue
	CLEFT*	External auditory canal		
	POUCH	Eustachian tube Middle ear cavity Mastoid air cells		
II	ARCH Stapedial artery Nerves VII and VIII	Stapes	Styloid process Hyoid (lesser horn and part of body)	Root of tongue Foramen cecum Thyroid gland
	POUCH	Palatine tonsil Supratonsilar fossa		
III	ARCH Internal carotid artery Nerve IX		Hyoid (greater horn and part of body) Part of epiglottis	
	POUCH	Inferior parathyroid Pyriform fossa	Thymus	
IV	ARCH Arch of aorta (left) Part of subclavian artery (right) Nerve X		Thyroid and cuneiform cartilages Part of epiglottis	
	POUCH	Superior parathyroid	Thymus (inconstant)	
V	ARCH	Transitory in humans		
	POUCH	Ultimobranchial body (C cells of thyroid)		
VI	ARCH Proximal: pulmonary artery Distal: ductus arteriosus (left) Nerve X (recurrent laryngeal)		Cricoid, arytenoid and corniculate cartilages	

* all other clefts normally disappear

PLATE 1-4
Anomalies of the Pharyngeal Derivatives

Some anomalies, such as a persistent thyroglossal duct, are common; others, such as a third cleft fistula, are very rare. Most cervical fistulas and sinuses are of second pouch and cleft origin.

The surgeon should be familiar with the relations of these cysts, sinuses or fistulas. They must be removed completely to prevent recurrence.

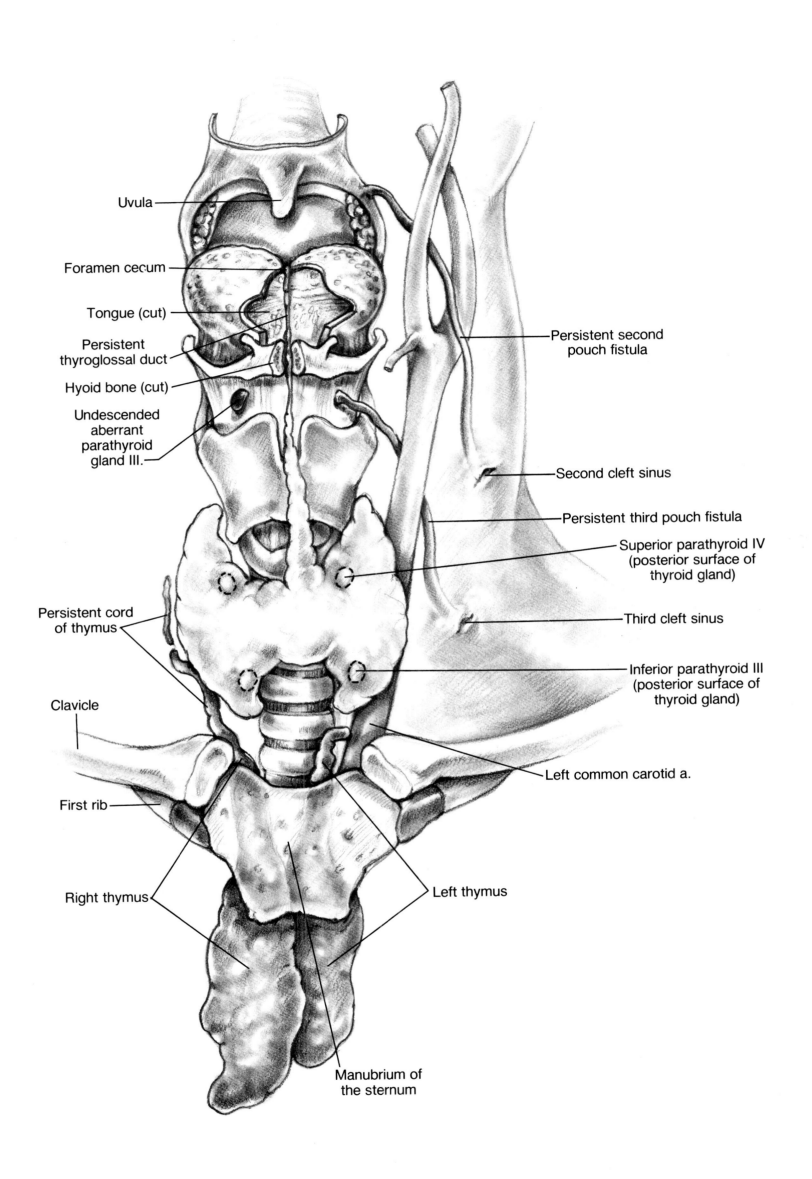

Uvula

Foramen cecum

Tongue (cut)

Persistent
thyroglossal duct

Hyoid bone (cut)

Undescended
aberrant
parathyroid
gland III.

Persistent cord
of thymus

Clavicle

Right thymus

First rib

Persistent second
pouch fistula

Second cleft sinus

Persistent third pouch fistula

Superior parathyroid IV
(posterior surface of
thyroid gland)

Third cleft sinus

Inferior parathyroid III
(posterior surface of
thyroid gland)

Left common carotid a.

Left thymus

Manubrium of
the sternum

PLATE 1-5
Cysts of Second Branchial Cleft or Pouch Origin

These are the most frequently encountered branchial malformations.

A. Superficial cyst of the neck representing persistence of the superficial portion of the second branchial cleft.

B. Larger second cleft cyst compressing the jugular vein.

C. Deep cyst of the second branchial cleft lying in the bifurcation of the carotid artery.

D. Cyst of the second branchial pouch lying deep to the carotid arteries, close to the pharyngeal wall.

Remember:

1) Superficial cysts become sinus tracts and eventually become infected. Aspiration or drainage is useless. All of the lining epithelium of cysts and sinuses must be removed surgically to prevent recurrence.

2) Second cleft cysts and fistulas lie near, or pass through, the crotch of the bifurcation of the carotid arteries exposing them to possible injury.

3) The following nerves should be protected: mandibular and cervical branches of the facial nerve, spinal accessory nerve, hypoglossal nerve, and vagus nerve.

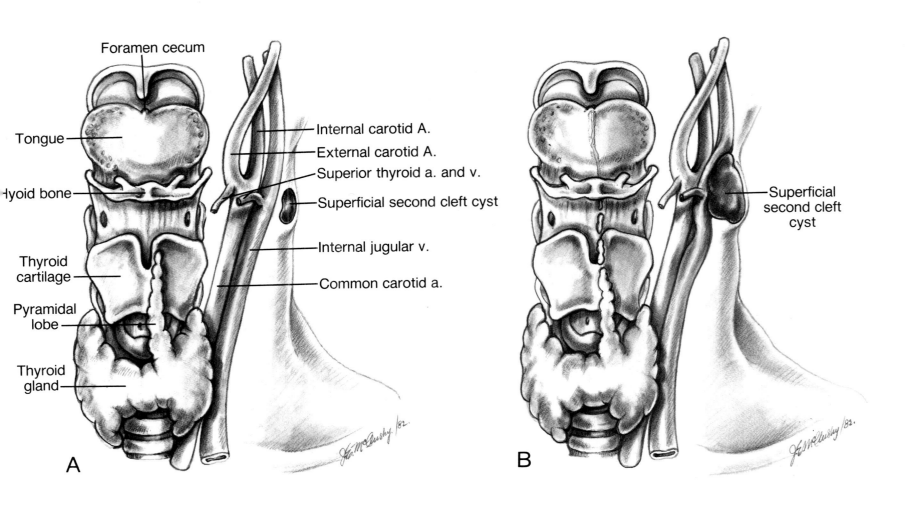

Foramen cecum

Tongue

Hyoid bone

Thyroid cartilage

Pyramidal lobe

Thyroid gland

Internal carotid A.

External carotid A.

Superior thyroid a. and v.

Superficial second cleft cyst

Internal jugular v.

Common carotid a.

A

Superficial second cleft cyst

B

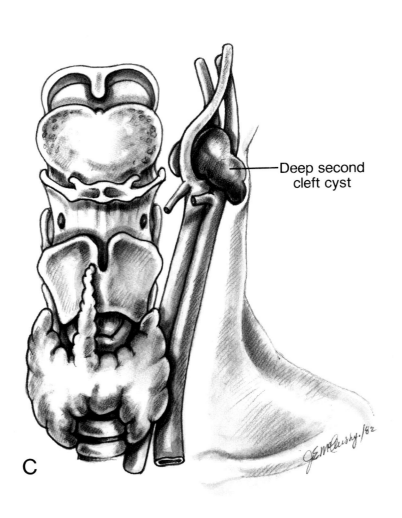

Deep second cleft cyst

C

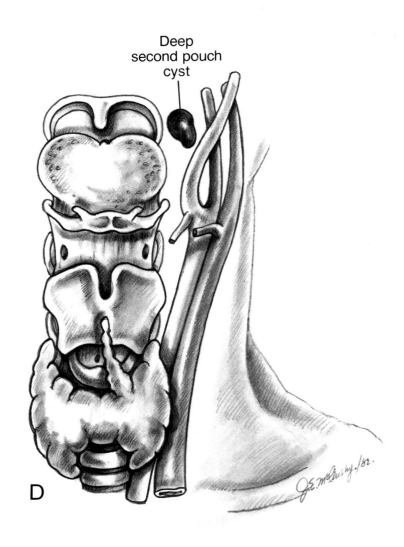

Deep second pouch cyst

D

PLATE 1-6
The Roof of the Submandibular Triangle

A. The platysma muscle lies in the superficial fascia, over the mandibular and cervical branches of the facial nerve.

B, C and D. The neural "hammocks" formed by the mandibular branch and the anterior ramus of the cervical branch of the facial nerve (measurements in cm). In B and C, both hammocks lie *below* the mandibular border. In D the mandibular branch is *above* the mandibular border. To ensure protection of these branches, the incision should be 4 cm *below* the mandibular border.

Remember:

1) Careful incision of the platysma muscle will reveal veins to be ligated or cauterized. The anterior cutaneous nerves (C_2-C_3) and the supraclavicular nerves may be cut.

2) Injury to the mandibular branch results in severe drooling at the corner of the mouth. Injury to the cervical branch results in minimal drooling that disappears in 4 to 6 months.

3) Be sure to approximate the cut edges of the platysma muscle for good cosmetic results following neck surgery.

For deeper exposure of the submandibular triangle, see Plate 1-20.

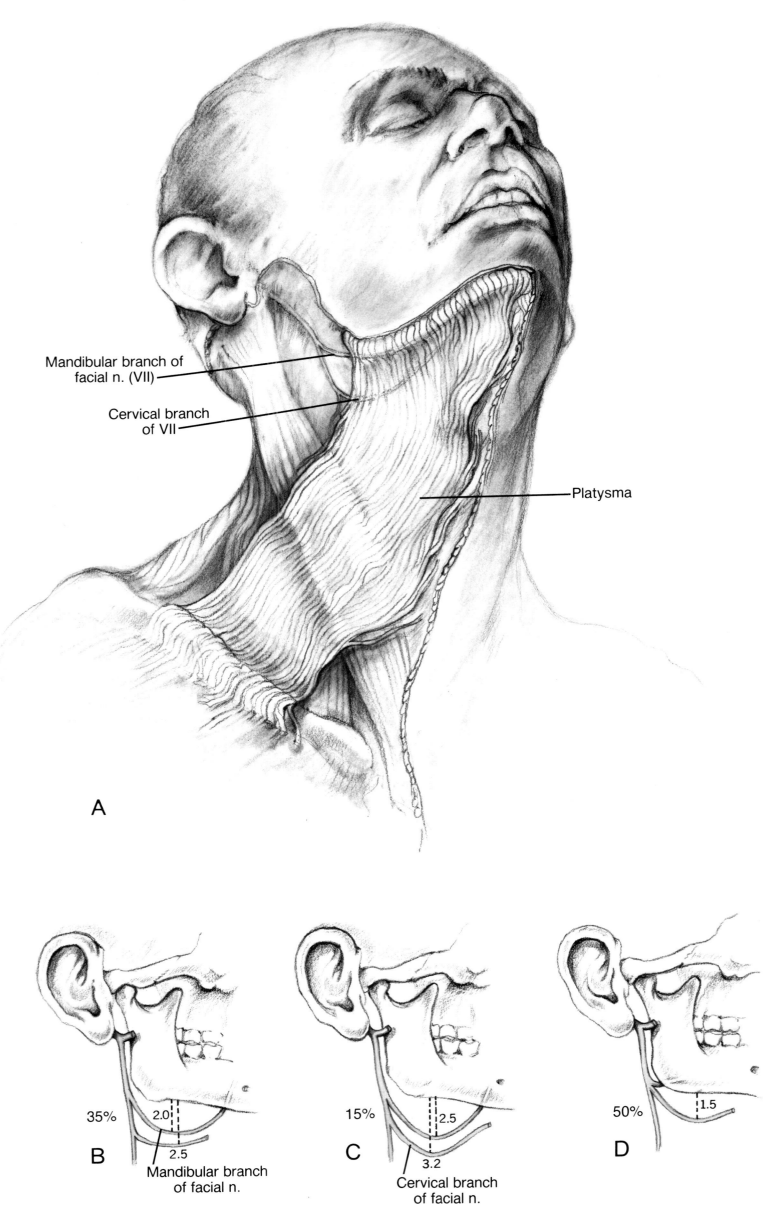

Mandibular branch of facial n. (VII)

Cervical branch of VII

Platysma

A

B

35%

2.0

2.5

Mandibular branch of facial n.

C

15%

2.5

3.2

Cervical branch of facial n.

D

50%

1.5

PLATE 1-7
The Fasciae of the Neck

Section through the neck showing the fascial planes at the level of the thyroid isthmus and the seventh cervical vertebra.

Inset: The superficial fascia of the neck lies between the skin and the investing layer of deep fascia. It contains the platysma muscle and some veins and arteries.

Remember:

1) The investing layer of the deep cervical fascia envelops *two* muscles (trapezius and sternocleidomastoid), *two* salivary glands (submandibular and parotid), and forms *two* spaces (supraclavicular and suprasternal). It gives rise to *two* fasciae (pretracheal and prevertebral) which form the carotid sheath.

2) The axillary sheath, formed by the prevertebral fascia, is associated with the scalene muscles and forms part of the floor of the posterior triangle.

3) In a radical neck dissection the whole of the deep cervical fascia must be removed because of its relation to the lymphatics of the neck. The carotid sheath and the internal jugular vein with its lymph nodes may be sacrificed.

4) Spare the hypoglossal, recurrent and superior laryngeal nerves, and the sympathetic trunk.

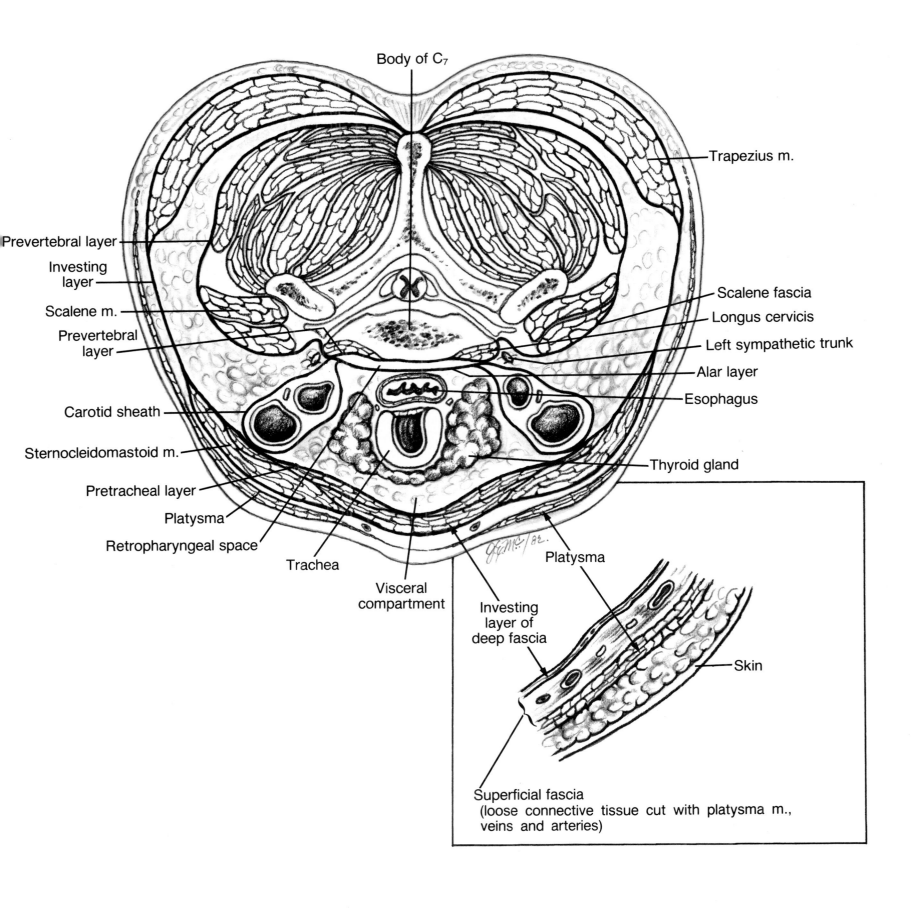

Body of C₇

Trapezius m.

Prevertebral layer

Investing layer

Scalene m.

Prevertebral layer

Scalene fascia

Longus cervicis

Left sympathetic trunk

Alar layer

Esophagus

Carotid sheath

Sternocleidomastoid m.

Thyroid gland

Pretracheal layer

Platysma

Retropharyngeal space

Trachea

Visceral compartment

Platysma

Investing layer of deep fascia

Skin

Superficial fascia
(loose connective tissue cut with platysma m., veins and arteries)

PLATE 1-8
The Anterior and Posterior Triangles of the Neck I (lateral view)

The anterior triangle may be divided into four smaller triangles. These, with their contents are:

1) Submental triangle: submental lymph nodes, branches of the submental artery and vein.

2) Submandibular triangle: see Plate 1-20.

3) Carotid triangle: carotid artery bifurcation and carotid body (see Plate 1-12), thyroid, occipital and ascending pharyngeal arteries, the vagus, hypoglossal, ansa cervicalis, and spinal accessory nerves, and part of the cervical sympathetic trunk.

4) Muscular triangle: trachea, esophagus, thyroid gland, parathyroid glands, ansa cervicalis nerve and sympathetic trunk.

Remember:

The posterior belly of the digastric muscle is an excellent landmark. Behind it lie the internal and external carotid arteries, the jugular vein, 10th, 11th and 12th nerves, and the superior horizontal chain of lymph nodes.

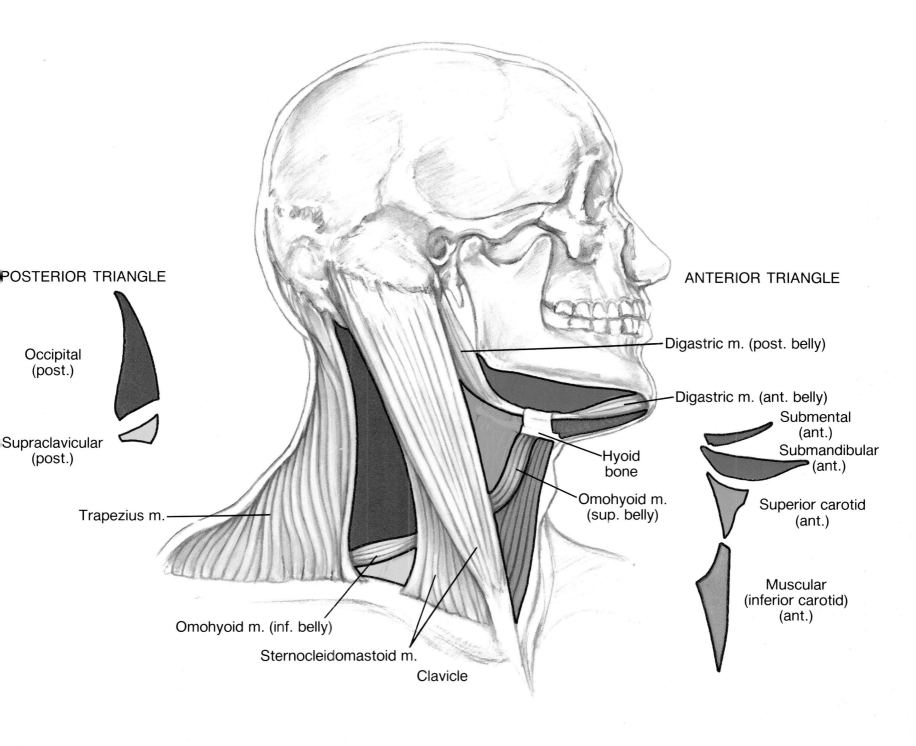

POSTERIOR TRIANGLE

Occipital
(post.)

Supraclavicular
(post.)

Trapezius m.

Omohyoid m. (inf. belly)

Sternocleidomastoid m.

Clavicle

ANTERIOR TRIANGLE

Digastric m. (post. belly)

Digastric m. (ant. belly)

Submental
(ant.)

Submandibular
(ant.)

Hyoid
bone

Superior carotid
(ant.)

Omohyoid m.
(sup. belly)

Muscular
(inferior carotid)
(ant.)

PLATE 1-9
The Anterior and Posterior Triangles of the Neck II (anterior view)

The contents of the anterior triangle are listed above (Plate 1-8). The contents of the posterior triangle are: subclavian artery and vein, cervical, phrenic, accessory phrenic, and spinal accessory nerves, brachial plexus and lymph nodes.

Remember:

1) The spinal accessory nerve is an excellent anatomical landmark in the posterior triangle.

2) The area between the clavicle and the spinal accessory nerve is the danger zone.

3) The surgeon should be familiar with the following anatomical entities in this danger zone: a) spinal accessory nerve; b) nerves to rhomboid and serratus muscles; c) internal jugular vein. This is the first vein to be injured in a radical neck dissection. It may be ligated; d) thoracic duct. It may be ligated; e) The cupula of the pleura projects 4 cm above the first rib deep in the root of the neck. The cupula is covered by the suprapleural membrane (Sibson's fascia). Perforation of the pleura, resulting in iatrogenic pneumothorax, hemothorax, or chylothorax, must be avoided.

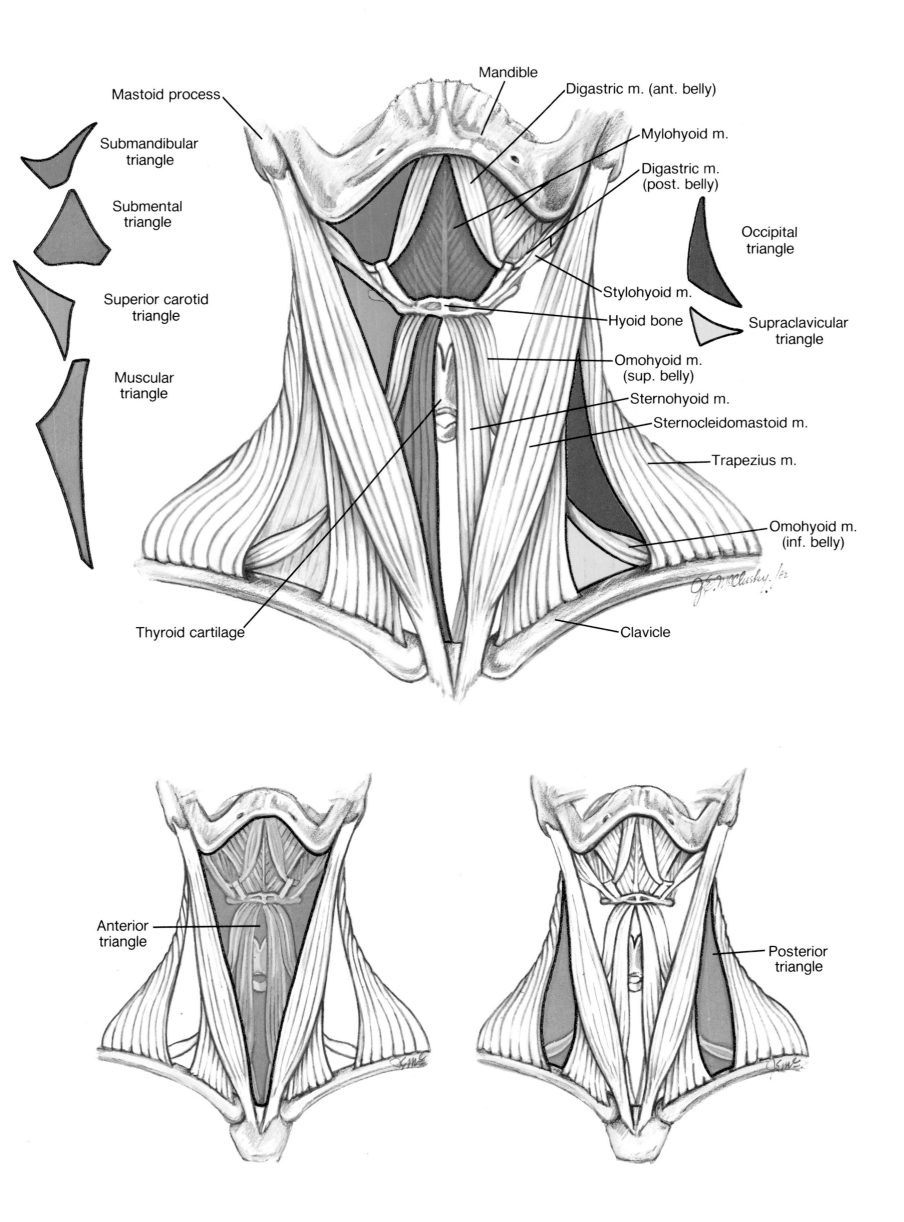

Mastoid process

Submandibular triangle

Submental triangle

Superior carotid triangle

Muscular triangle

Mandible

Digastric m. (ant. belly)

Mylohyoid m.

Digastric m. (post. belly)

Occipital triangle

Stylohyoid m.

Hyoid bone

Supraclavicular triangle

Omohyoid m. (sup. belly)

Sternohyoid m.

Sternocleidomastoid m.

Trapezius m.

Omohyoid m. (inf. belly)

Thyroid cartilage

Clavicle

Anterior triangle

Posterior triangle

PLATE 1-10
General Anterior View of the Neck

A. On the right side of the neck, the separation between the fibers of the clavicular and of the sternal portions of the sternocleidomastoid muscle has been exaggerated to show the underlying carotid sheath.

On the left side of the neck the sternocleidomastoid muscle and the medial portion of the clavical have been removed.

Inset: The relationship of the cupula of the left pleura with the first rib and the subclavian artery and vein.

Remember:

1) The carotid sheath contains the common carotid artery, the internal jugular vein and the vagus nerve.

2) The sternocleidomastoid muscle protects the carotid sheath.

3) The deep cervical lymph nodes (intermediate vertical chain) are located within the sheath medial and lateral to the internal jugular vein.

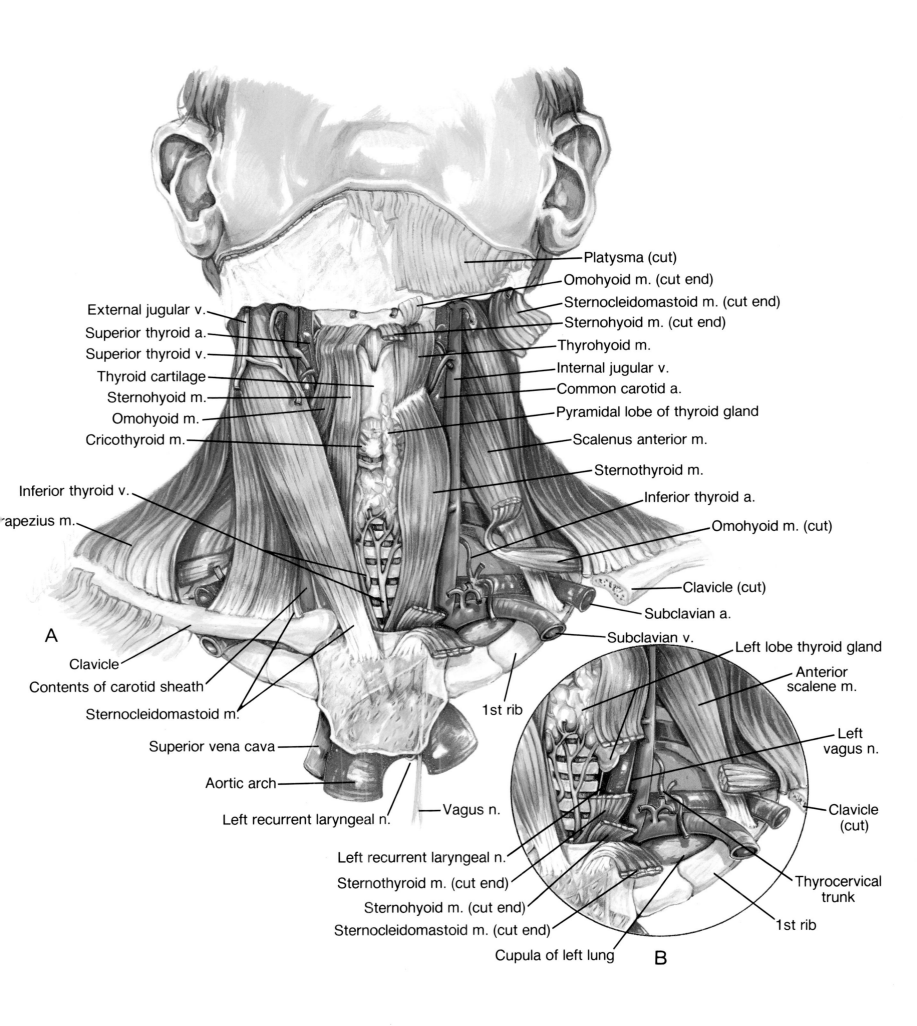

External jugular v.

Superior thyroid a.

Superior thyroid v.

Thyroid cartilage

Sternohyoid m.

Omohyoid m.

Cricothyroid m.

Inferior thyroid v.

Trapezius m.

A

Clavicle

Contents of carotid sheath

Sternocleidomastoid m.

Superior vena cava

Aortic arch

Left recurrent laryngeal n.

Platysma (cut)

Omohyoid m. (cut end)

Sternocleidomastoid m. (cut end)

Sternohyoid m. (cut end)

Thyrohyoid m.

Internal jugular v.

Common carotid a.

Pyramidal lobe of thyroid gland

Scalenus anterior m.

Sternothyroid m.

Inferior thyroid a.

Omohyoid m. (cut)

Clavicle (cut)

Subclavian a.

Subclavian v.

1st rib

Vagus n.

Left recurrent laryngeal n.

Sternothyroid m. (cut end)

Sternohyoid m. (cut end)

Sternocleidomastoid m. (cut end)

Cupula of left lung

Left lobe thyroid gland

Anterior scalene m.

Left vagus n.

Clavicle (cut)

Thyrocervical trunk

1st rib

B

PLATE 1-11
Deep Anterior View of the Neck

Center: The sternocleidomastoid, the strap muscles and the clavicles have been removed to expose the thyroid gland.

Left *inset*: The right lobe of the thyroid gland has been retracted medially; the superior thyroid artery and vein, and the middle thyroid vein, have been cut. The inferior thyroid artery has been preserved. Two parathyroid glands are visible.

Right *inset*: The left subclavian vein has been retracted to show the entrance of the thoracic duct. The duct may enter as one or as several trunks. If injured the duct may be ligated safely.

Remember:

1) Do not stretch the recurrent laryngeal nerve by pulling on the thyroid gland.

2) The superior thyroid artery and the middle thyroid vein may retract when cut; ligate carefully. The superior artery enters the gland superficially and the inferior artery enters posteriorly.

3) The superior artery and the external laryngeal branch of the superior laryngeal nerve travel together at the upper pole of the thyroid gland. Ligate the artery, including a small part of the thyroid pole in benign disease, to avoid injury to the external laryngeal nerve with paralysis or the cricothyroid muscle.

4) The thoracic duct reaches the level of the seventh cervical vertebra and turns down to terminate in the angle formed by the subclavian and internal jugular veins.

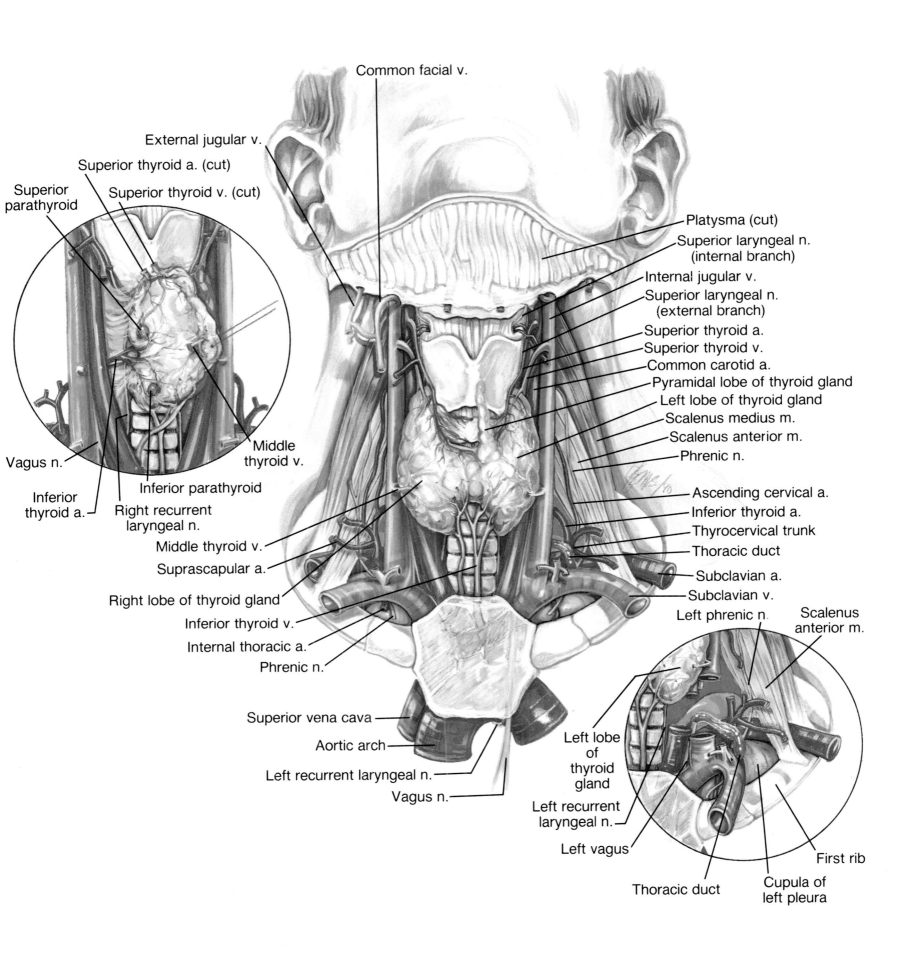

Common facial v.

External jugular v.

Superior thyroid a. (cut)

Superior thyroid v. (cut)

Superior parathyroid

Vagus n.

Inferior thyroid a.

Inferior parathyroid

Right recurrent laryngeal n.

Middle thyroid v.

Middle thyroid v.

Suprascapular a.

Right lobe of thyroid gland

Inferior thyroid v.

Internal thoracic a.

Phrenic n.

Superior vena cava

Aortic arch

Left recurrent laryngeal n.

Vagus n.

Platysma (cut)

Superior laryngeal n. (internal branch)

Internal jugular v.

Superior laryngeal n. (external branch)

Superior thyroid a.

Superior thyroid v.

Common carotid a.

Pyramidal lobe of thyroid gland

Left lobe of thyroid gland

Scalenus medius m.

Scalenus anterior m.

Phrenic n.

Ascending cervical a.

Inferior thyroid a.

Thyrocervical trunk

Thoracic duct

Subclavian a.

Subclavian v.

Left phrenic n.

Scalenus anterior m.

Left lobe of thyroid gland

Left recurrent laryngeal n.

Left vagus

Thoracic duct

Cupula of left pleura

First rib

PLATE 1-12
Some Nerves of the Neck

A. and B. The innervation of the strap muscles of the neck by the cervical plexus and the hypoglossal nerve. The broken line indicates the level at which these muscles and their nerves may be sectioned to preserve their function, as well as possible, and to expose the thyroid gland.

C. The bifurcation of the right carotid artery, the carotid body and its nerve supply. Manipulation, or pressure from an instrument, during a radical neck procedure may produce a fall in blood pressure.

Remember:

1) The ansa hypoglossi is formed by cervical nerves 1, 2 and 3 which join the hypoglossal nerve.

2) The superior cervical sympathetic ganglion participates in the formation of the cervical plexus with gray rami communicantes to the first four cervical nerves.

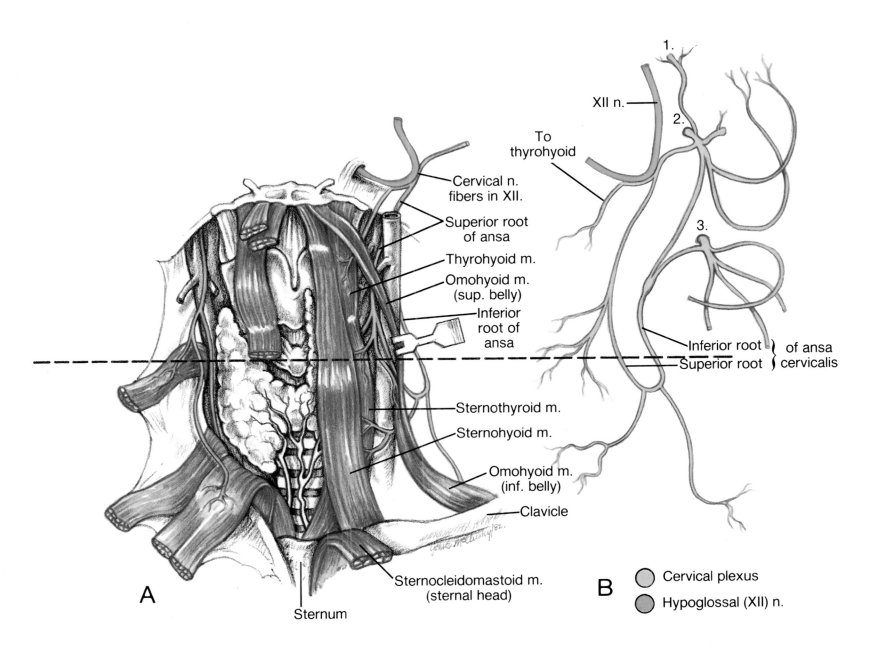

A

Cervical n. fibers in XII.
Superior root of ansa
Thyrohyoid m.
Omohyoid m. (sup. belly)
Inferior root of ansa
Sternothyroid m.
Sternohyoid m.
Omohyoid m. (inf. belly)
Clavicle
Sternocleidomastoid m. (sternal head)
Sternum

B

1.
XII n.
To thyrohyoid
2.
3.
Inferior root } of ansa
Superior root } cervicalis

○ Cervical plexus
● Hypoglossal (XII) n.

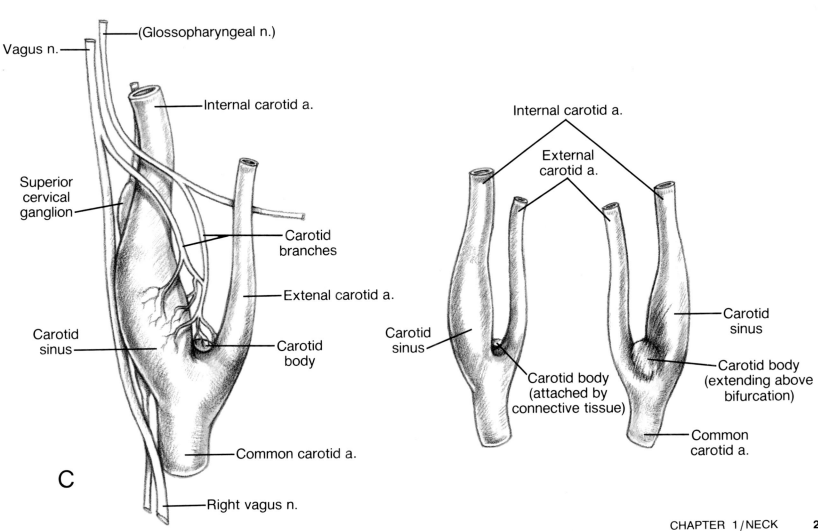

C

Vagus n.
(Glossopharyngeal n.)
Internal carotid a.
Superior cervical ganglion
Carotid branches
Extenal carotid a.
Carotid sinus
Carotid body
Common carotid a.
Right vagus n.

Internal carotid a.
External carotid a.
Carotid sinus
Carotid body (attached by connective tissue)
Carotid sinus
Carotid body (extending above bifurcation)
Common carotid a.

PLATE 1-13
Vessels, Lymph Nodes and Parathyroid Glands

A. The thyroid gland has been removed to show the veins and arteries. Lymph nodes are shown at the most common sites. Notice the retrothyroid tracheal nodes that must not be mistaken for parathyroid glands or for sympathetic ganglia.

B. As in preceding figure but with thyroid and parathyroid glands in place. The extreme superior and inferior locations of the latter are shown.

Remember:

1) Most parathyroid glands will lie between the false and the true capsule of the thyroid gland, about 2.5 cm above to 2.5 cm below the entrance of the inferior thyroid artery into the thyroid. The inferior thyroid artery may be absent (2 to 5%).

2) Absence of the inferior thyroid artery increases the risk of injury to the recurrent laryngeal nerve.

3) The highest reported location of a parathyroid gland is at the upper pole of the thyroid gland; the lowest is in the thymus.

4) Four glands are present in 80% of subjects. More than four glands are found in 6%, fewer than four in 14%. Do not remove normal glands.

5) Deep lymph nodes must be identified to avoid accidental removal of sympathetic ganglia with resulting Horner's syndrome. Any "lymph node" near the vertebral artery in front of the transverse process of the seventh cervical vertebra may prove to be a ganglion.

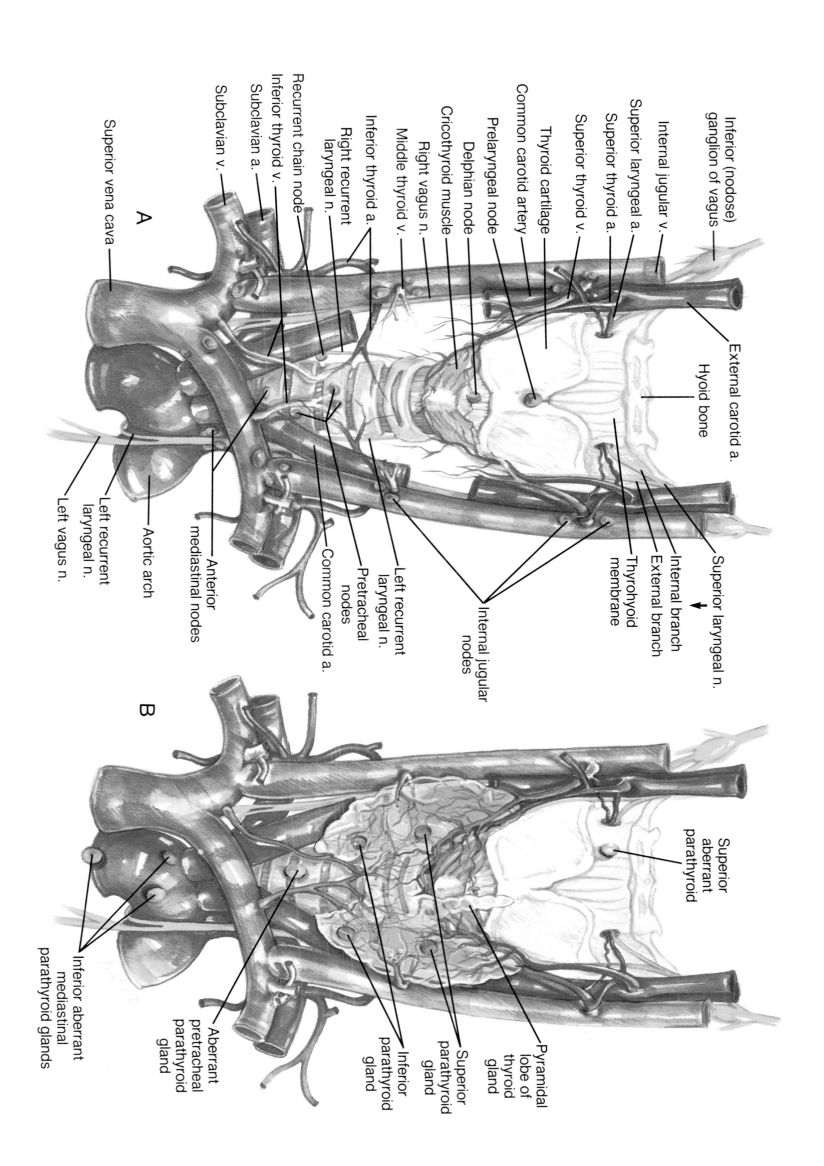

A

Inferior (nodose) ganglion of vagus

Internal jugular v.

Superior laryngeal a.

Superior thyroid a.

Superior thyroid v.

Thyroid cartilage

Common carotid artery

Prelaryngeal node

Delphian node

Cricothyroid muscle

Right vagus n.

Middle thyroid v.

Inferior thyroid a.

Right recurrent laryngeal n.

Recurrent chain node

Inferior thyroid v.

Subclavian a.

Subclavian v.

Superior vena cava

Left recurrent laryngeal n.

Aortic arch

Anterior mediastinal nodes

Common carotid a.

Pretracheal nodes

Left recurrent laryngeal n.

Internal jugular nodes

Left vagus n.

External carotid a.

Hyoid bone

Superior laryngeal n.

Internal branch

External branch

Thyrohyoid membrane

B

Superior aberrant parathyroid

Inferior aberrant mediastinal parathyroid glands

Aberrant pretracheal parathyroid gland

Inferior parathyroid gland

Superior parathyroid gland

Pyramidal lobe of thyroid gland

CHAPTER 1 / NECK   27

PLATE 1-14
Lymphatic Drainage of the Neck I

A. The 300 lymph nodes of the neck (out of 800 in the human body) have been arbitrarily grouped by Healey in two horizontal and three vertical chains of communicating nodes. Their drainage is described in Plate 1-15.

B. Most of the lymphatic drainage enters the right lymphatic duct or, on the left, the thoracic duct. Lymphatic trunks may enter the subclavian veins or the internal jugular veins separately. There is considerable variation in their pattern.

C. The tonsilar ring of Waldeyer. The components of the ring are shown in the coronal section through the nasal cavity above, the pharynx, and the esophagus below.

Inset: In addition to the chains of cervical lymph nodes, the tonsilar region of the pharynx is provided with subepithelial lymphoid organs that drain to some nodes in the neck. They produce lymphocytes that pass in large numbers directly into the pharynx.

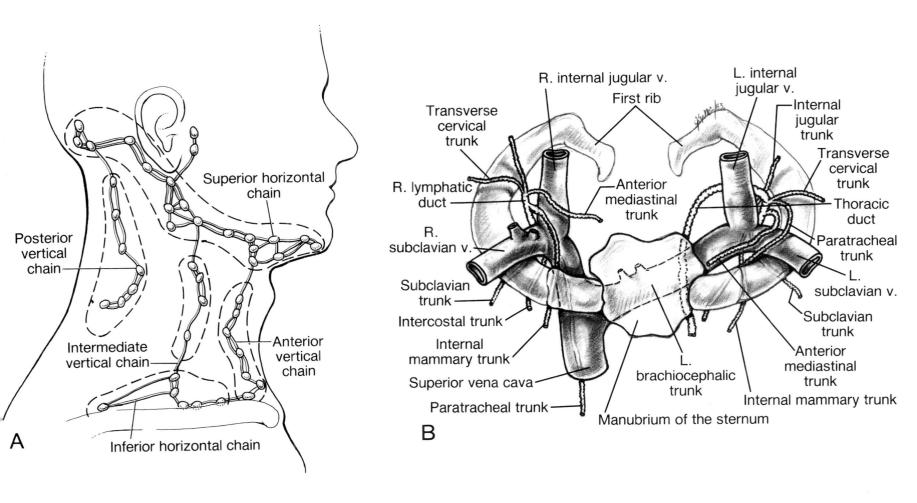

A

Posterior
vertical
chain

Superior horizontal
chain

Intermediate
vertical chain

Anterior
vertical
chain

Inferior horizontal chain

B

R. internal jugular v.

First rib

L. internal
jugular v.

Internal
jugular
trunk

Transverse
cervical
trunk

R. lymphatic
duct

R.
subclavian v.

Anterior
mediastinal
trunk

Transverse
cervical
trunk

Thoracic
duct

Paratracheal
trunk

L.
subclavian v.

Subclavian
trunk

Intercostal trunk

Internal
mammary trunk

Superior vena cava

Paratracheal trunk

L.
brachiocephalic
trunk

Manubrium of the sternum

Subclavian
trunk

Anterior
mediastinal
trunk

Internal mammary trunk

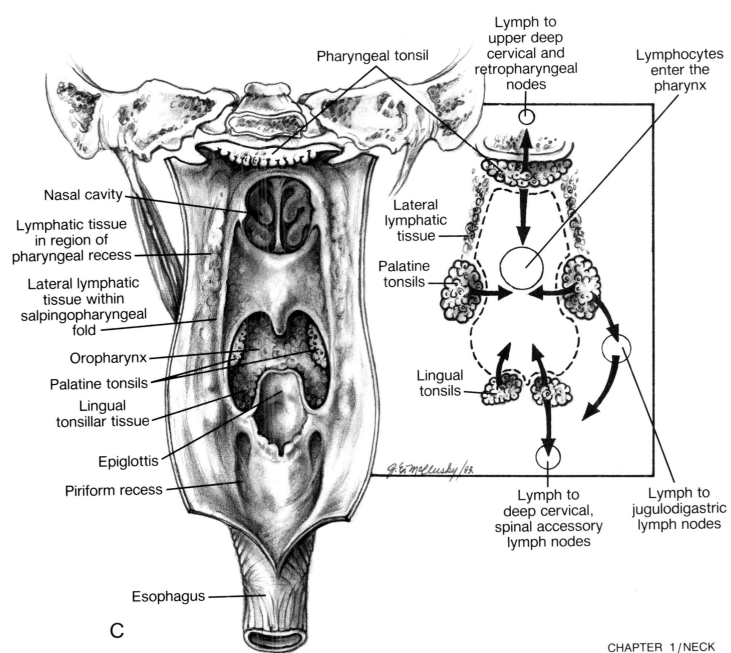

Pharyngeal tonsil

Lymph to
upper deep
cervical and
retropharyngeal
nodes

Lymphocytes
enter the
pharynx

Nasal cavity

Lymphatic tissue
in region of
pharyngeal recess

Lateral
lymphatic
tissue

Lateral lymphatic
tissue within
salpingopharyngeal
fold

Oropharynx

Palatine tonsils

Lingual
tonsillar tissue

Palatine
tonsils

Lingual
tonsils

Epiglottis

Piriform recess

Esophagus

C

Lymph to
deep cervical,
spinal accessory
lymph nodes

Lymph to
jugulodigastric
lymph nodes

G.E.McClusky/93.

PLATE 1-15
Lymphatic Drainage of the Neck II

A. The Two Horizontal Chains of Nodes

	Location	Lymphatics From	To
1. Superior Horizontal Chain			
Submental nodes	Submental triangle	Skin of chin and lip; Floor of mouth, tip of tongue	Submandibular nodes or jugular chain
Submandibular nodes	Submandibular triangle	Submental nodes, oral cavity; face (except forehead and part of lower lip)	Intermediate jugular nodes; deep posterior cervical nodes
Preauricular (parotid) nodes	In front of tragus	Lateral surface of pinna, side of scalp, forehead, part of eyelids	Submandibular nodes
Postauricular (mastoid) nodes	Mastoid process	Medial surface of pinna, temporal scalp; external auditory meatus	Deep cervical nodes
Occipital nodes	Between mastoid process and external occipital protuberance	Back of scalp	Deep cervical nodes
2. Inferior Horizontal Chain			
Supraclavicular and scalene nodes	Subclavian triangle	Axilla, thorax, vertical chain	Jugular or subclavian trunks to right lymphatic duct and thoracic duct

PLATE 1-15
Lymphatic Drainage of the Neck III

B. The Three Vertical Chains of Nodes

| | | Lymphatics | |
	Location	From	To
3. Posterior Vertical Chain (posterior triangle) nodes		Subparotid nodes, jugular chain, occipital and mastoid area	Supraclavicular and deep cervical nodes
a) Superficial	Along external jugular vein		
b) Deep	Along spinal accessory nerve		
4. Intermediate (jugular) Vertical Chain		All other nodes of neck	Lymphatic trunks to left and right thoracic ducts
a) Juguloparotid (subparotid) nodes	Angle of mandible near parotid gland	Parotid gland	Same as above
b) Jugulodigastric (subdigastric) nodes	Junction of common facial and internal jugular veins	Palatine tonsils	Same as above
c) Jugulocarotid (bifurcation) nodes	Bifurcation of common carotid artery close to carotid body	Tongue, except tip	Same as above
d) Jugulo-omohyoid (omohyoid) nodes	Crossing of omohyoid and internal jugular vein	Tip of tongue	Same as above
5. Anterior (visceral) Vertical Chain			
a) Parapharyngeal nodes	Lateral and posterior wall of pharynx	Deep face and esophagus	Intermediate nodes
b) Paralaryngeal nodes	Lateral wall of larynx	Larynx and thyroid gland	Deep cervical nodes
c) Paratracheal nodes	Lateral wall of trachea	Thyroid gland, trachea, esophagus	Deep cervical and mediastinal nodes
d) Prelaryngeal (Delphian) nodes	Cricothyroid ligament	Thyroid gland, and pharynx	Deep cervical nodes
e) Pretracheal nodes	Anterior wall of trachea below isthmus of thyroid gland	Thyroid gland, trachea, esophagus	Deep cervical and mediastinal nodes

PLATE 1-16
Retrosternal Goiter I

A. Diagram of retrosternal goiter and its relation to the mediastinal pleura.

B. Course of the thyroid ima artery (inconstant, 1.5 to 12.2%). The thyroid ima artery may arise from the brachiocephalic artery, the right common carotid artery or the aortic arch. It may be as large as the inferior thyroid artery or be a mere twig. Its presence is important in performing a tracheostomy.

C. Diagram of pretracheal (anterior mediastinal) and posttracheal (posterior mediastinal) pathways which may be taken by a retrosternal goiter.

Remember:

1) Intrathoracic thyroid may descend into the superior, anterior or posterior mediastinum, and may be attached to the mediastinal pleurae.

2) Pneumothorax or pneumomediastinum can occur during the removal of such goiter.

3) The recurrent laryngeal nerve and the inferior thyroid arteries and veins are posterior to the gland when the goiter is in the anterior mediastinum, and anterior to the gland when the goiter is in the posterior mediastinum. Be careful.

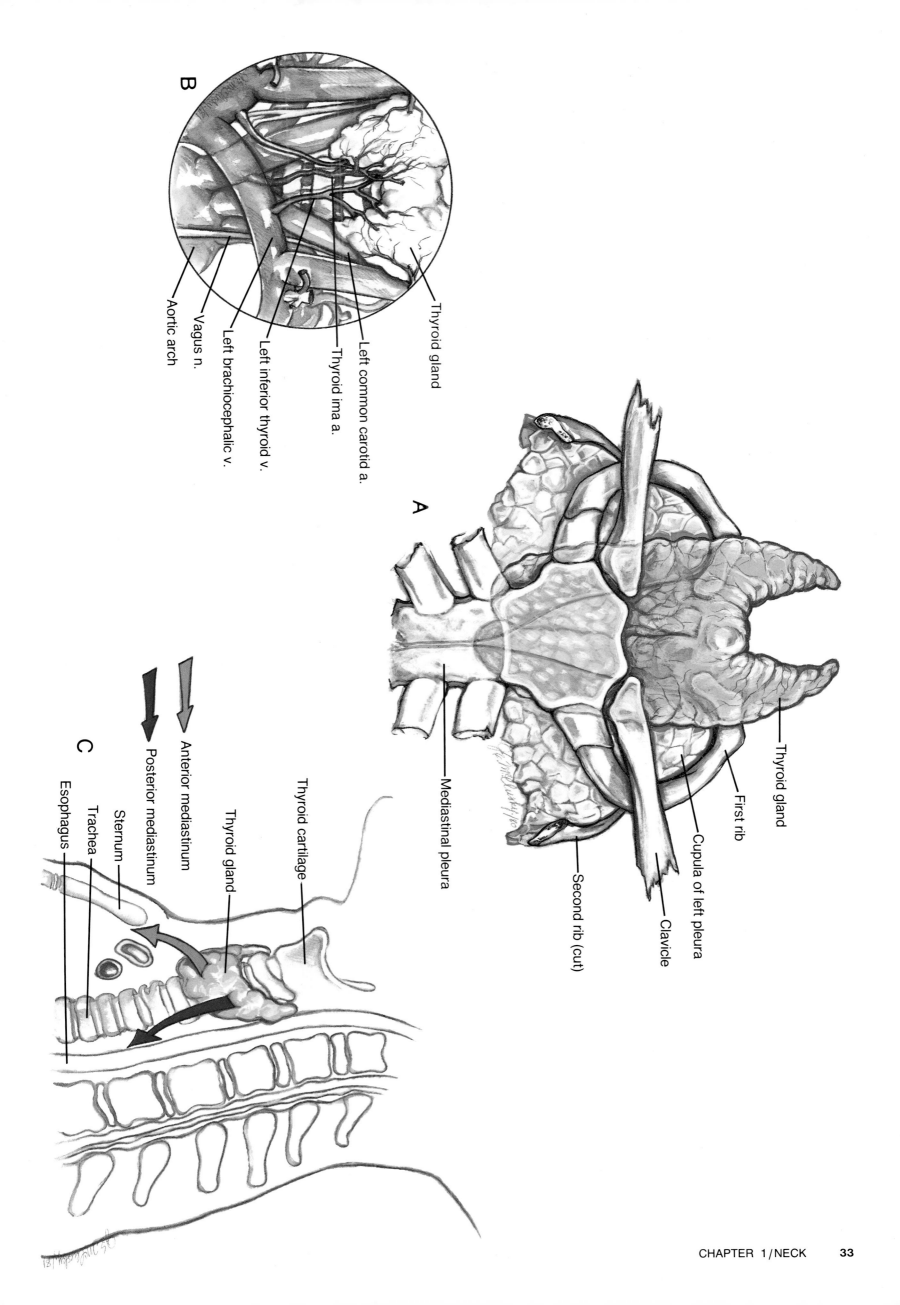

B

Aortic arch

Vagus n.

Left brachiocephalic v.

Left inferior thyroid v.

Thyroid ima a.

Left common carotid a.

Thyroid gland

A

Mediastinal pleura

Second rib (cut)

Thyroid gland

First rib

Cupula of left pleura

Clavicle

C

Posterior mediastinum

Anterior mediastinum

Thyroid gland

Thyroid cartilage

Sternum

Trachea

Esophagus

PLATE 1-17
Retrosternal Goiter II

A. Asymmetrical retrosternal goiter. The left lobe is normal; the right lobe is invading the anterior superior mediastinum.

B. Diagram of anterior retrosternal goiter seen from the right side. The recurrent laryngeal nerve and the inferior thyroid artery are posterior to the gland.

C. Retrosternal goiter, anterior view. The left lobe is normal; the right lobe is invading the posterior superior mediastinum. Compare with A above.

D. Diagram of posterior retrosternal goiter seen from the right side. The recurrent laryngeal nerve and the inferior thyroid artery are anterior to the gland. Compare with B above.

Remember:

1) Be gentle trying to separate the goiter from the pleurae.

2) Do not cut or ligate blindly; the recurrent nerve is very close to the inferior thyroid vessels.

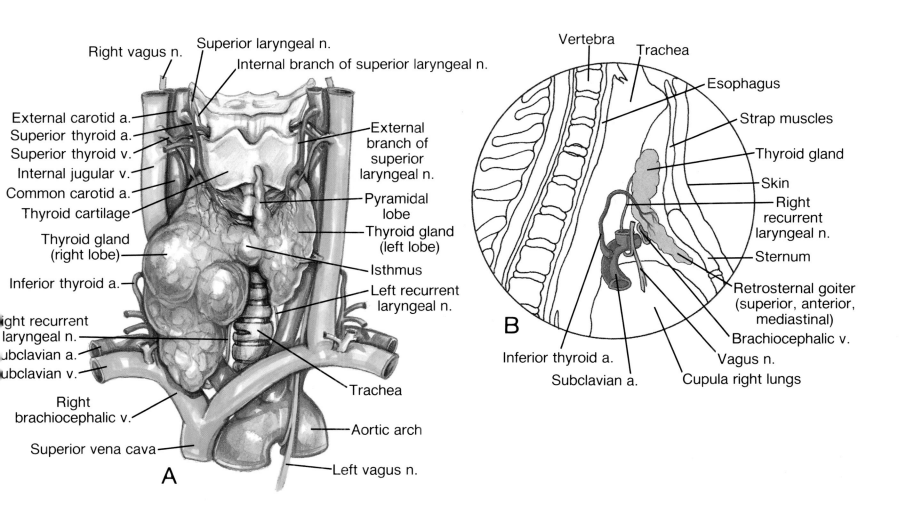

A

Right vagus n.
Superior laryngeal n.
Internal branch of superior laryngeal n.
External carotid a.
Superior thyroid a.
Superior thyroid v.
Internal jugular v.
Common carotid a.
Thyroid cartilage
Thyroid gland (right lobe)
Inferior thyroid a.
Right recurrent laryngeal n.
Subclavian a.
Subclavian v.
Right brachiocephalic v.
Superior vena cava
External branch of superior laryngeal n.
Pyramidal lobe
Thyroid gland (left lobe)
Isthmus
Left recurrent laryngeal n.
Trachea
Aortic arch
Left vagus n.

B

Vertebra
Trachea
Esophagus
Strap muscles
Thyroid gland
Skin
Right recurrent laryngeal n.
Sternum
Retrosternal goiter (superior, anterior, mediastinal)
Brachiocephalic v.
Vagus n.
Cupula right lungs
Inferior thyroid a.
Subclavian a.

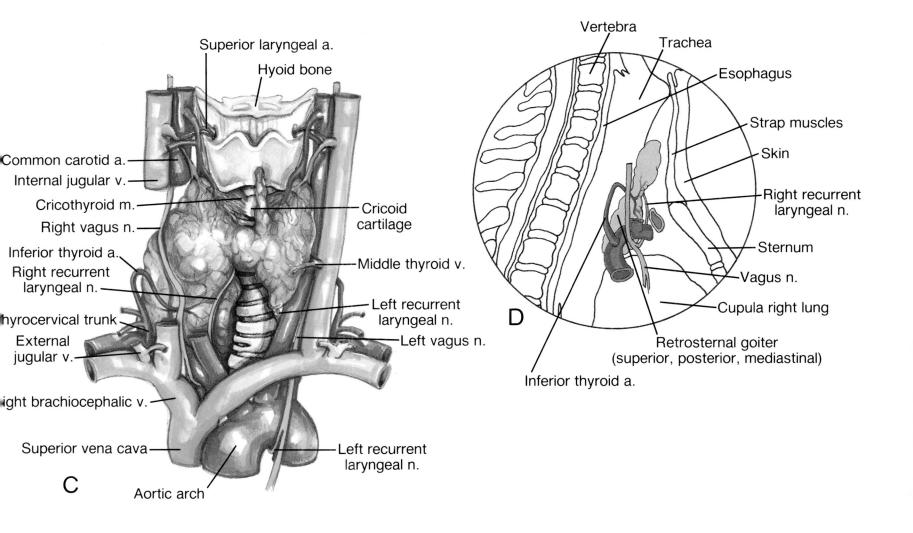

C

Superior laryngeal a.
Hyoid bone
Common carotid a.
Internal jugular v.
Cricothyroid m.
Right vagus n.
Inferior thyroid a.
Right recurrent laryngeal n.
Thyrocervical trunk
External jugular v.
Right brachiocephalic v.
Superior vena cava
Cricoid cartilage
Middle thyroid v.
Left recurrent laryngeal n.
Left vagus n.
Left recurrent laryngeal n.
Aortic arch

D

Vertebra
Trachea
Esophagus
Strap muscles
Skin
Right recurrent laryngeal n.
Sternum
Vagus n.
Cupula right lung
Retrosternal goiter (superior, posterior, mediastinal)
Inferior thyroid a.

PLATE 1-18
The Course of the Recurrent Right Inferior Laryngeal Nerve I

A. Anterior view of the great arteries, the vagi and the superior and inferior laryngeal nerves in the neck. The right recurrent laryngeal nerve passes between branches of the artery. The right vagus nerve lies anterior to the inferior thyroid artery. These relations of nerves and artery are subject to variations illustrated in B to F below.

B. The right laryngeal nerve is nonrecurrent. This indicates the presence of a retroesophageal subclavian artery. The vagus nerve passes anterior to the inferior thyroid artery.

C. The recurrent right laryngeal nerve is anterior to the inferior thyroid artery and the vagus nerve is posterior to the artery.

D. Both the recurrent laryngeal nerve and the vagus lie posterior to the inferior thyroid artery.

E. The right laryngeal nerve is nonrecurrent and the vagus lies posterior to the inferior thyroid artery.

F. The right laryngeal nerve is recurrent around the inferior thyroid artery, passing anterior, then posterior to the artery. The vagus lies posterior to the artery.

Remember:

1) The surgeon must identify both the recurrent laryngeal nerve and the inferior thyroid artery.

2) The recurrent laryngeal nerve enters the larynx at the joint between the thyroid and cricoid cartilages. Do not clamp or ligate blindly in this area. The inferior cornu of the thyroid cartilage is useful for identification of the nerve.

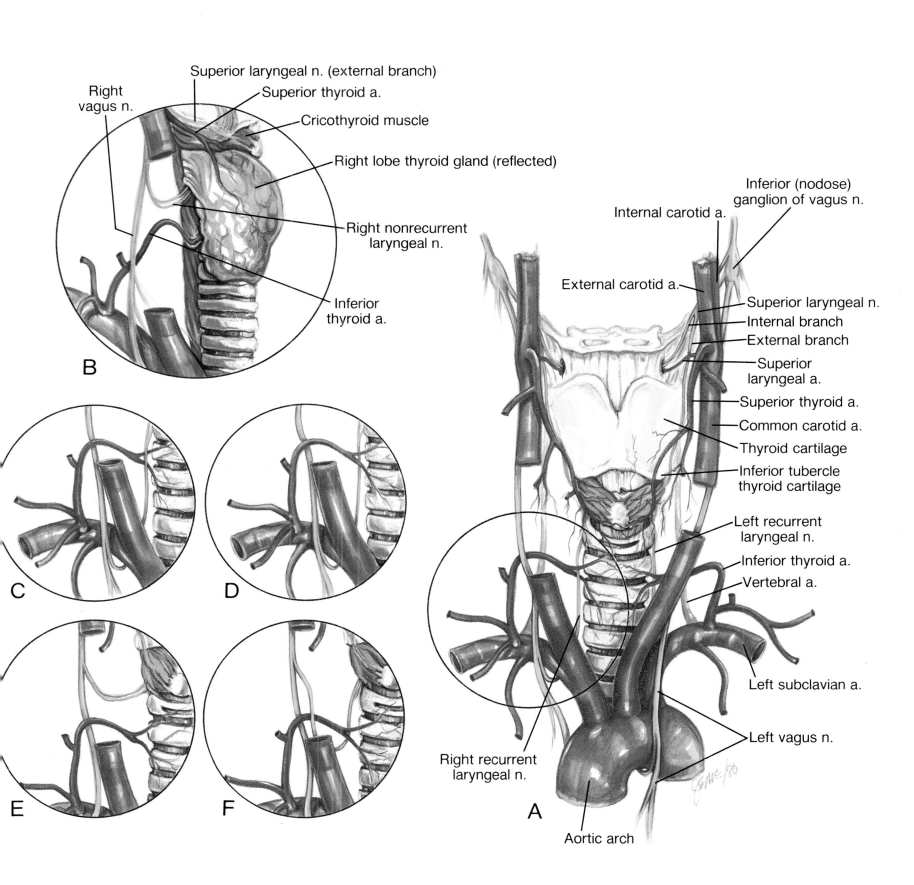

Right
vagus n.

Superior laryngeal n. (external branch)

Superior thyroid a.

Cricothyroid muscle

Right lobe thyroid gland (reflected)

Right nonrecurrent
laryngeal n.

Inferior
thyroid a.

B

Internal carotid a.

External carotid a.

Inferior (nodose)
ganglion of vagus n.

Superior laryngeal n.
Internal branch
External branch
Superior
laryngeal a.
Superior thyroid a.
Common carotid a.
Thyroid cartilage
Inferior tubercle
thyroid cartilage

Left recurrent
laryngeal n.

Inferior thyroid a.

Vertebral a.

Left subclavian a.

Left vagus n.

C

D

E

F

Right recurrent
laryngeal n.

A

Aortic arch

PLATE 1-19
The Course of the Recurrent Right Inferior Laryngeal Nerve II

A. Lateral view of the possible courses of the right recurrent laryngeal nerve in relation to the thyroid gland. The relative frequency of each course in 204 cases is shown.

   Inset: Same in cross-sectional view.

B. The dangerous middle one third of the thyroid gland (in red). In this region the following structures may be injured:
   Recurrent laryngeal nerve (phonation)
   Inferior thyroid artery (bleeding)
   Sympathetic ganglia (Horner's syndrome)

Remember:

   1) Always expose and identify the recurrent laryngeal nerve if possible.

   2) If the nerve cannot be found, and the disease is benign, perform a subtotal intracapsular thyroidectomy leaving thyroid parenchyma in the tracheoesophageal grooves.

   3) The best protected location of the nerve is posterior to the tracheoesophageal groove; the least protected location of the nerve is within the substance of the thyroid gland.

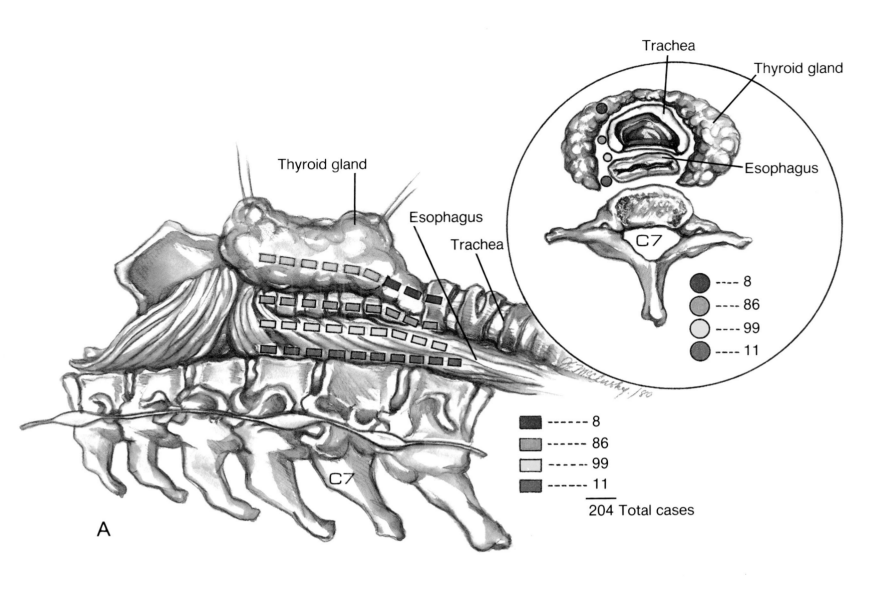

Thyroid gland

Esophagus

Trachea

Trachea

Thyroid gland

Esophagus

C7

---- 8

---- 86

---- 99

---- 11

C7

■ ------ 8

▨ ------ 86

□ ------ 99

▨ ------ 11

204 Total cases

A

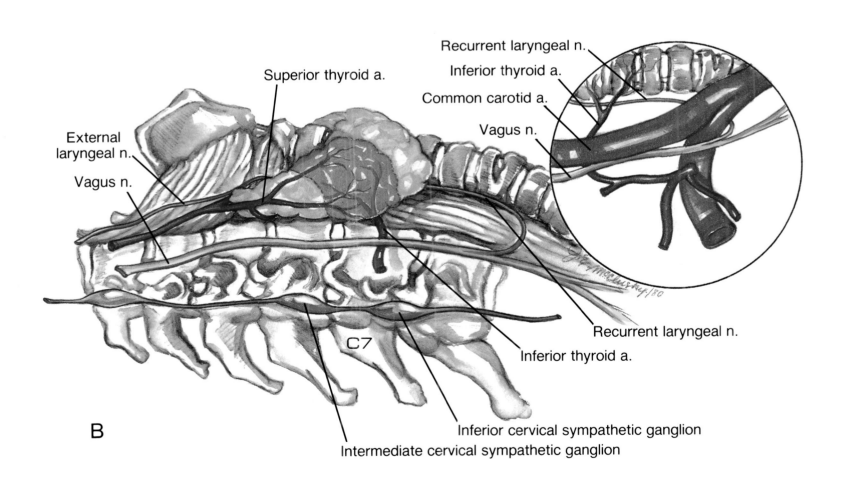

Superior thyroid a.

Recurrent laryngeal n.

Inferior thyroid a.

Common carotid a.

Vagus n.

External
laryngeal n.

Vagus n.

Recurrent laryngeal n.

C7

Inferior thyroid a.

Inferior cervical sympathetic ganglion

Intermediate cervical sympathetic ganglion

B

PLATE 1-20
Surgical Planes of the
Submandibular Triangle

A. The first surgical plane: the roof of the triangle.

Contents: skin, superficial fascia (with platysma muscle), mandibular branch and cervical branch of the facial nerve. In 50% of subjects the mandibular branch is above the mandibular border. In all subjects, the anterior ramus of the cervical branch is below the border (see Plate 1–6).

B. The second surgical plane.

Contents (from superficial to deep): facial vein and artery, submental branch of facial artery, deep cervical fascia (investing layer), lymph nodes, superficial portion of the submandibular gland, deep cervical fascia (deep layer) and hypoglossal nerve.

C. The third surgical plane.

Contents (from superficial to deep): mylohyoid, stylohyoid, hyoglossus, middle constrictor, styloglossus muscles and deep portions of the submandibular gland.

D. The fourth surgical plane: the basement of the triangle.

Contents: deep portion of submandibular gland, submandibular duct (of Wharton), lingual nerve, lingual artery and vein, sublingual gland, hypoglossal nerve and submandibular ganglion.

Remember:

1) Protect cervical and mandibular branches of the facial nerve.

2) In radical neck dissection excise *in toto* the submaxillary gland and its lymph nodes.

3) Protect the hypoglossal and lingual nerves.

4) The submandibular duct (of Wharton) is located above the hypoglossal nerve and below the lingual nerve.

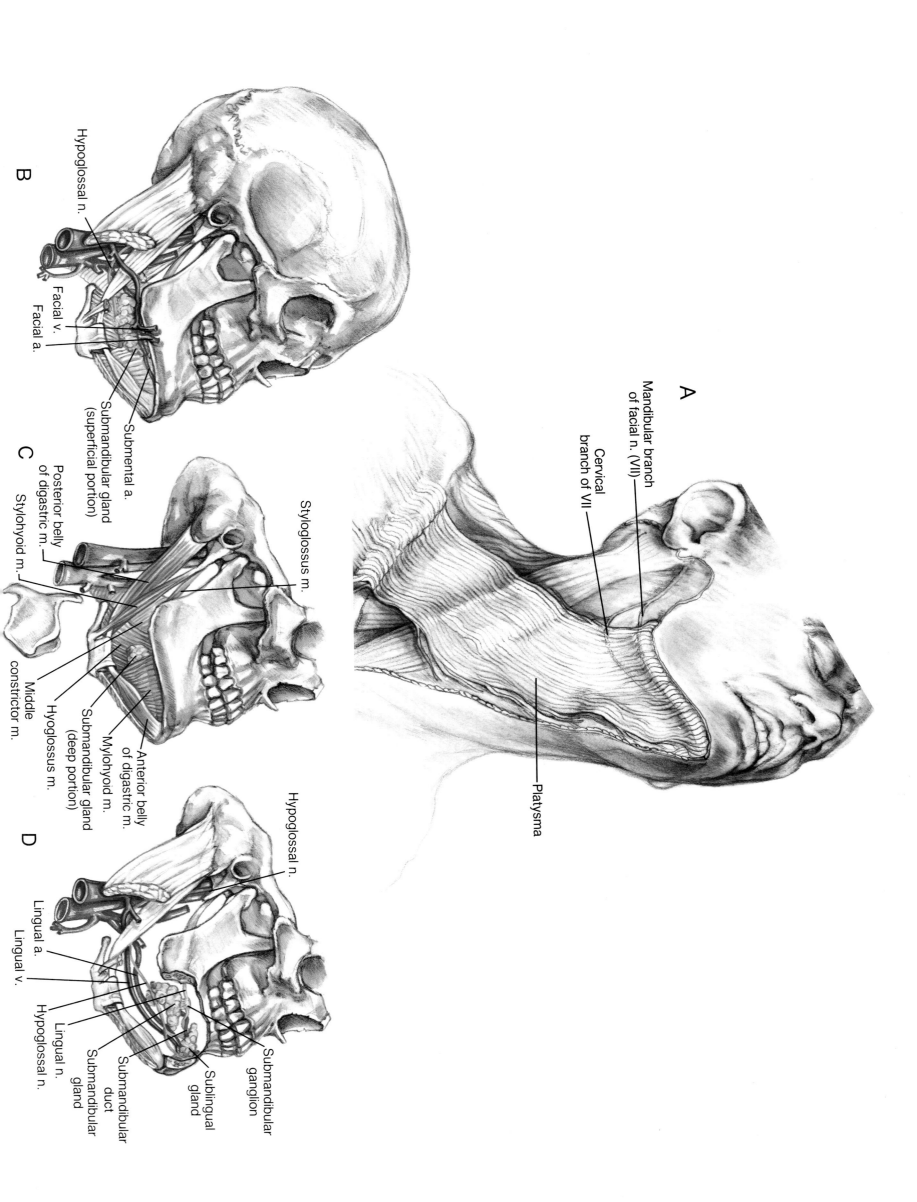

B

Hypoglossal n.

Facial v.

Facial a.

Submental a.

Submandibular gland
(superficial portion)

A

Mandibular branch
of facial n. (VII)

Cervical
branch of VII

Platysma

C

Stylohyoid m.

Posterior belly
of digastric m.

Styloglossus m.

Middle
constrictor m.

Hyoglossus m.

Submandibular gland
(deep portion)

Mylohyoid m.

Anterior belly
of digastric m.

D

Hypoglossal n.

Lingual a.

Lingual v.

Lingual n.

Hypoglossal n.

Submandibular
gland

Submandibular
duct

Sublingual
gland

Submandibular
ganglion

PLATE 1-21
The Salivary Glands and the Facial Nerve

A. Superficial relationships of the salivary glands.

B. Deep relationships of the parotid gland and facial nerve.

Remember:

1) The main trunk of the facial nerve lies within a triangle formed by the mastoid process, the cartilage of the auditory canal and the ramus of the mandible (see Plate 1–22).

2) The nerve, from its emergence from the skull to its division into branches, has a length of about 2 cm. It is anterior and superficial to the veins.

3) A beautiful and constant anatomical landmark for finding the facial nerve is the mastoid process. A fingertip on the lateral surface of the mastoid is just above the danger zone. The facial nerve is located deep and slightly anterior to the center of the fingertip. Go slowly, dissect with hemostat or Kelly forceps and test any white cord-like structure.

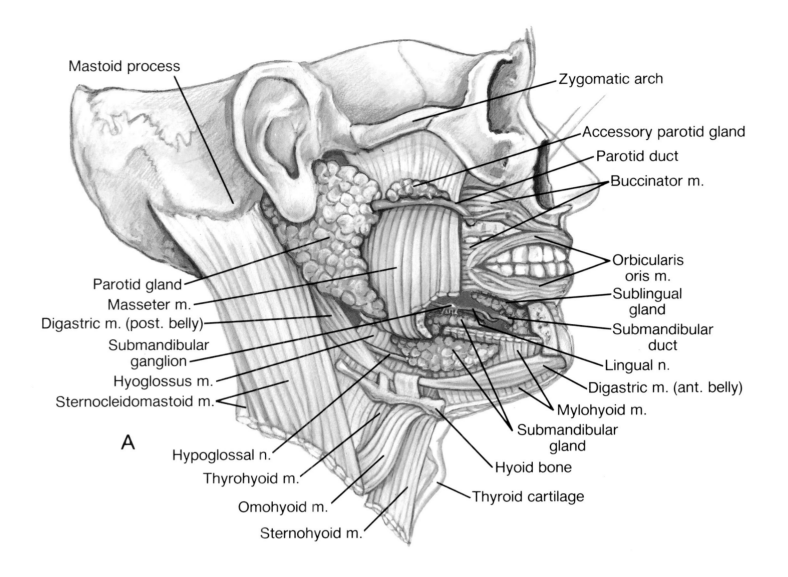

Mastoid process

Zygomatic arch

Accessory parotid gland

Parotid duct

Buccinator m.

Orbicularis oris m.

Sublingual gland

Submandibular duct

Lingual n.

Digastric m. (ant. belly)

Mylohyoid m.

Submandibular gland

Hyoid bone

Thyroid cartilage

Parotid gland

Masseter m.

Digastric m. (post. belly)

Submandibular ganglion

Hyoglossus m.

Sternocleidomastoid m.

A

Hypoglossal n.

Thyrohyoid m.

Omohyoid m.

Sternohyoid m.

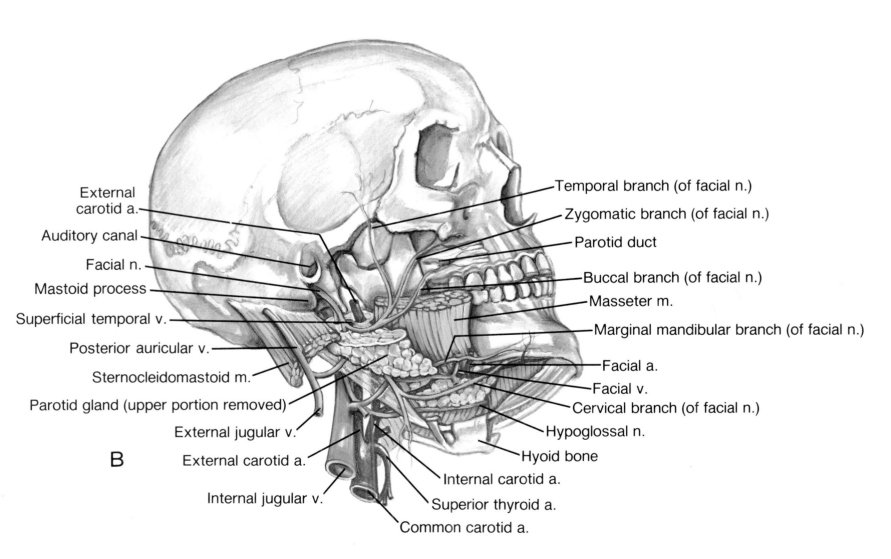

External carotid a.

Auditory canal

Facial n.

Mastoid process

Superficial temporal v.

Posterior auricular v.

Sternocleidomastoid m.

Parotid gland (upper portion removed)

External jugular v.

External carotid a.

Internal jugular v.

B

Internal carotid a.

Superior thyroid a.

Common carotid a.

Temporal branch (of facial n.)

Zygomatic branch (of facial n.)

Parotid duct

Buccal branch (of facial n.)

Masseter m.

Marginal mandibular branch (of facial n.)

Facial a.

Facial v.

Cervical branch (of facial n.)

Hypoglossal n.

Hyoid bone

PLATE 1-22
The Parotid Gland and the Facial Nerve

A. The parotid gland and the branches of the facial nerve.

B. The right parotid gland is partially retracted laterally to show the parotid duct (green) and the facial nerve (yellow) with its extracranial distribution.

C. Lateral view of the skull. The components of the right carotid sheath showing portions of cranial nerves VII, X, XI, XII.

D and E. The last four cranial nerves and their relationships to the vascular and bony landmarks.

Remember:

After total parotidectomy, the following structures will be found in the parotid bed. The acronym VANS may be helpful.

V = one Vein (internal jugular)

A = two Arteries (external and internal carotid)

N = four Nerves (glossopharyngeal, vagus, spinal accessory, hypoglossal)

S = Styloid process and three muscles (stylohyoid, styloglossus, stylopharyngeus). The last two muscles are not illustrated.

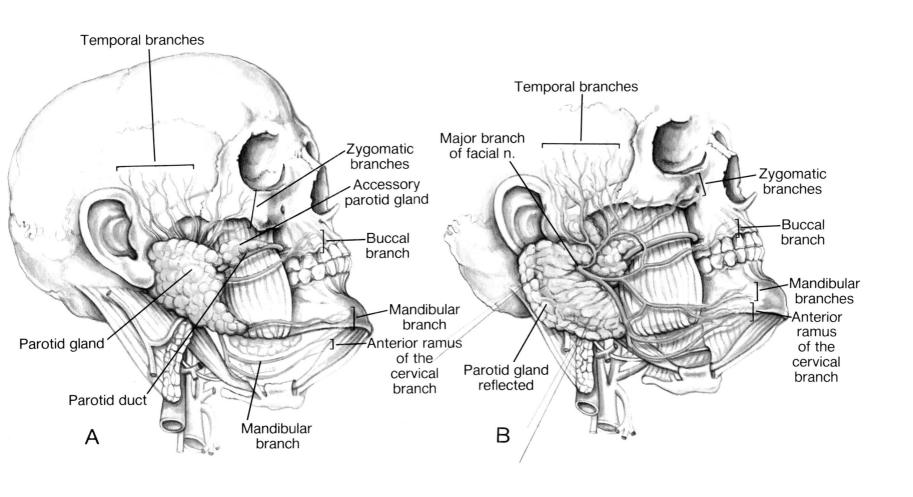

Temporal branches

Zygomatic branches

Accessory parotid gland

Buccal branch

Mandibular branch

Anterior ramus of the cervical branch

Parotid gland

Parotid duct

Mandibular branch

A

Temporal branches

Major branch of facial n.

Zygomatic branches

Buccal branch

Mandibular branches

Anterior ramus of the cervical branch

Parotid gland reflected

B

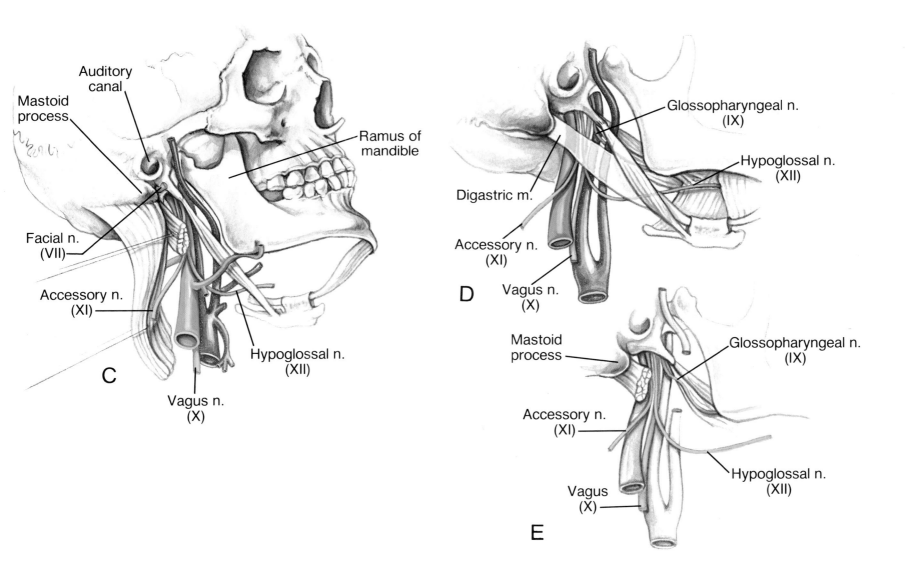

Auditory canal

Mastoid process

Ramus of mandible

Facial n. (VII)

Accessory n. (XI)

Hypoglossal n. (XII)

Vagus n. (X)

C

Glossopharyngeal n. (IX)

Hypoglossal n. (XII)

Digastric m.

Accessory n. (XI)

Vagus n. (X)

D

Mastoid process

Glossopharyngeal n. (IX)

Accessory n. (XI)

Hypoglossal n. (XII)

Vagus (X)

E

PLATE 2-1
Superficial Thoracic Muscles

The muscles involved in surgery of the breast. Superficial thoracic muscles of the right side, anterior view:

A. Pectoralis major   Deltoid
    Serratus anterior   Latissimus dorsi

B. Pectoralis minor   External oblique (not shown)
    Subscapularis   Rectus abdominis

Remember:

1) The base of the adult female breast extends from the second to the sixth or seventh rib and from the medial sternal border to the midaxillary line.

2) Good skin marking of the periphery of the breast prior to surgery is essential to avoid unnecessary dissection in the infraclavicular area and the lateral chest wall.

3) Two thirds of the base of the breast lies on pectoralis major, and one third lies on serratus anterior muscle.

4) The pectoralis major and minor may be saved in breast surgery, but the pectoral deep fascia which covers the pectoralis major should be removed, since it is the host of a rich lymphatic network.

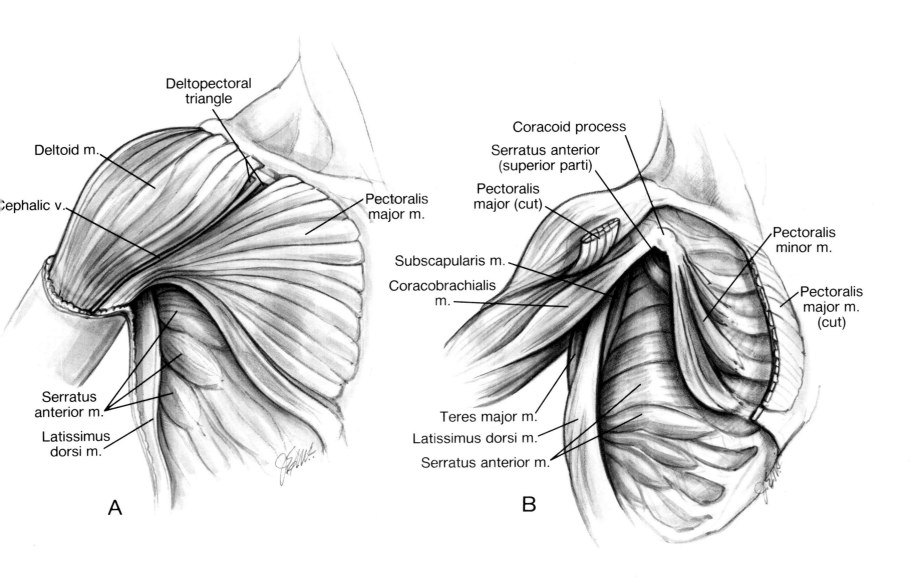

Deltopectoral
triangle

Deltoid m.

Cephalic v.

Pectoralis
major m.

Serratus
anterior m.

Latissimus
dorsi m.

A

Coracoid process

Serratus anterior
(superior parti)

Pectoralis
major (cut)

Subscapularis m.

Coracobrachialis
m.

Pectoralis
minor m.

Pectoralis
major m.
(cut)

Teres major m.

Latissimus dorsi m.

Serratus anterior m.

B

PLATE 2-2
Arteries and Nerves of the Breast

Remember:

The following nerves should be spared if possible: long thoracic nerve, thoracodorsal nerve, lateral pectoral nerve, medial pectoral nerve, subscapular nerve (not shown).

1) The long thoracic nerve can be found and protected at the point where the axillary vein passes over the second rib. Cutting this nerve will result in "winged scapula" due to paralysis of serratus anterior.

2) The thoracodorsal nerve can be found near the medial border of the latissimus dorsi. If cut, weakness of abduction and internal rotation will result.

3) The medial anterior pectoral nerve is superficial to the axillary vein and lateral to the pectoralis minor muscle.

4) The lateral anterior pectoral nerve lies at the medial edge of the pectoralis minor muscle and superficial to the axillary vein.

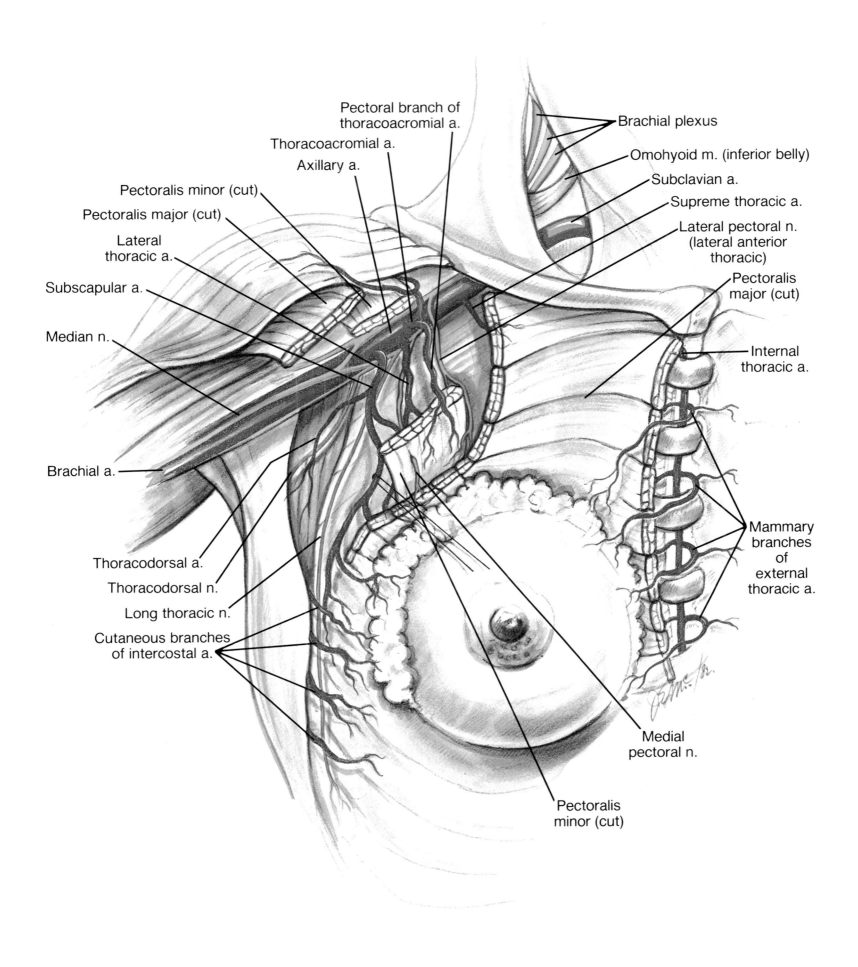

Pectoral branch of
thoracoacromial a.

Thoracoacromial a.

Axillary a.

Pectoralis minor (cut)

Pectoralis major (cut)

Lateral
thoracic a.

Subscapular a.

Median n.

Brachial a.

Thoracodorsal a.

Thoracodorsal n.

Long thoracic n.

Cutaneous branches
of intercostal a.

Brachial plexus

Omohyoid m. (inferior belly)

Subclavian a.

Supreme thoracic a.

Lateral pectoral n.
(lateral anterior
thoracic)

Pectoralis
major (cut)

Internal
thoracic a.

Mammary
branches
of
external
thoracic a.

Medial
pectoral n.

Pectoralis
minor (cut)

PLATE 2-3
The Breast in Longitudinal Section

A. Longitudinal section through a normal breast and thoracic wall.
   Secretory acini, ducts and fat lobules lie within the superficial fascia.

B. Three common patterns of the arterial supply to the breast and their relative frequency.

Arteries may arise from the internal thoracic artery *medially*, the axillary artery *superiorly* and the intercostal arteries *laterally* and *inferiorly.* Only the internal thoracic branches are always present. In most breasts, the arteries anastomose freely with one another. In a few, the arterial sources remain separate.

Remember:

1) The skin has veins and superficial lymphatic vessels. There is no fat beneath the areola.

2) Blockage of superficial lymphatics results in edema and the "peau d'orange" appearance.

3) If invaded by cancer, the ligaments of Cooper shorten, and the overlying skin becomes fixed.

4) Cancer of the lactiferous ducts products inversion of the nipple.

5) If the pectoralis major fascia is invaded by cancer, the breast takes an upward tilt.

6) Phlebitis of a superficial vein (Mondor's disease) is self limiting and is not precancerous.

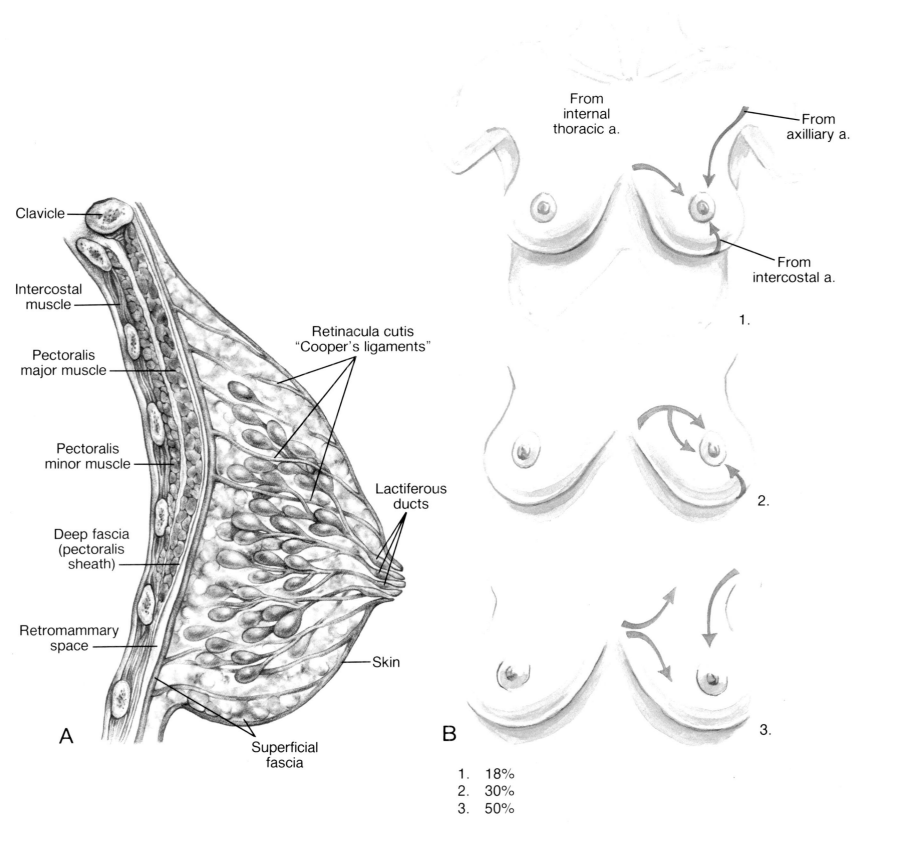

Clavicle

Intercostal muscle

Pectoralis major muscle

Pectoralis minor muscle

Deep fascia (pectoralis sheath)

Retromammary space

A

Superficial fascia

Retinacula cutis "Cooper's ligaments"

Lactiferous ducts

Skin

From internal thoracic a.

From axilliary a.

From intercostal a.

1.

2.

3.

B

1.   18%
2.   30%
3.   50%

PLATE 2-4
The Lymph Nodes and Lymphatic Drainage of the Breast

The terminology of the lymph nodes is that of Haagensen. The groups are somewhat arbitrary. The number of lymph nodes and the groups which they form are inconstant. Many axillary nodes are very small and readily overlooked by the pathologist.

Inset: The usual direction of lymphatic spread through the groups of lymph nodes. About three fourths of the drainage is to axillary nodes and one fourth is to internal mammary nodes.

Remember:

1) Breast cancer spreads by lymphatics in 30% of patients, by veins in 50%, and by local infiltration in 20%.

2) Venous drainage of the breast is *medial*, from internal thoracic veins to the right heart, *superior* from branches of the axillary vein to the right heart, and *posterior*, through intercostal veins to the vertebral plexus, and superior epigastric veins to the portal vein.

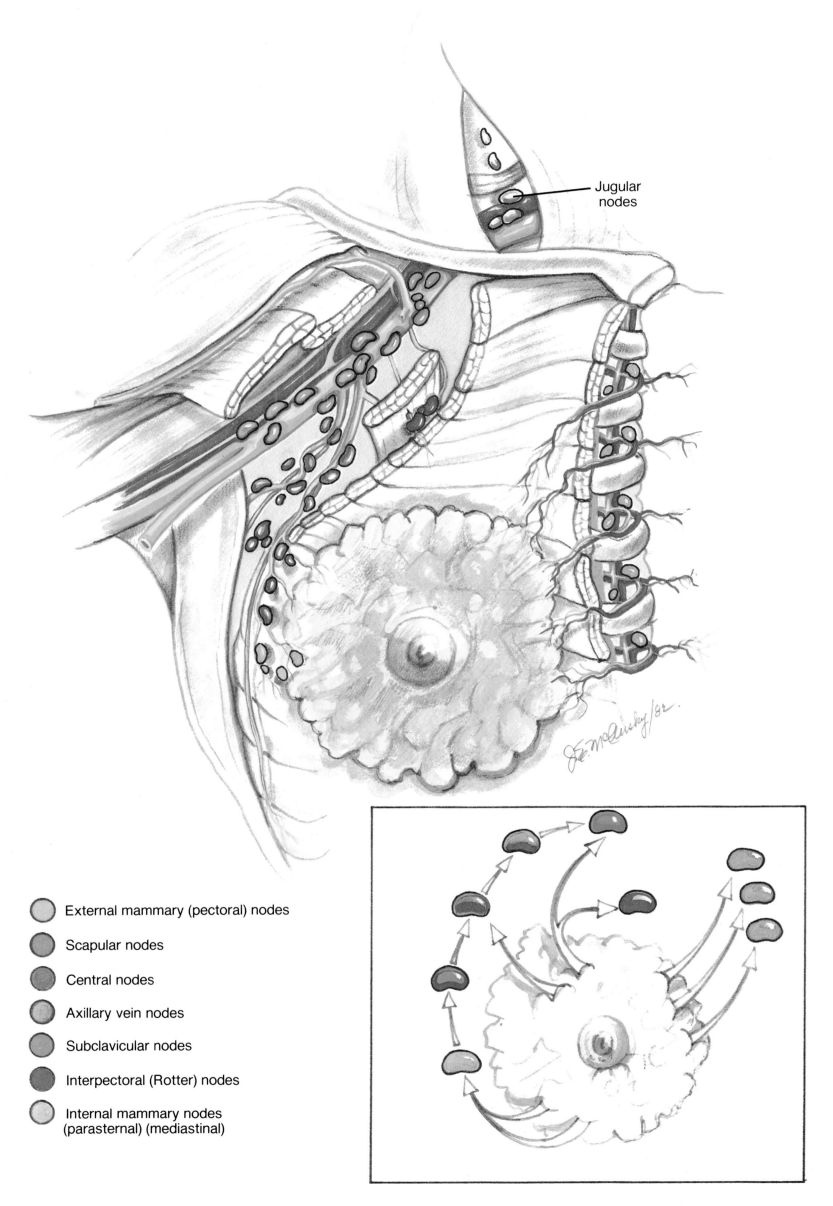

Jugular
nodes

External mammary (pectoral) nodes

Scapular nodes

Central nodes

Axillary vein nodes

Subclavicular nodes

Interpectoral (Rotter) nodes

Internal mammary nodes
(parasternal) (mediastinal)

PLATE 2-5
Mastectomy

A. The bed of modified radical mastectomy. In this illustration the pectoralis major muscle has been retracted medially and the pectoralis minor muscle has been removed to show the thoracodorsal and long thoracic nerves.

B. *Inset:* In actual surgery, both pectoralis major and minor are retracted without being cut.

C. The bed of radical mastectomy. Both pectoralis muscles have been cut.

Remember:

Good axillary dissection may be done easily leaving both pectoralis muscles *in situ* in a modified radical mastectomy.

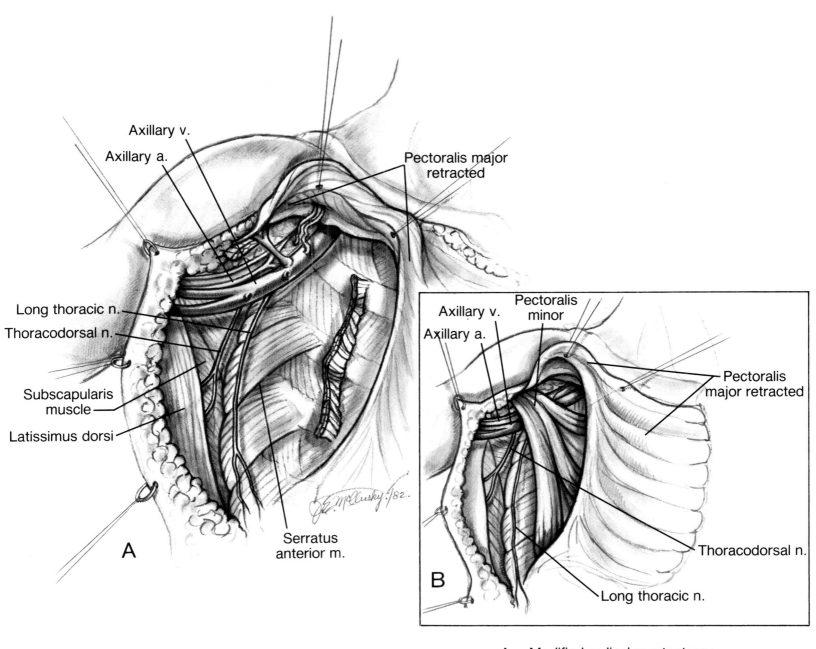

Axillary v.

Axillary a.

Pectoralis major
retracted

Long thoracic n.

Thoracodorsal n.

Subscapularis
muscle

Latissimus dorsi

Serratus
anterior m.

A

Axillary v.

Axillary a.

Pectoralis
minor

Pectoralis
major retracted

Thoracodorsal n.

Long thoracic n.

B

A.   Modified radical mastectomy
     (pectoralis minor removed)

B.   Modified radical with pectoralis minor intact

C.   Radical mastectomy (pectoralis
     major and minor m. removed)

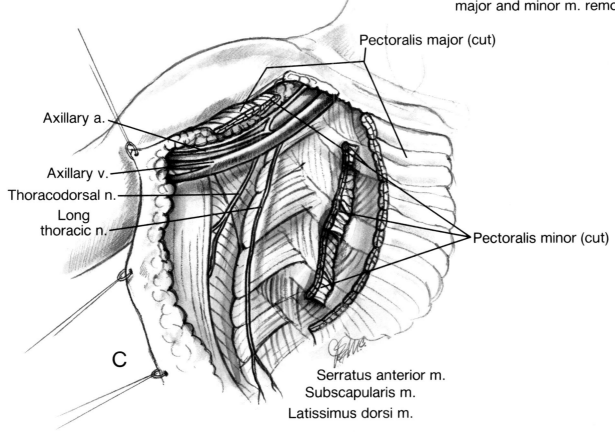

Pectoralis major (cut)

Axillary a.

Axillary v.

Thoracodorsal n.

Long
thoracic n.

Pectoralis minor (cut)

C

Serratus anterior m.
Subscapularis m.
Latissimus dorsi m.

PLATE 3-1
Development of the Diaphragm

A. The embryonic components of the diaphragm. The diaphragm is formed by the primitive septum transversum, the dorsal mesentery (mediastinum), the pleuroperitoneal membrane and the posterolateral wall of the thorax. The pleuroperitoneal canal is closed chiefly by the expansion of surrounding tissues. The pleuroperitoneal membrane makes only a small contribution.

B. The diaphragm of the newborn showing the sites of the posterolateral "foramina" of Bochdalek in blue. These potential defects do not arise from failure of the pleuroperitoneal canals to close, but are areas of weakness in the posterolateral musculature of the diaphragm. The left foramen of Bochdalek is the most frequent site of diaphragmatic hernia in infants and children. The right foramen is protected by the liver.

Remember:

Most diaphragmatic defects are the results of failure of fusion rather than failure of formation of the components.

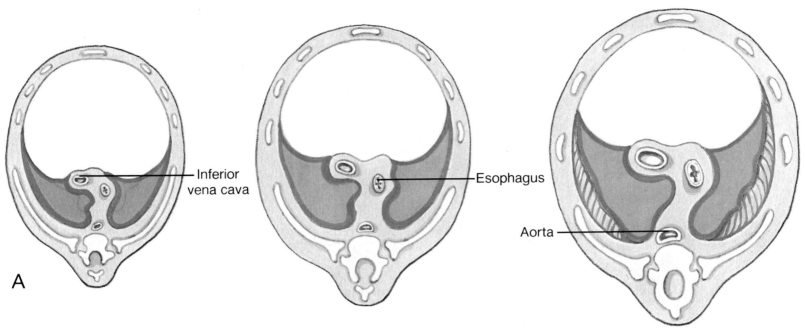

Inferior vena cava

Esophagus

Aorta

A

○ Septum transversum

◐ Dorsal mesentery

● Pleuroperitoneal membranes

▨ Body wall

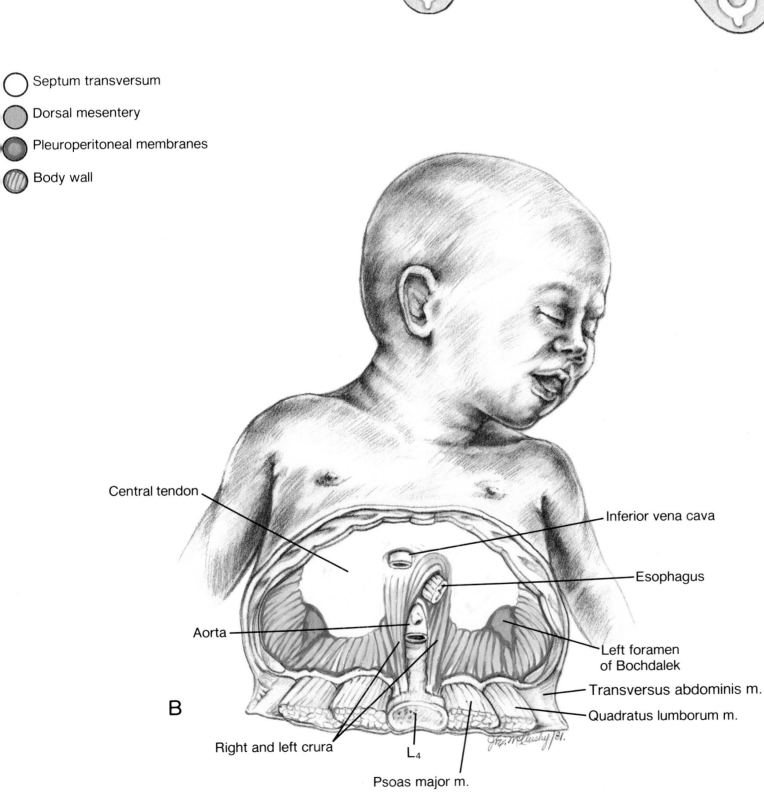

Central tendon

Inferior vena cava

Esophagus

Aorta

Left foramen of Bochdalek

Transversus abdominis m.

Quadratus lumborum m.

B

Right and left crura

L₄

Psoas major m.

PLATE 3-2
Diaphragmatic Hernias

A. Hernia through the left foramen of Bochdalek. The stomach, spleen, large and small intestine may enter the defect. A hernial sac is usually absent. The mediastinum is shifted to the right. The ipsilateral lung is compressed and the contralateral lung is reduced in size. After reduction and repair of the hernia, the lungs will assume their normal size.

B. The diaphragm from below showing sites of congenital hernias. In order of frequency they are: hernia through the left foramen of Bochdalek and hernia through the right foramen of Morgagni (space of Larrey). In adults, hiatal hernia is the most frequently encountered.

C. The diaphragm from above. Sites of hernias are indicated by dashed lines.

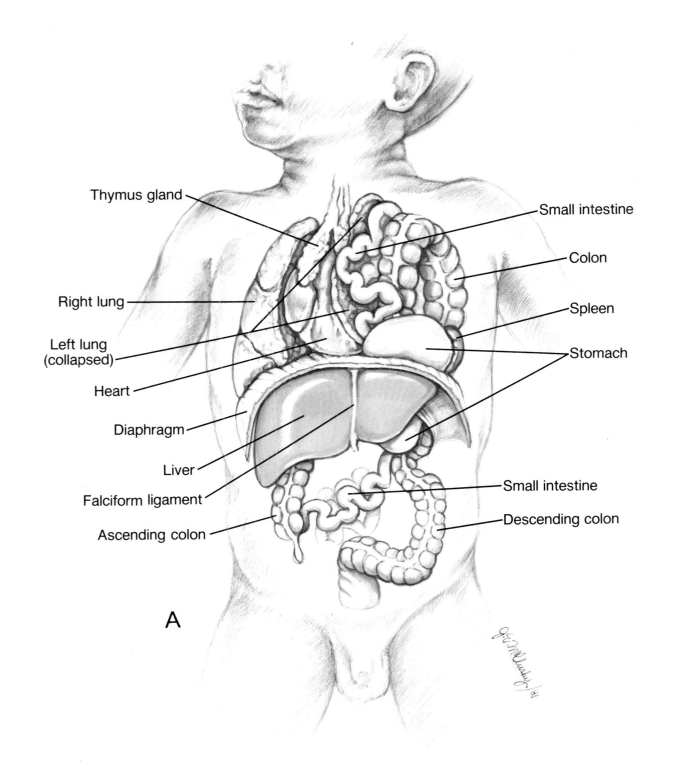

Thymus gland

Right lung

Left lung
(collapsed)

Heart

Diaphragm

Liver

Falciform ligament

Ascending colon

Small intestine

Colon

Spleen

Stomach

Small intestine

Descending colon

A

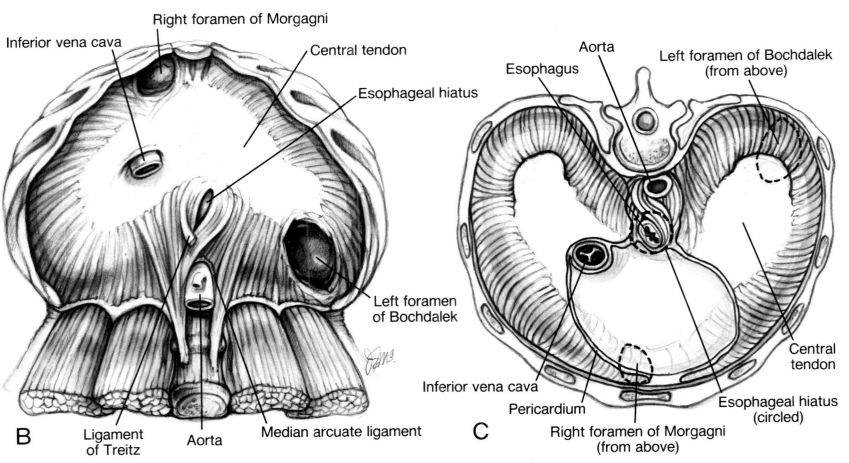

Inferior vena cava

Right foramen of Morgagni

Central tendon

Esophageal hiatus

Left foramen
of Bochdalek

Ligament
of Treitz

Aorta

Median arcuate ligament

B

Aorta

Esophagus

Left foramen of Bochdalek
(from above)

Central
tendon

Esophageal hiatus
(circled)

Inferior vena cava

Pericardium

Right foramen of Morgagni
(from above)

C

PLATE 3-3
Eventration of the Diaphragm

This is a congenital absence, or a great reduction, of the normal muscular component of one or both leaves of the diaphragm. The phrenic nerves are normal. The eventrated leaf is composed of pleura, fascia and peritoneum only. It forms the hernial sac. Malrotation of the intestines accompanies the diaphragmatic defect, and the mediastinum may be shifted toward the unaffected side. The radiological findings are similar to those of herniation through the foramen of Bochdalek (see Plate 3-2A).

Remember:

This pathological entity is not a true hernia.

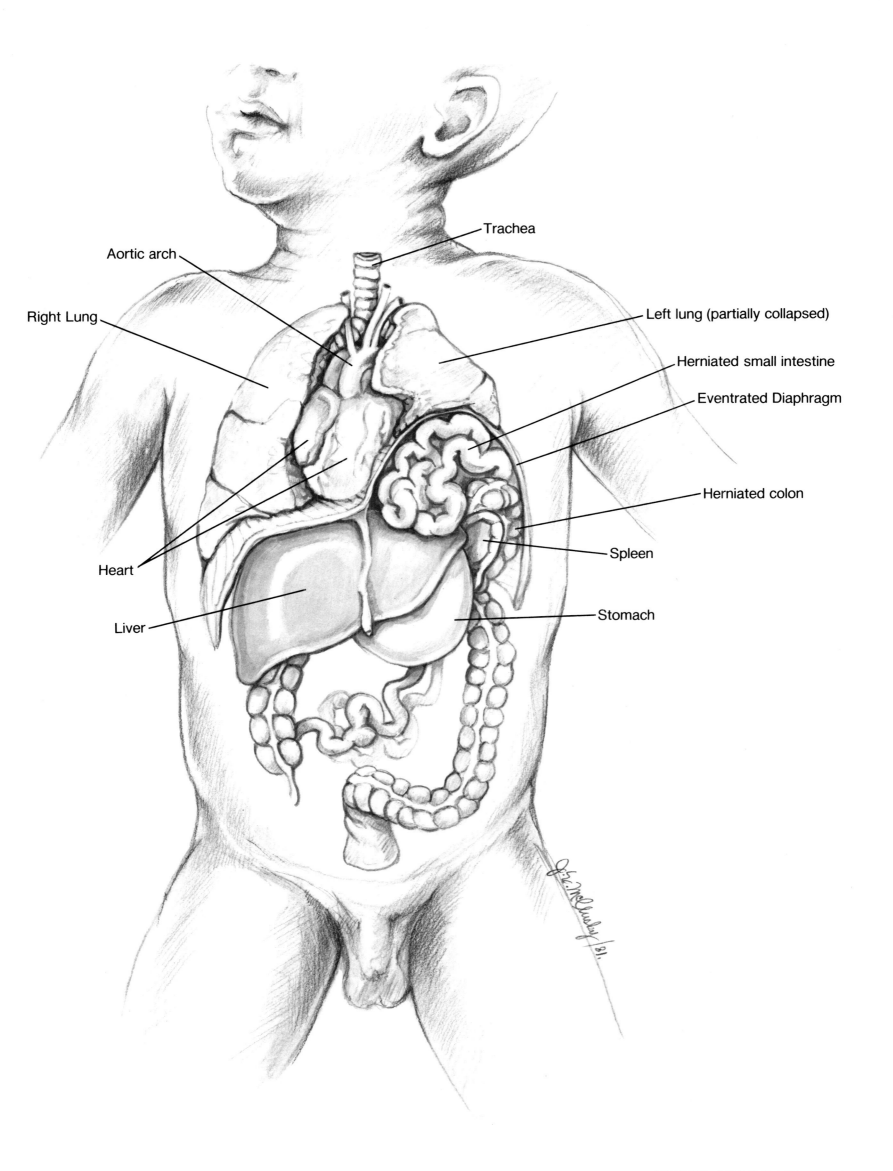

Trachea

Aortic arch

Right Lung

Left lung (partially collapsed)

Herniated small intestine

Eventrated Diaphragm

Herniated colon

Heart

Spleen

Liver

Stomach

PLATE 3-4
Congenital Hernias of the Diaphragm

Congenital Hernias	Anatomy	Sac and Herniated Organs	Remarks
Eventration of the diaphragm.	Congenital hernia. Diaphragm is thin with sparsely distributed, but normal muscle fibers. Either or both sides may be affected. Phrenic nerve appears normal.	"Sac" is formed by the attenuated diaphragm. Contents: Normal abdominal organs under elevated dome of hemidiaphragm.	Heart and mediastinum shifted to contralateral side. Ipsilateral lung collapsed, but normal. Malrotation and inversion of abdominal viscera are common.
Hernia through the foramen of Bochdalek. Posterolateral hernia of the diaphragm.	Congenital hernia through the lumbocostal trigone. May expand to include almost whole hemidiaphragm. More common on left.	Sac present in 10 to 15%. Contents: Small intestine, usual; stomach, colon, spleen, frequent. Pancreas and liver, rare. Liver only in right-sided hernia.	Heart and mediastinum shifted to contralateral side. Ipsilateral lung collapsed but usually not hypoplastic. Secondary malrotation is common. Craniorrhachischisis, tracheoesophageal fistula and heart defects are common.
Hernia through the foramen of Morgagni. Retrosternal hernia. Parasternal hernia. Anterior diaphragmatic hernia.	Congenital potential hernia through muscular hiatus on either side of the xiphoid process. Usually on the right; bilateral cases are known. Actual herniation usually the result of postnatal trauma.	Sac present at first. May rupture later, leaving no trace. Contents: Infants: Liver. Adults: Omentum. May be followed by colon and stomach later.	Rare in infants and children.
Peritoneopericardial hernia. Defect of the central tendon. Defect of the transverse septum.	Congenital hernia through central tendon and pericardium	Sac rarely present. Contents: Stomach, colon.	Has been seen in newborns and in adults. Perhaps traumatic in adults. Very rare.

PLATE 3-4
Acquired Hernias of the Diaphragm

Acquired Hernias	Anatomy	Sac and Herniated Organs	Remarks
Hiatal hernia. Sliding hiatal hernia. Fixed hiatal hernia	Congenital potential hernia. The enlarged esophageal hiatus of the diaphragm permits the cardia of the stomach to enter the mediastinum above the diaphragm. The phrenoesophageal ligament is attenuated and stretched. The gastroesophageal junction may be freely movable or fixed in the thorax.	Sac lies anterior and lateral to the herniated stomach. Contents: Cardiac stomach.	A large hiatus (admitting three fingers) may be a predisposing factor; actual herniation usually occurs in late adult life. It has been seen in newborn infants.
Paraesophageal hernia.	Congenital potential hernia. The cardia is in the normal position. The fundus has herniated through the hiatus, into the thorax.	Sac lies anterior to the esophagus and posterior to the pericardium. Contents: Fundus of stomach. Body of stomach, transverse colon, omentum and spleen may enter the sac later.	An esophageal hiatus larger than normal may be the predisposing factor. Actual herniation occurs in later adult life.
Acquired eventration	Paralysis of normal muscle resulting from phrenic nerve injury.	Diaphragm elevated. No true hernial sac.	Heart and mediastinum shifted to contralateral side. Ipsilateral lung collapsed but normal. No malrotation.
Traumatic hernia.	Acquired hernia. Tear, usually from esophageal hiatus across dome to left costal attachment of diaphragm.	There is no sac. Herniated organs: None at first. Spleen, splenic flexure of colon, stomach, left lobe of liver later.	

PLATE 3-5
The Superior Surface of the Diaphragm

The superior surface of the diaphragm at the level of the 10th thoracic vertebra. The pericardium has been cut to show its relation to the pleura and to the superior surface of the diaphragm. The phrenic nerves and the pericardiacophrenic arteries lie between the pericardium and the pleura.

Remember:

1) The inferior vena cava at the caval hiatus is accompanied by branches of the right phrenic nerve. The hiatus is in the central tendon and lies at the level of the eighth thoracic vertebra.

2) The esophageal opening is at the level of the 10th thoracic vertebra. The esophagus is accompanied by the vagus nerve and some branches of the left gastric vessels (see Plate 3–9).

3) The aortic hiatus lies at the level of the 12th thoracic vertebra. The aorta is accompanied by the azygos vein and the thoracic duct.

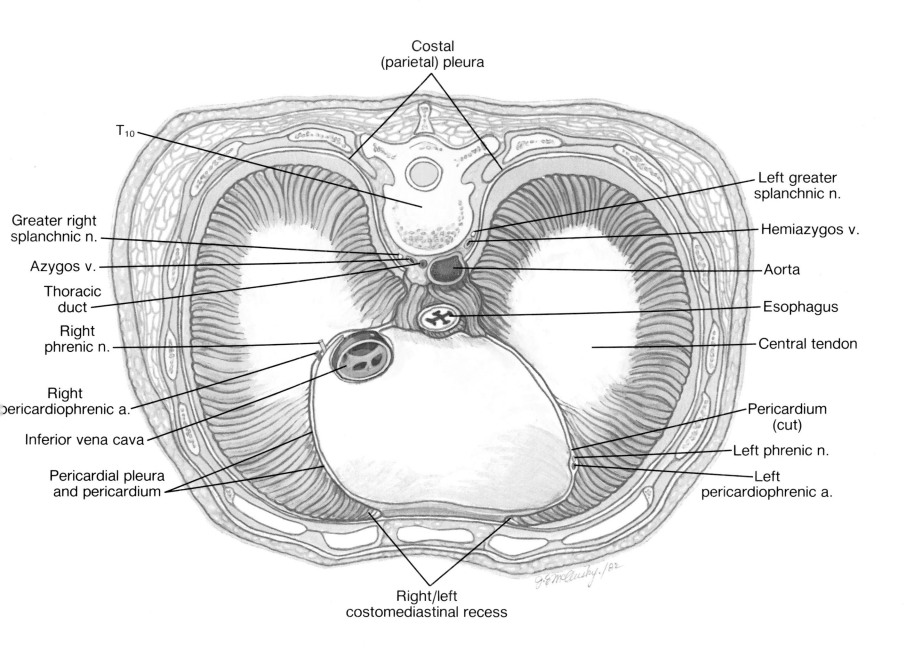

Costal
(parietal) pleura

T_{10}

Left greater
splanchnic n.

Greater right
splanchnic n.

Hemiazygos v.

Azygos v.

Aorta

Thoracic
duct

Esophagus

Right
phrenic n.

Central tendon

Right
pericardiophrenic a.

Pericardium
(cut)

Inferior vena cava

Left phrenic n.

Pericardial pleura
and pericardium

Left
pericardiophrenic a.

Right/left
costomediastinal recess

PLATE 3-6
The Diaphragm and the Mediastinum I

A. The diaphragm and mediastinum seen from the right. This is the "venous" side, so called because of the predominance of venous structures: superior and inferior venae cavae, the azygos vein and the right atrium.

B. Structures in the vicinity of the right side of the esophageal hiatus. The right vagal trunk may be seen passing through the esophageal hiatus posterior and lateral to the esophagus.

Remember:

1) The valveless inferior vena cava accepts tributaries from the gastrointestinal tract, liver, spleen, pancreas, kidneys, adrenal glands and gonads, as well as veins of the anterior body wall (see Plate 13–1).

2) The most important veins of collateral circulation after ligation of the inferior vena cava are the lumbar, vertebral and azygos veins.

3) Survival of patients with acute ligation of the inferior vena cava above the renal veins is extremely rare.

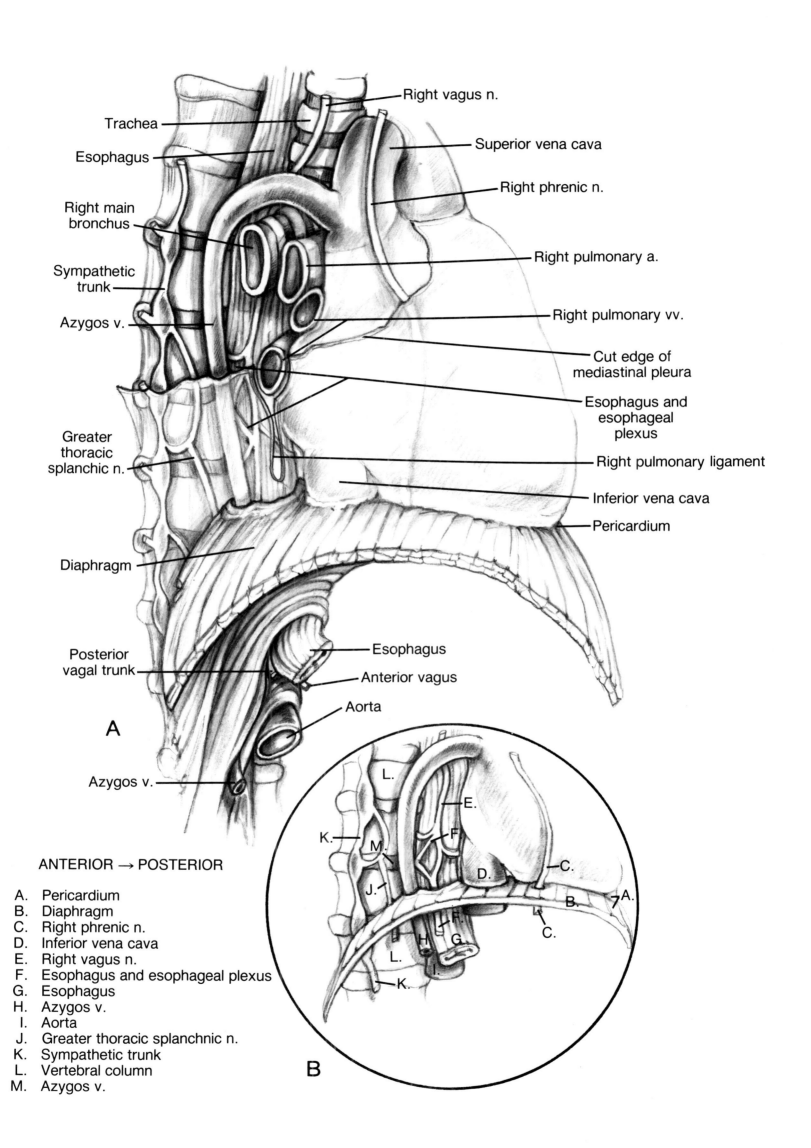

Trachea

Esophagus

Right main
bronchus

Sympathetic
trunk

Azygos v.

Greater
thoracic
splanchic n.

Diaphragm

Posterior
vagal trunk

Azygos v.

Right vagus n.

Superior vena cava

Right phrenic n.

Right pulmonary a.

Right pulmonary vv.

Cut edge of
mediastinal pleura

Esophagus and
esophageal
plexus

Right pulmonary ligament

Inferior vena cava

Pericardium

Esophagus

Anterior vagus

Aorta

A

ANTERIOR → POSTERIOR

A. Pericardium
B. Diaphragm
C. Right phrenic n.
D. Inferior vena cava
E. Right vagus n.
F. Esophagus and esophageal plexus
G. Esophagus
H. Azygos v.
I. Aorta
J. Greater thoracic splanchnic n.
K. Sympathetic trunk
L. Vertebral column
M. Azygos v.

B

PLATE 3-7
The Diaphragm and the Mediastinum II

A. The diaphragm and mediastinum seen from the left. This is the "arterial" side because of the predominance of arterial structures: ascending aorta, aortic arch and pulmonary arch.

B. Structures in the vicinity of the left side of the esophageal hiatus. The left vagal trunk passes through the hiatus anterior and lateral to the esophagus.

Remember:

The esophagus at the hiatus is accompanied by the anterior and posterior vagal trunks in 88% of subjects. In 9%, the trunks divide above the hiatus, and in 3%, the esophageal plexus passes through the hiatus to form the vagal trunks below the diaphragm (see Plate 5-7).

2) Small islands of gastric mucosa (columnar epithelium) in the esophagus are common, especially in the upper one third. Chronic peptic ulcers of the esophagus may be related to these areas of gastric mucosa.

3) A congenital short esophagus with a portion of the stomach above the diaphragm is rare. It differs from hiatal hernia in that there is no peritoneal sac in the mediastinum and the left gastric artery does not extend above the diaphragm.

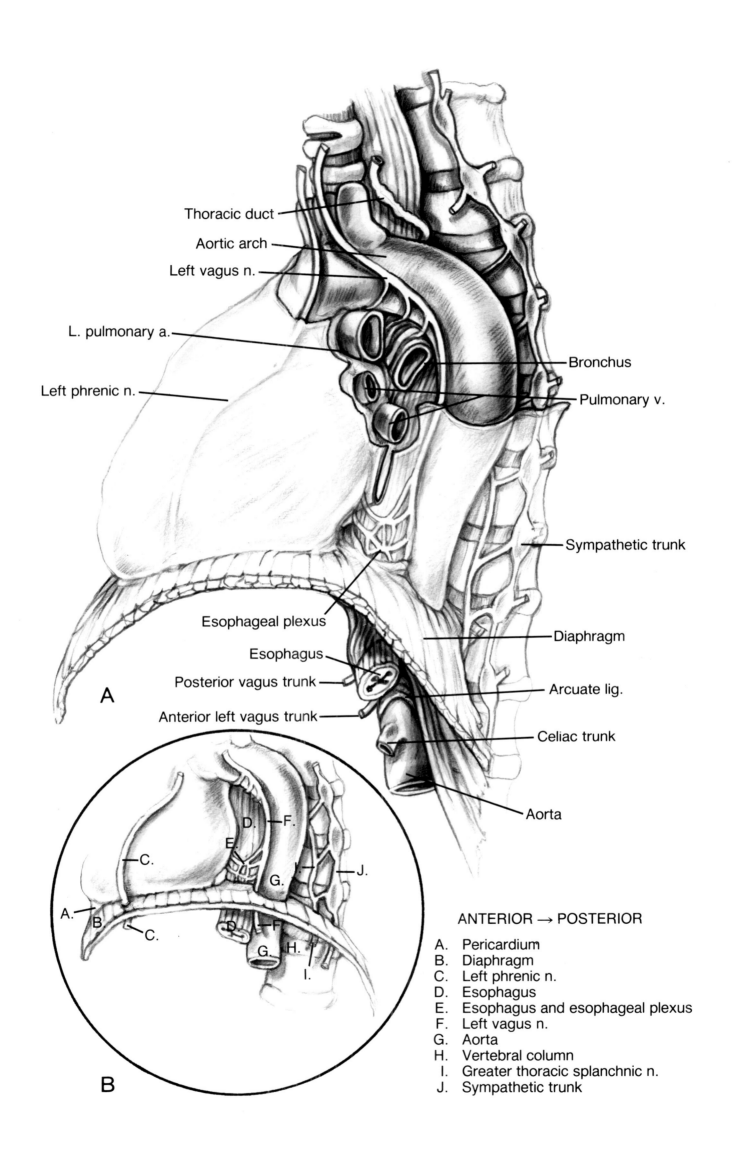

Thoracic duct

Aortic arch

Left vagus n.

L. pulmonary a.

Left phrenic n.

Bronchus

Pulmonary v.

Sympathetic trunk

Esophageal plexus

Esophagus

Posterior vagus trunk

Anterior left vagus trunk

Diaphragm

Arcuate lig.

Celiac trunk

Aorta

A

B

ANTERIOR → POSTERIOR

A. Pericardium
B. Diaphragm
C. Left phrenic n.
D. Esophagus
E. Esophagus and esophageal plexus
F. Left vagus n.
G. Aorta
H. Vertebral column
I. Greater thoracic splanchnic n.
J. Sympathetic trunk

PLATE 3-8
Vascular Relations of the Inferior Surface of the Diaphragm and Crura

A. Arteries and veins of the inferior surface of the diaphragm. The left phrenic vein may enter the inferior vena cava, the left adrenal vein, or both.

B. The relations of the cisterna chyli and lymphatic trunks to the diaphragmatic crura, aorta and inferior vena cava. The aorta over the cisterna has been removed. The cisterna may be single (as shown), multiple or absent.

   Inset: Relations of the vessels anterior to the cisterna chyli.

Remember:

1) The cisterna chyli is located between the aorta and right crus of the diaphragm in front of the first and second lumbar vertebrae.

2) The thoracic duct and cisterna chyli may be ligated with impunity.

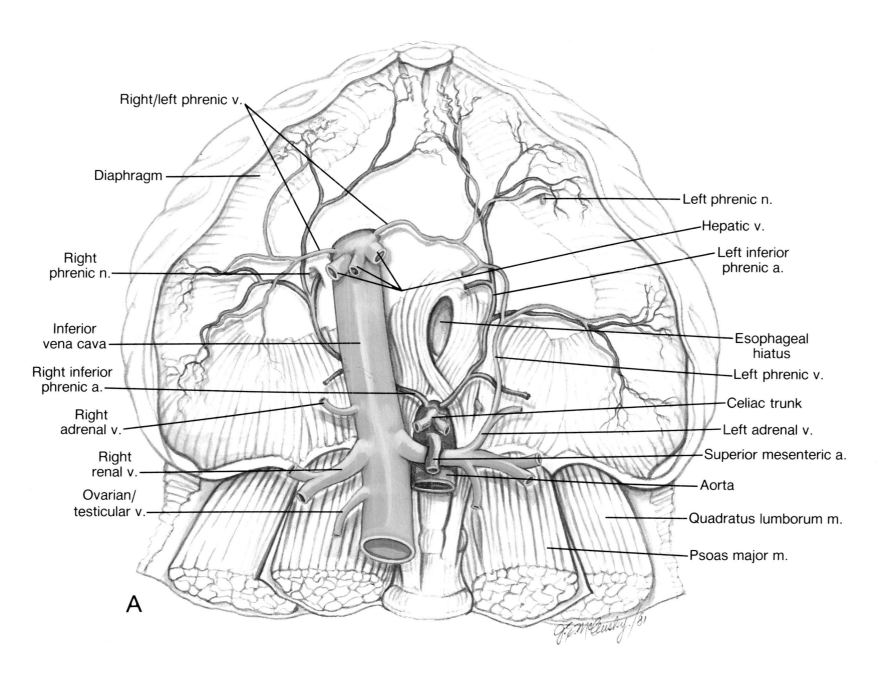

Right/left phrenic v.

Diaphragm

Right phrenic n.

Inferior vena cava

Right inferior phrenic a.

Right adrenal v.

Right renal v.

Ovarian/ testicular v.

Left phrenic n.

Hepatic v.

Left inferior phrenic a.

Esophageal hiatus

Left phrenic v.

Celiac trunk

Left adrenal v.

Superior mesenteric a.

Aorta

Quadratus lumborum m.

Psoas major m.

A

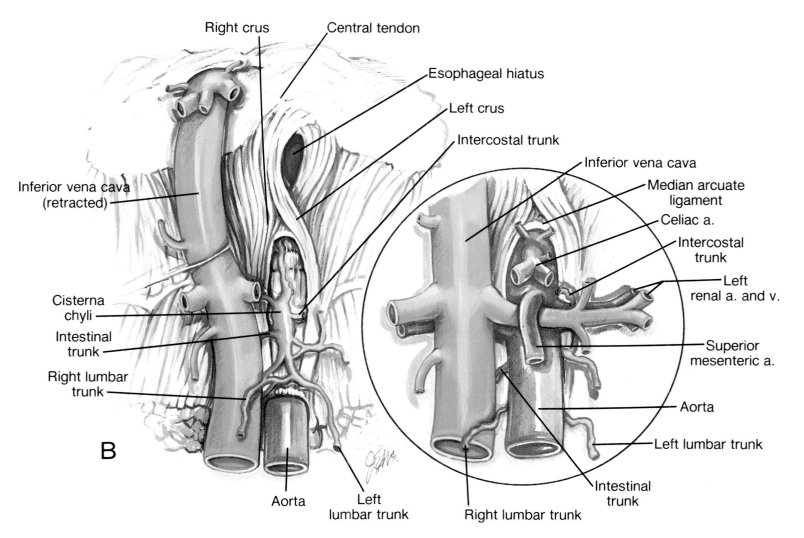

Right crus

Central tendon

Esophageal hiatus

Left crus

Intercostal trunk

Inferior vena cava (retracted)

Cisterna chyli

Intestinal trunk

Right lumbar trunk

Aorta

Left lumbar trunk

Inferior vena cava

Median arcuate ligament

Celiac a.

Intercostal trunk

Left renal a. and v.

Superior mesenteric a.

Aorta

Left lumbar trunk

Intestinal trunk

Right lumbar trunk

B

PLATE 3-9
Variations of the Blood Supply to the Gastroesophageal Junction and the Esophageal Hiatus

A. The right inferior phrenic artery arises from the aorta; the left inferior phrenic artery arises from the left gastric artery. An esophageal branch arises from the left phrenic artery only.

B. Both inferior phrenic arteries arise from the aorta just above the celiac trunk. Esophageal branches arise from both phrenic arteries.

C. Origin of phrenic arteries as in A, but with esophageal branches arising from both phrenic arteries.

Remember:

1) The left phrenic artery with its esophageal branch, together with the short gastric arteries and the posterior gastric artery, if present, are responsible for the blood supply of the gastric remnant after gastrectomy.

2) Mobilize the left lobe of the liver carefully to avoid bleeding. Keep in mind the variations of the blood supply to the abdominal esophagus and the inferior surface of the diaphragm.

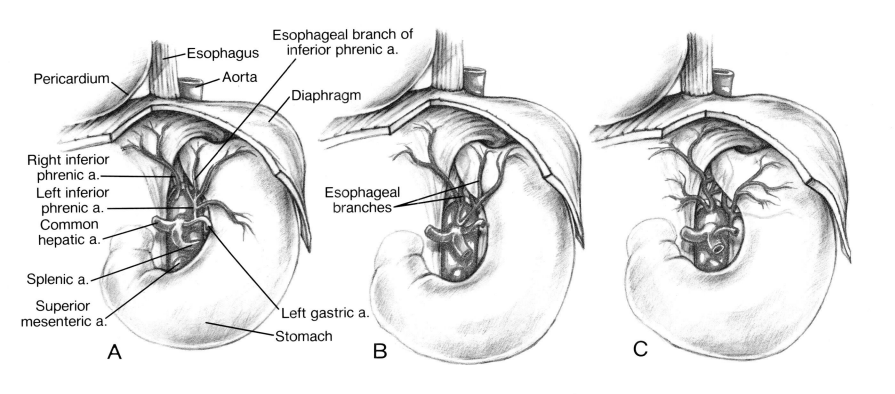

PLATE 3-10
Lymphatics of the Diaphragm

A. Lymph nodes of the superior surface of the diaphragm. They are usually placed in three groups: anterior, middle and posterior.

B. Diagram of the lymphatic drainage of the diaphragm seen from above. This system receives a large contribution from the superior surface of the liver (see Plate 8-7) and probably from the left adrenal glands (see Plate 11-5).

Remember:

All diaphragmatic lymph nodes lie on the superior surface of the diaphragm.

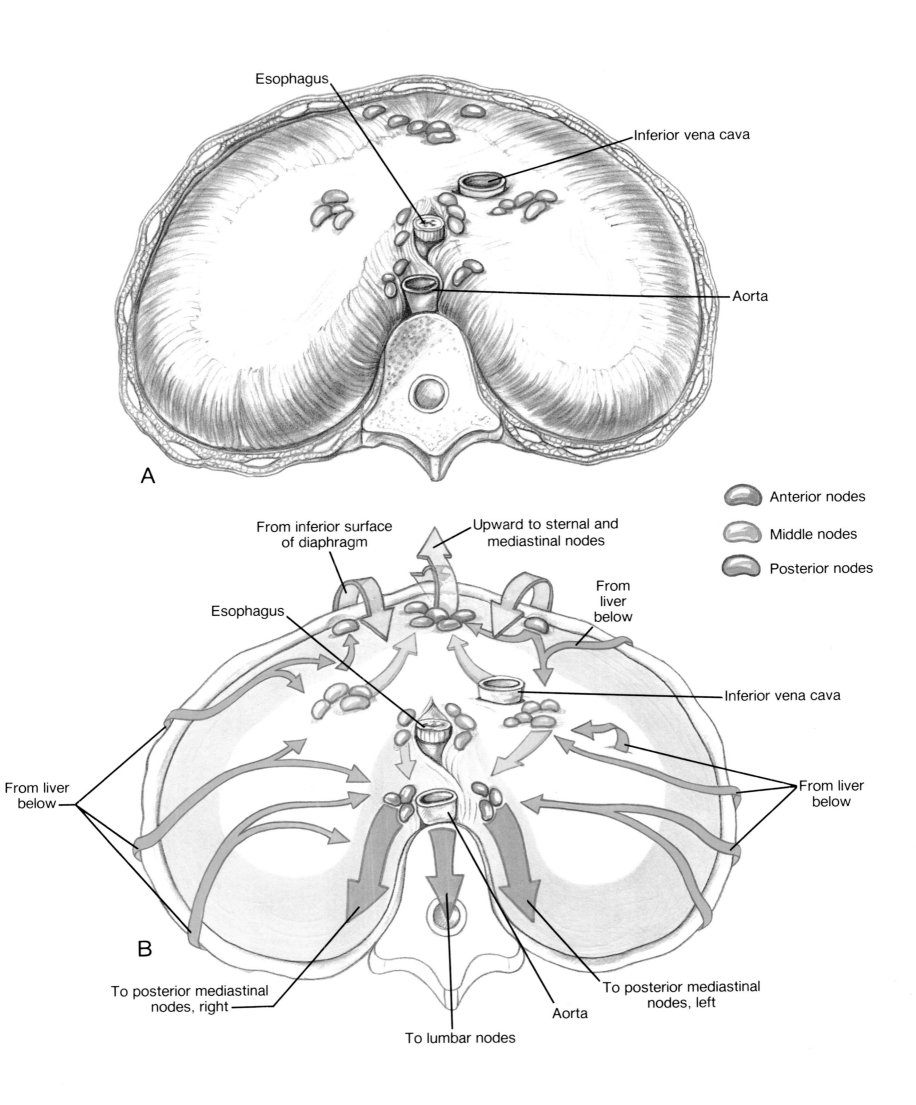

Esophagus

Inferior vena cava

Aorta

A

Anterior nodes

Middle nodes

Posterior nodes

From inferior surface
of diaphragm

Upward to sternal and
mediastinal nodes

From
liver
below

Esophagus

Inferior vena cava

From liver
below

From liver
below

B

To posterior mediastinal
nodes, right

To posterior mediastinal
nodes, left

Aorta

To lumbar nodes

PLATE 3-11
The Normal Constrictions of the Esophagus

A bolus that is not stopped at the cricopharyngeal or aortic constrictions will probably pass the constriction at the esophageal hiatus of the diaphragm.

Remember:

1) The three curvatures: to the left at T_1; to the right at T_6; to the left at T_8.

2) The four constrictions: cricopharyngeal at C_6; aortic arch at T_4; left primary bronchus at T_5; diaphragm at T_{10}.

3) Most esophageal pathology occurs at these constrictions.

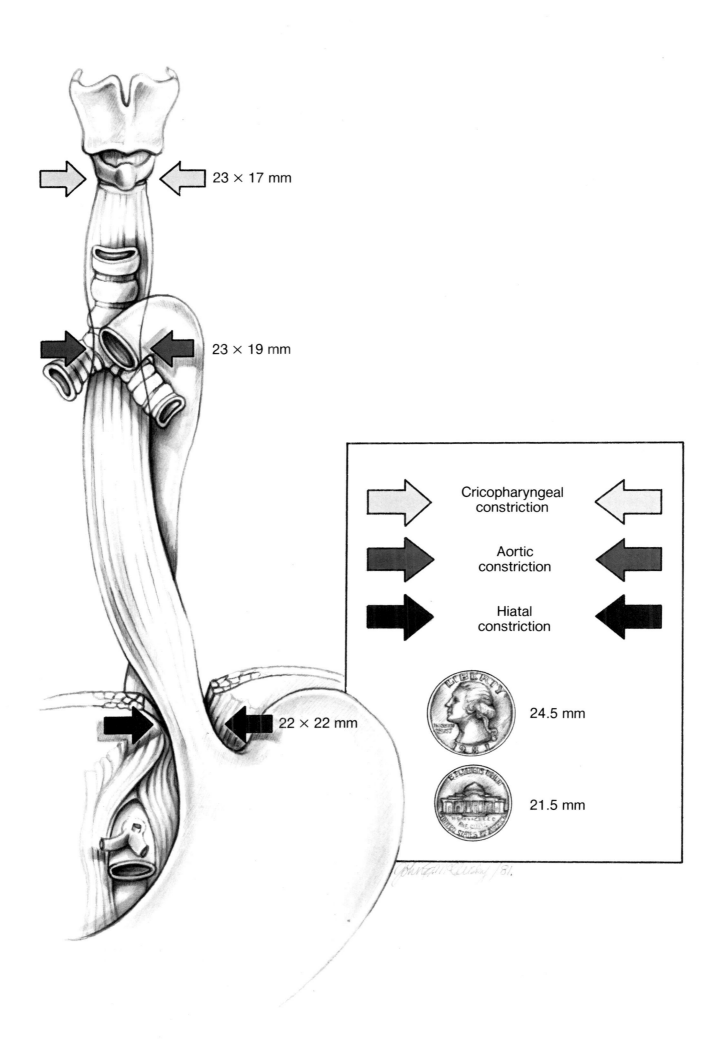

23 × 17 mm

23 × 19 mm

22 × 22 mm

Cricopharyngeal
constriction

Aortic
constriction

Hiatal
constriction

24.5 mm

21.5 mm

PLATE 3-12
Hiatal Hernia I

A. The normal distal esophagus and proximal stomach. The thickness of the phrenoesophageal ligament (purple) is exaggerated.

B. The gastroesophageal junction according to the endoscopist, the surgeon, the anatomist and the radiologist!

C. Diagram of the gastroesophageal junction and the phrenoesophageal ligament in the newborn.

D. The same area in the adult without hiatal hernia. The range of movement of the esophagus has increased.

E. The same area in the adult with hiatal hernia. The phrenoesophageal ligament is difficult and often impossible to identify.

Remember:

The phrenoesophageal ligament is present in newborn infants; it is attenuated in normal adults, and it usually cannot be found in adults with hiatal hernia.

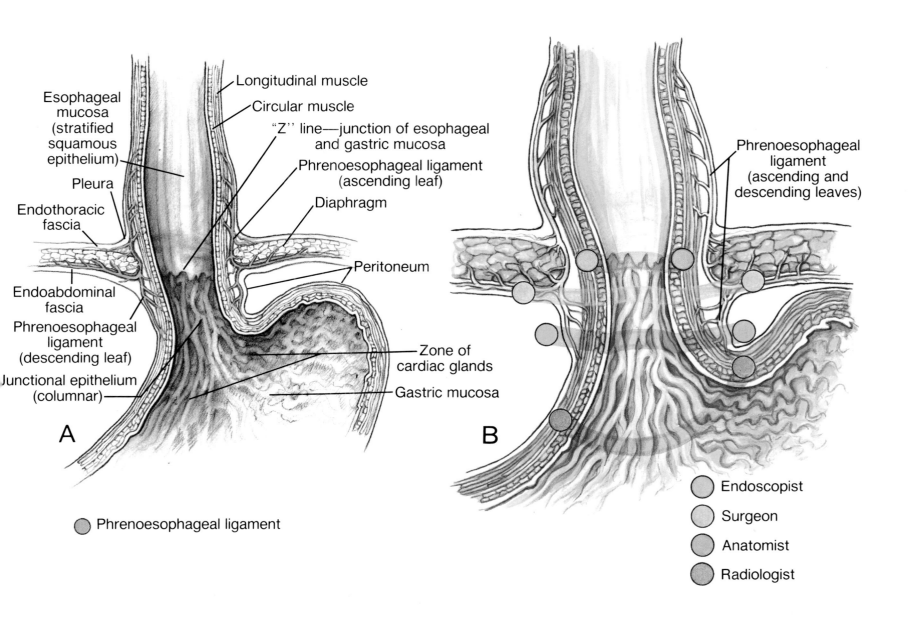

Esophageal mucosa (stratified squamous epithelium)

Pleura

Endothoracic fascia

Endoabdominal fascia

Phrenoesophageal ligament (descending leaf)

Junctional epithelium (columnar)

Longitudinal muscle

Circular muscle

"Z" line—junction of esophageal and gastric mucosa

Phrenoesophageal ligament (ascending leaf)

Diaphragm

Peritoneum

Zone of cardiac glands

Gastric mucosa

A

● Phrenoesophageal ligament

Phrenoesophageal ligament (ascending and descending leaves)

B

● Endoscopist

● Surgeon

● Anatomist

● Radiologist

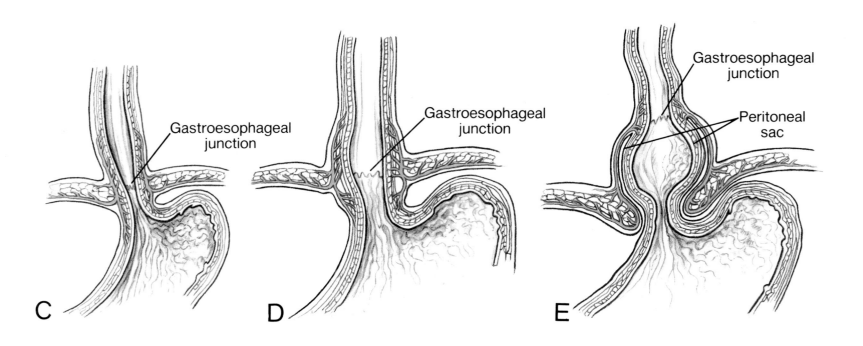

Gastroesophageal junction

Gastroesophageal junction

Gastroesophageal junction

Peritoneal sac

C

D

E

C Newborn

D Adult without hernia

E Adult with hernia

Phrenoesophageal ligament

PLATE 3-13
Hiatal Hernia II

A. Diagram of a sliding hiatal hernia in anterior view. The gastroesophageal junction and the phrenoesophageal ligament, if present, have been carried upward into the thorax. This is the most frequent type of hiatal hernia.

B. Paraesophageal hiatal hernia in anterior view. The gastroesophageal junction remains at the normal level; the fundus of the stomach has herniated anterior to the esophagus. This type is rare.

Remember:

1) The philosophy behind the repair of sliding hiatal hernia is the formation of a competent gastroesophageal junction in the abdomen. This is achieved by four steps: a) reduction of the hernia; b) obliteration of the hernial sac; c) contraction of the hiatus; d) fixation of the esophagus.

2) Repair of paraesophageal hernia requires reduction of the stomach and anatomic repair of the hiatus. Occasionally, the entire procedure for repair of sliding hernia may be required.

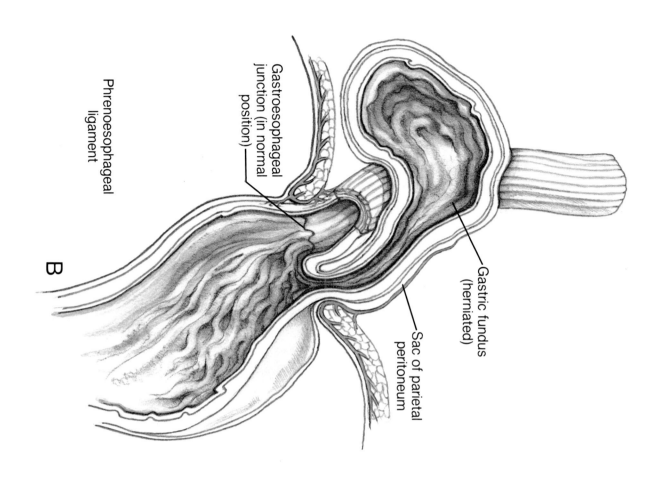

Gastroesophageal
junction (in normal
position)

Phrenoesophageal
ligament

B

Gastric fundus
(herniated)

Sac of parietal
peritoneum

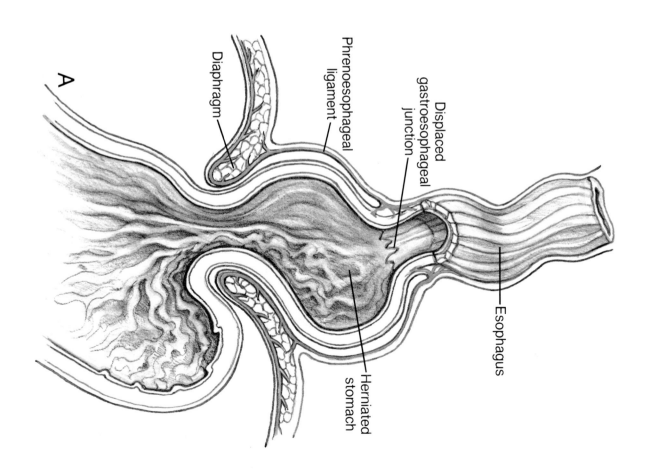

Diaphragm

Phrenoesophageal
ligament

Displaced
gastroesophageal
junction

A

Esophagus

Herniated
stomach

PLATE 3-14
The Hiatus and the Crura I

A. Crura and the esophageal hiatus seen from below. In over one half of subjects, both arms of the hiatal ring arise from the right crus; in over one third of subjects the right arm arises from the left crus and the left arm arises from the right crus. In the remainder of subjects there is a variety of other configurations. There appears to be no relation between the crural pattern and hiatal hernia.

B. The esophageal hiatus seen from above. Two muscle patterns are associated with each of the types of crura seen on the inferior surface (see Plate 3–14A above).

C. Lateral view of the diaphragm showing its relations to the inferior vena cava, the esophagus and the aorta.

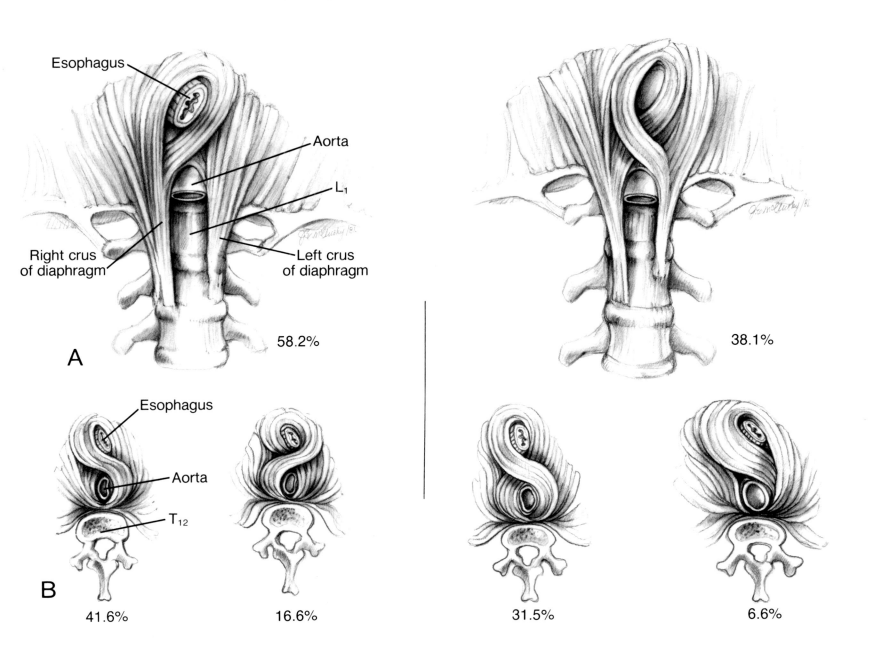

Esophagus

Aorta

L_1

Right crus
of diaphragm

Left crus
of diaphragm

A   58.2%

38.1%

Esophagus

Aorta

T_{12}

B

41.6%   16.6%   31.5%   6.6%

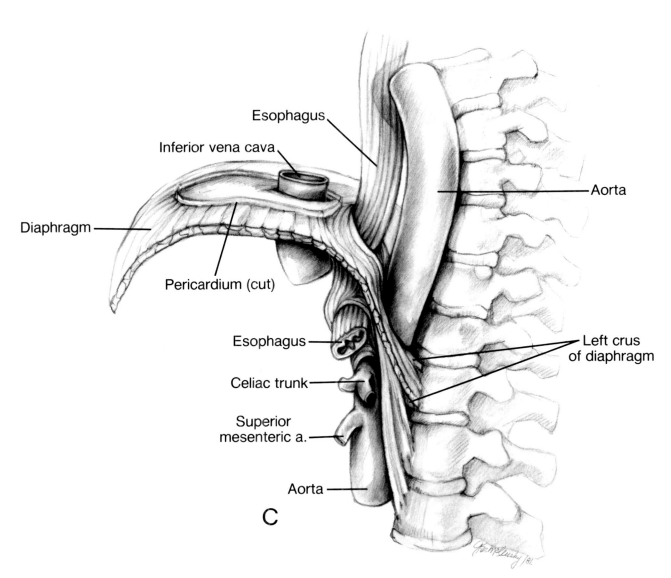

Esophagus

Inferior vena cava

Aorta

Diaphragm

Pericardium (cut)

Esophagus

Left crus
of diaphragm

Celiac trunk

Superior
mesenteric a.

Aorta

C

PLATE 3-15
The Hiatus and Crura II

Mobilization of the abdominal esophagus.

A. The forefinger is passed gently beneath the abdominal esophagus.

B. The forefinger has passed too deep and has entered and perforated the pleura as indicated by the appearance of air bubbles.

C. Diagram of the esophageal hiatus of the diaphragm showing the right and left arms of the right crus and the median arcuate ligament. The median arcuate ligament is a region of fusion of the tendinous portions of the crura above the aorta. It is present in only 50% of patients. In 16%, it partially covers the origin of the celiac trunk from the aorta.

D, E and F. Other variations of the muscular arms forming the esophageal hiatus (see also Plate 3-14).

Remember:

1) The abdominal esophagus lies between the two layers of the gastrohepatic ligament.

2) The gastrosplenic ligament contains the short gastric vessels and left gastroepiploic vessels.

3) Approach the gastroesophageal junction by perforating the avascular upper part of the gastrophrenic ligament (see Plate 3-15A).

4) Both mediastinal pleurae are close to the esophagus at the hiatus. Be careful during mobilization of the esophagus not to produce pneumo- or hemopneumothorax (see Plate 3-15B).

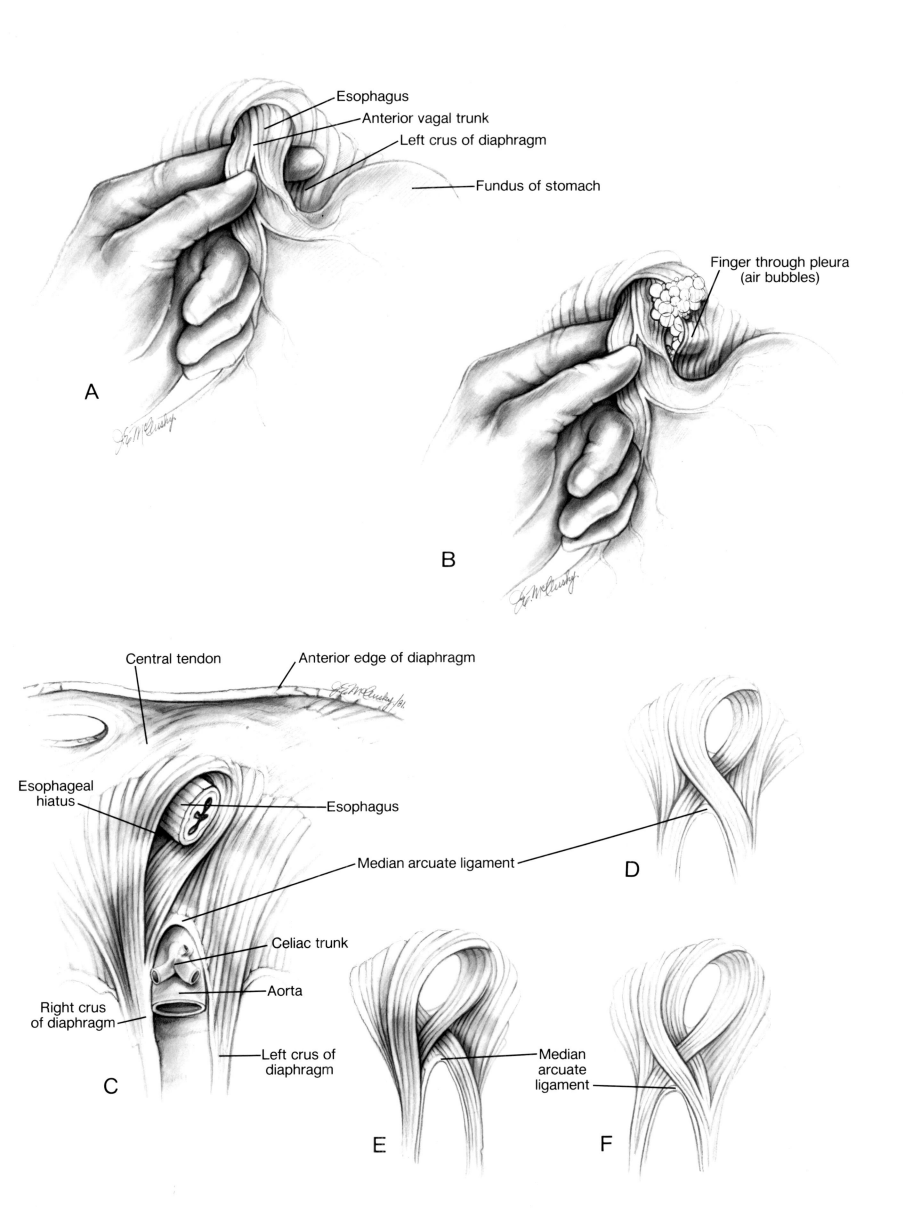

Esophagus
Anterior vagal trunk
Left crus of diaphragm
Fundus of stomach

A

Finger through pleura (air bubbles)

B

Central tendon
Anterior edge of diaphragm

Esophageal hiatus
Esophagus
Median arcuate ligament

D

Celiac trunk

Aorta

Right crus of diaphragm

Left crus of diaphragm

C

Median arcuate ligament

E

F

PLATE 3-16
The Hiatus and Crura III

A. The crura are composed of a tendinous, posterior portion and a muscular, anterior portion. The latter will not hold sutures well.

B. The right crus and its continuation as the suspensory muscle of the duodenum (ligament of Treitz).

C. Variations of the duodenal attachment of the suspensory muscle to the duodenum.

Remember:

1) In 90% of subjects the crura are tendinous posteriorly and medially, from their vertebral origins to the level of the 10th thoracic vertebra. Sutures for crural approximation should always be placed deep, and through the tendinous parts.

2) Sutures to approximate the crura must be placed above the celiac ganglia and behind the celiac division of the posterior vagal trunk.

3) The ligament of Treitz passes posterior to the pancreas and the splenic vein, and anterior to the left renal vein.

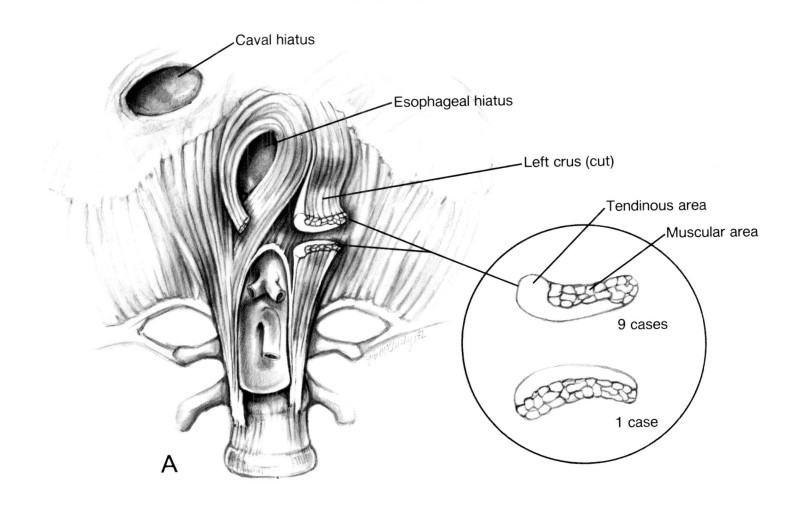

Caval hiatus

Esophageal hiatus

Left crus (cut)

Tendinous area

Muscular area

9 cases

1 case

A

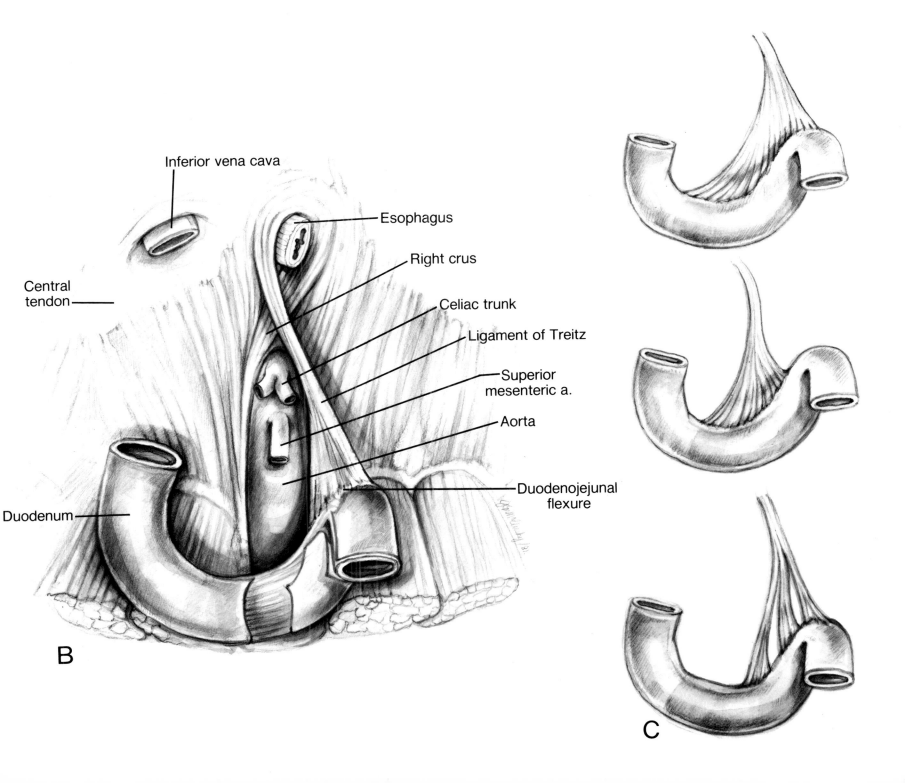

Inferior vena cava

Esophagus

Right crus

Celiac trunk

Ligament of Treitz

Superior mesenteric a.

Aorta

Duodenojejunal flexure

Central tendon

Duodenum

B

C

PLATE 3-17
Nerves of the Diaphragm

A. The adult diaphragm from below showing nerves and blood vessels passing through it.

B. The distribution of the phrenic nerves on the inferior surface of the diaphragm.

Inset: Incisions along the dotted lines will cause the least injury to the phrenic nerves, according to Merendino.

Remember:

The phrenic nerve supplies not only the diaphragm but also the three P's: pleura, peritoneum and pericardium.

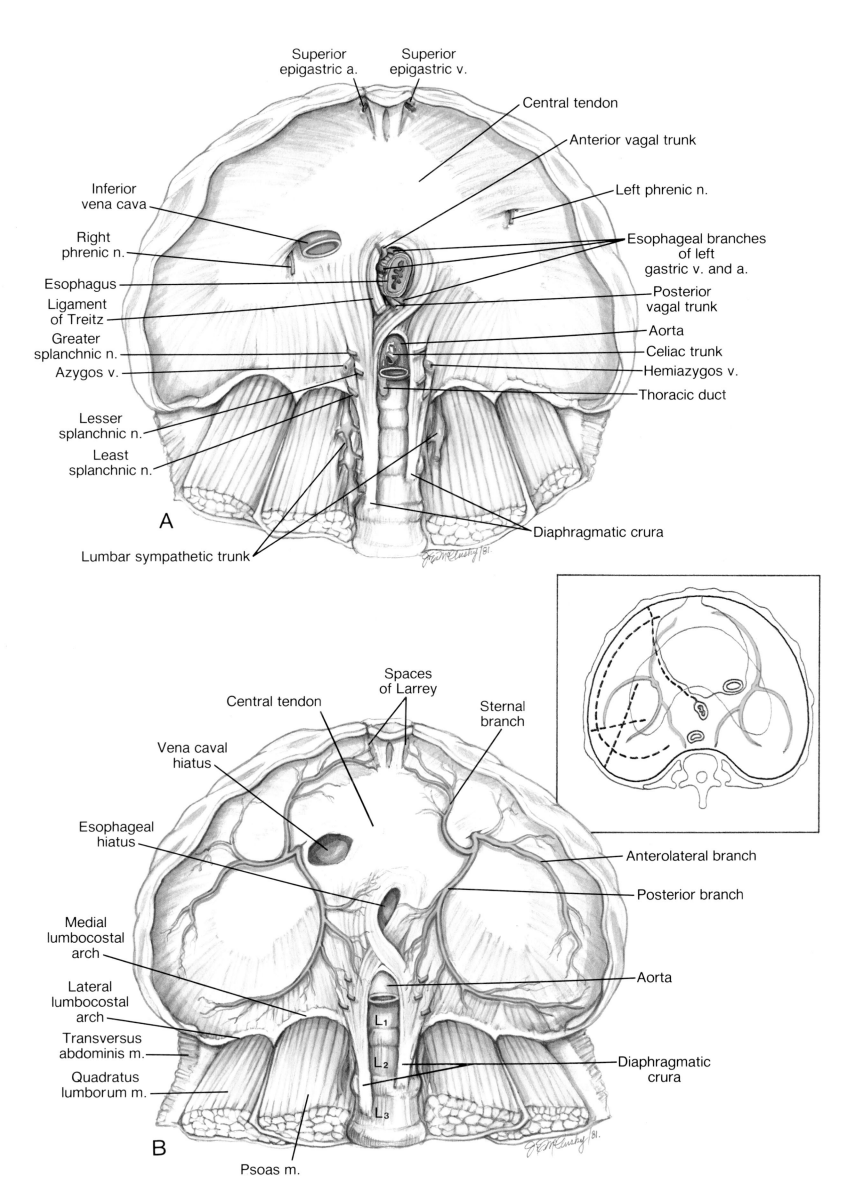

Superior
epigastric a.

Superior
epigastric v.

Central tendon

Anterior vagal trunk

Left phrenic n.

Inferior
vena cava

Right
phrenic n.

Esophageal branches
of left
gastric v. and a.

Esophagus

Posterior
vagal trunk

Ligament
of Treitz

Aorta

Greater
splanchnic n.

Celiac trunk

Azygos v.

Hemiazygos v.

Thoracic duct

Lesser
splanchnic n.

Least
splanchnic n.

Diaphragmatic crura

Lumbar sympathetic trunk

A

Spaces
of Larrey

Central tendon

Sternal
branch

Vena caval
hiatus

Esophageal
hiatus

Anterolateral branch

Posterior branch

Medial
lumbocostal
arch

Lateral
lumbocostal
arch

Aorta

Transversus
abdominis m.

Diaphragmatic
crura

Quadratus
lumborum m.

L₁

L₂

L₃

B

Psoas m.

PLATE 4-1
The Anterior Abdominal Wall

The anterior abdominal wall, its layers, and the composition of the rectus sheath in sections through the wall at two levels.

Robert Maingot stated three requirements for an abdominal incision: accessibility, extensibility and security. These may be achieved by the following rules.

1. The incision should be long enough for a good exposure with room to work, and short enough to avoid complications.

2. Skin incisions should follow Langer's lines where possible.

3. Avoid incisions parallel to existing scars. Excise the scar and proceed.

4. Muscles, except the rectus abdominis, should be split in the direction of their fibers rather than transected. The rectus muscle may be transected without risk of denervation because it has a segmental nerve supply.

5. Openings formed through the different layers of the abdominal wall should not be superimposed.

6. Avoid cutting nerves wherever possible.

7. Muscles and abdominal organs should be retracted toward their neurovascular supply.

8. Drainage tubes should be inserted through separate incisions; in the main incision they may weaken the wound.

9. Cosmetic considerations must be given close attention, but Maingot's principles must not be sacrificed.

Remember:

1) An upper midline incision should open the peritoneum slightly to the left of the midline to avoid the round ligament.

2) Do not cut more than one thoracic nerve.

3) Suture linea alba to linea alba. Anatomical approximation is paramount. To avoid dehiscence, use closely spaced sutures with big bites.

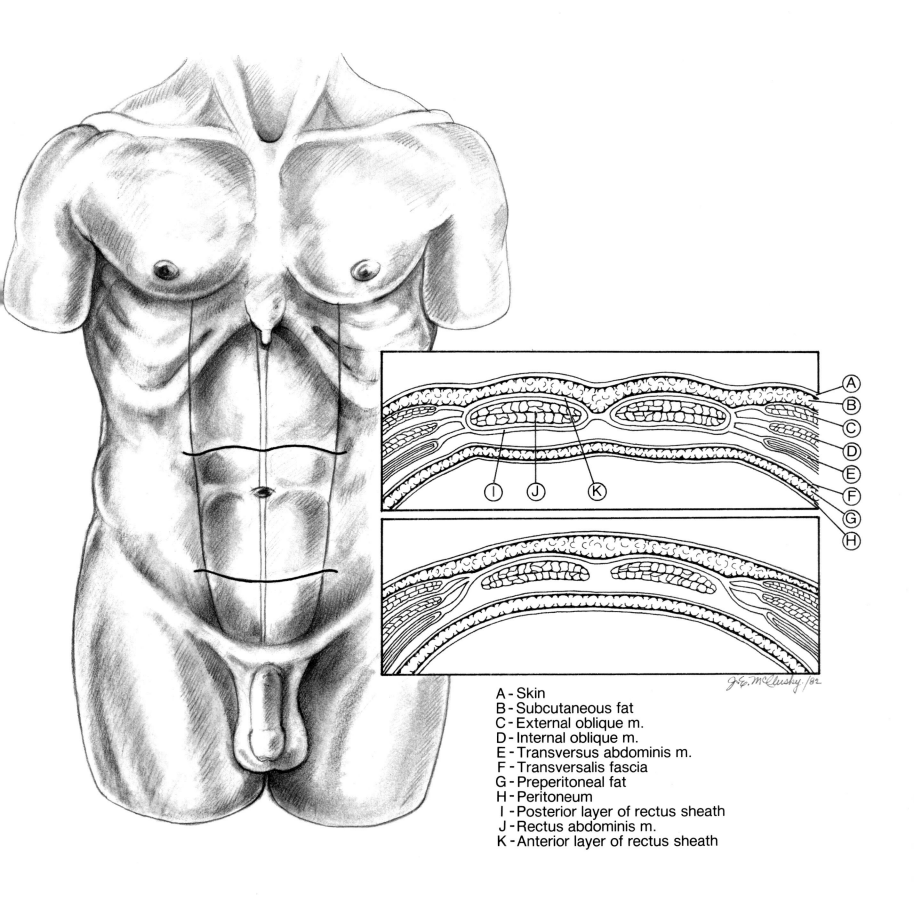

A - Skin
B - Subcutaneous fat
C - External oblique m.
D - Internal oblique m.
E - Transversus abdominis m.
F - Transversalis fascia
G - Preperitoneal fat
H - Peritoneum
I - Posterior layer of rectus sheath
J - Rectus abdominis m.
K - Anterior layer of rectus sheath

PLATE 4-2
Development of the Mesenteries I

A. Schematic cross section through the upper abdomen of an embryo at the end of the first month of gestation. The primitive dorsal and ventral mesenteries (dorsal and ventral mesogastria) are present.

B. Schematic cross section through the upper abdomen in later embryonic life showing the movements of the stomach, pancreas and spleen in the dorsal mesogastrium.

Remember:

1) The only remaining parts of the primitive ventral mesentery are the hepatic, falciform, coronary, triangular and gastrohepatic ligaments all derived from the ventral mesogastrium.

2) The duodenum, ascending and descending colon do not retain the primitive dorsal mesentery.

3) The first portion of the duodenum is related to both mesenteries.

4) The adult greater omentum is part of the embryonic dorsal mesogastrium.

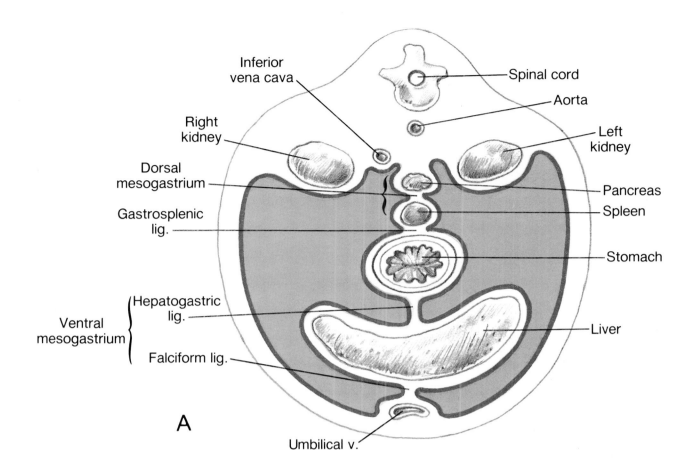

Inferior vena cava

Spinal cord

Aorta

Right kidney

Left kidney

Dorsal mesogastrium

Pancreas

Gastrosplenic lig.

Spleen

Stomach

Ventral mesogastrium

Hepatogastric lig.

Liver

Falciform lig.

Umbilical v.

A

A. Early stage
B. Late fetal stage

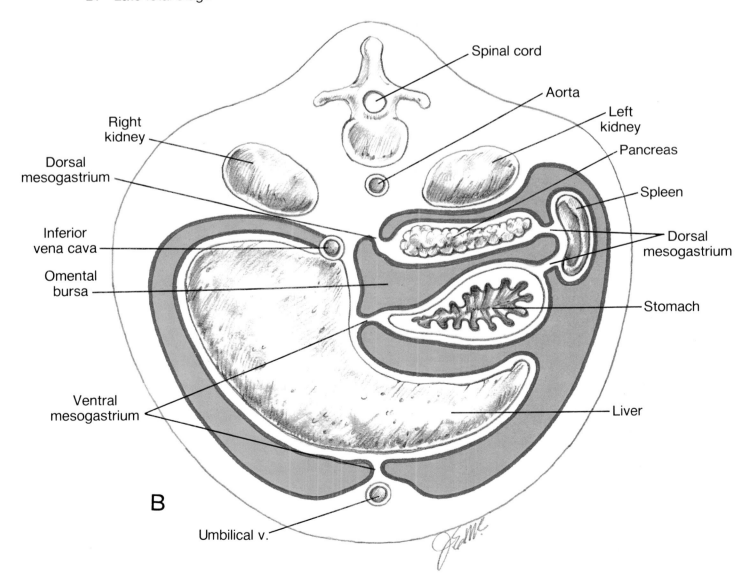

Spinal cord

Aorta

Right kidney

Left kidney

Dorsal mesogastrium

Pancreas

Spleen

Inferior vena cava

Dorsal mesogastrium

Omental bursa

Stomach

Ventral mesogastrium

Liver

B

Umbilical v.

PLATE 4-3
Development of the Mesenteries II

A. Schematic sagittal section through the abdomen of a fetus at about 2 months gestation. The dorsal mesentery, containing duodenum and pancreas, is still unattached to the posterior wall. The omental bursa (lesser sac) is outlined with a black line.

B. Similar section of a fetus at 4 months gestation. The dorsal mesogastrium, containing the duodenum and pancreas, has fused with the abdominal wall; the plane of fusion is avascular. The greater omentum is elongating.

C. Newborn infant. The layers of the greater omentum have fused. A red arrow indicates the epiploic foramen (of Winslow).

Remember:

1) The omentum is not well developed in children. In adults it is well developed in most subjects.

2) Occasionally in children and adults, the fusion of the leaves does not take place and a cavity exists below the transverse colon from which the omentum hangs.

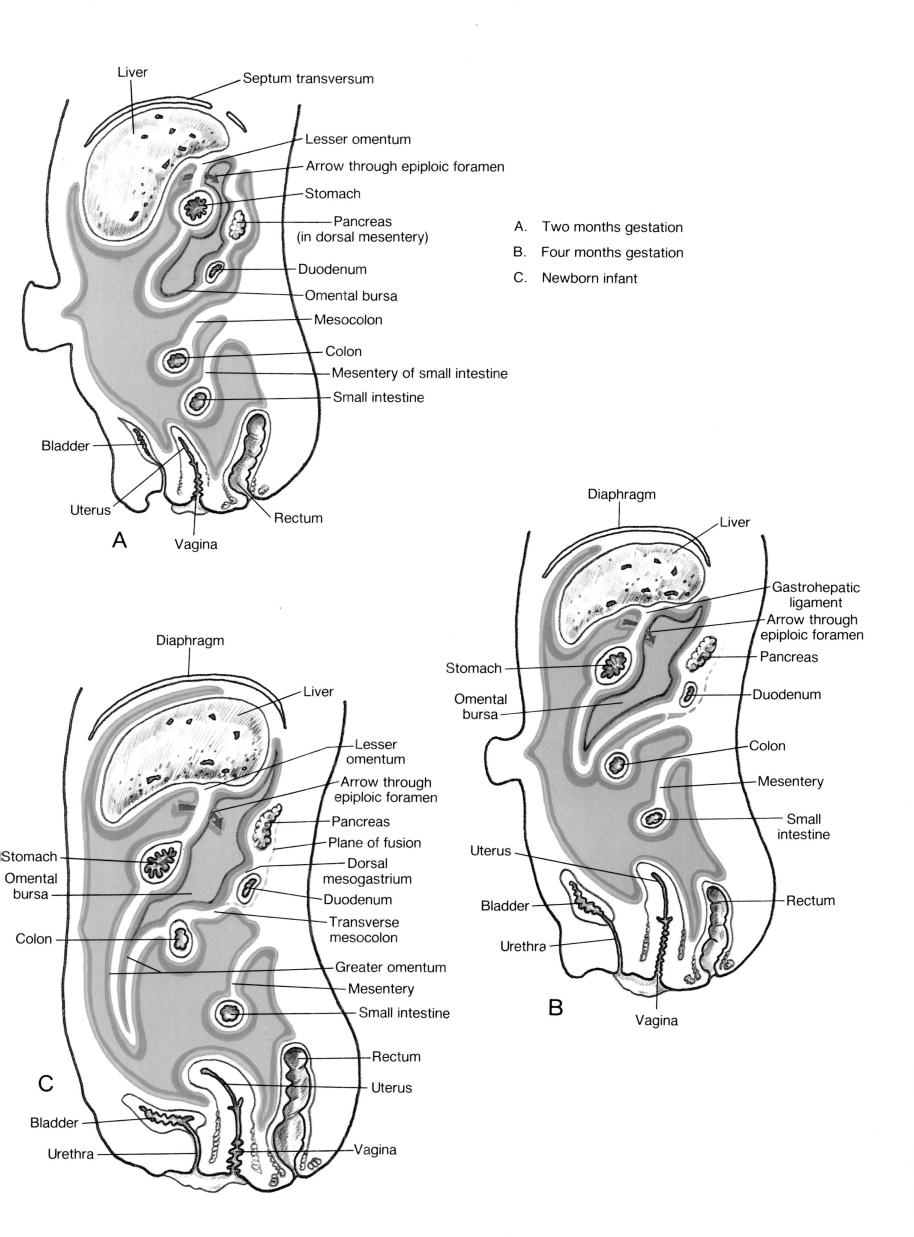

Liver

Septum transversum

Lesser omentum

Arrow through epiploic foramen

Stomach

Pancreas
(in dorsal mesentery)

Duodenum

Omental bursa

Mesocolon

Colon

Mesentery of small intestine

Small intestine

Bladder

Uterus

Vagina

Rectum

A

A. Two months gestation

B. Four months gestation

C. Newborn infant

Diaphragm

Liver

Gastrohepatic ligament

Arrow through epiploic foramen

Pancreas

Duodenum

Colon

Mesentery

Small intestine

Stomach

Omental bursa

Uterus

Bladder

Urethra

Rectum

Vagina

B

Diaphragm

Liver

Lesser omentum

Arrow through epiploic foramen

Pancreas

Plane of fusion

Dorsal mesogastrium

Duodenum

Transverse mesocolon

Greater omentum

Mesentery

Small intestine

Rectum

Uterus

Vagina

Stomach

Omental bursa

Colon

Bladder

Urethra

C

PLATE 4-4
Development of the Mesenteries III

The greater omentum and its relationships.

Inset: The primitive cavity of the greater omentum is obliterated by the fusion of the four primitive layers of peritoneum derived from the dorsal mesogastrium. The arrow passes between the fused layers.

Remember:

1) The greater omentum, with its blood vessels and lymphatics, is attached to the first portion of the duodenum, greater curvature of the stomach and the abdominal esophagus.

2) The outer leaf of the greater sac envelops the spleen; the inner leaf is related to the lesser sac.

3) Idiopathic infarction of the greater omentum is rare.

4) The greater omentum has been called the "policeman" of the abdomen. We believe it provides police protection not police brutality.

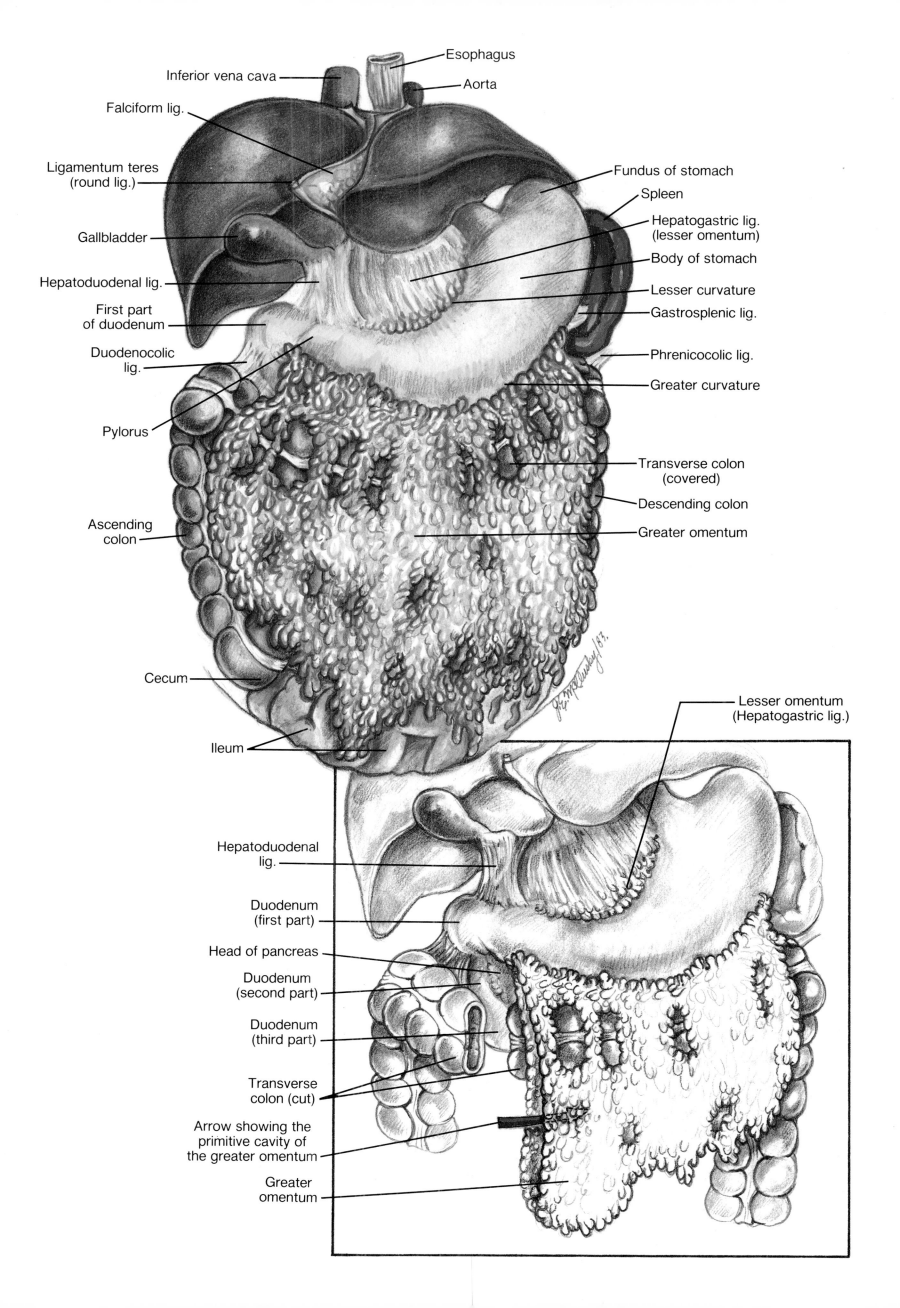

Inferior vena cava

Esophagus

Aorta

Falciform lig.

Ligamentum teres
(round lig.)

Fundus of stomach

Spleen

Hepatogastric lig.
(lesser omentum)

Gallbladder

Body of stomach

Hepatoduodenal lig.

Lesser curvature

First part
of duodenum

Gastrosplenic lig.

Duodenocolic
lig.

Phrenicocolic lig.

Greater curvature

Pylorus

Ascending
colon

Transverse colon
(covered)

Descending colon

Greater omentum

Cecum

Ileum

Lesser omentum
(Hepatogastric lig.)

Hepatoduodenal
lig.

Duodenum
(first part)

Head of pancreas

Duodenum
(second part)

Duodenum
(third part)

Transverse
colon (cut)

Arrow showing the
primitive cavity of
the greater omentum

Greater
omentum

PLATE 4-5
Attachments of the Transverse Mesocolon

A. The stomach and the transverse colon have been removed to show the relation of the transverse mesocolon to the duodenum, pancreas and the mesentery.

B. Schematic sagittal section showing the relations of the mesocolon, pancreas and superior mesenteric artery.

Remember:

1) The splenic (left) flexure of the colon is attached to the diaphragm by the phrenocolic ligament. The hepatic flexure of the colon on the right has no such attachment. Thus, the right peritoneal gutter is uninterrupted from the pelvis to the diaphragm, whereas the left gutter is blocked at the phrenocolic ligament.

2) Free the omentum carefully from the transverse colon. Don't forget the middle colic artery.

3) The omentum has a rich blood supply from the right and left gastroepiploic arteries, the pancreatic arteries and branches of the middle colic artery. All together they form the avascular arc of Barkow, which prevents omental necrosis following separation of the omentum from the greater curvature of the stomach and transverse colon.

4) By preservation of the omental blood supply, postoperative omental infarction and fever "of unknown origin" may be avoided.

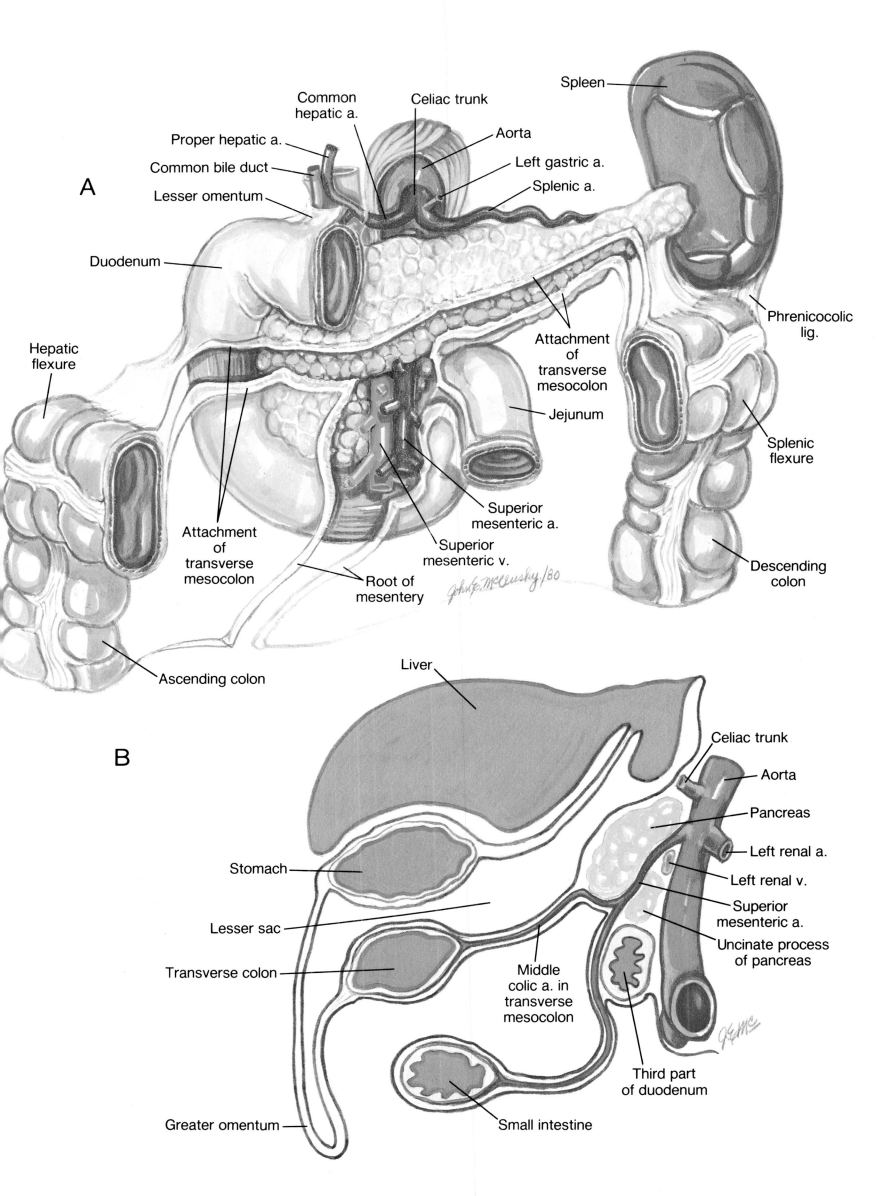

A

Common
hepatic a.

Celiac trunk

Proper hepatic a.

Aorta

Common bile duct

Left gastric a.

Lesser omentum

Splenic a.

Spleen

Duodenum

Hepatic
flexure

Attachment
of
transverse
mesocolon

Phrenicocolic
lig.

Jejunum

Attachment
of
transverse
mesocolon

Root of
mesentery

Superior
mesenteric a.

Superior
mesenteric v.

Splenic
flexure

Descending
colon

John E. McCleusky/80

Ascending colon

B

Liver

Celiac trunk

Aorta

Pancreas

Stomach

Left renal a.

Left renal v.

Lesser sac

Superior
mesenteric a.

Transverse colon

Uncinate process
of pancreas

Middle
colic a. in
transverse
mesocolon

Third part
of duodenum

Greater omentum

Small intestine

PLATE 4-6
Pitfalls of Entering the Lesser Sac

A. Normal anatomy. The hemostat, directed upward, has entered the lesser sac by perforation of the omentum just beneath the stomach.

B. Inflammatory fixation of the omentum, stomach wall and transverse mesocolon may result in the perforating instrument passing through the mesocolon with risk of injury to the middle colic artery.

C. Normal anatomy, but inferiorly directed instrument may endanger the middle colic artery.

Remember:

1) By carefully incising and ligating the vessels of the gastrocolic ligament, the posterior gastric surface can be freed from the omental bursa.

2) Separate the transverse mesocolon carefully to avoid injuring the middle colic artery.

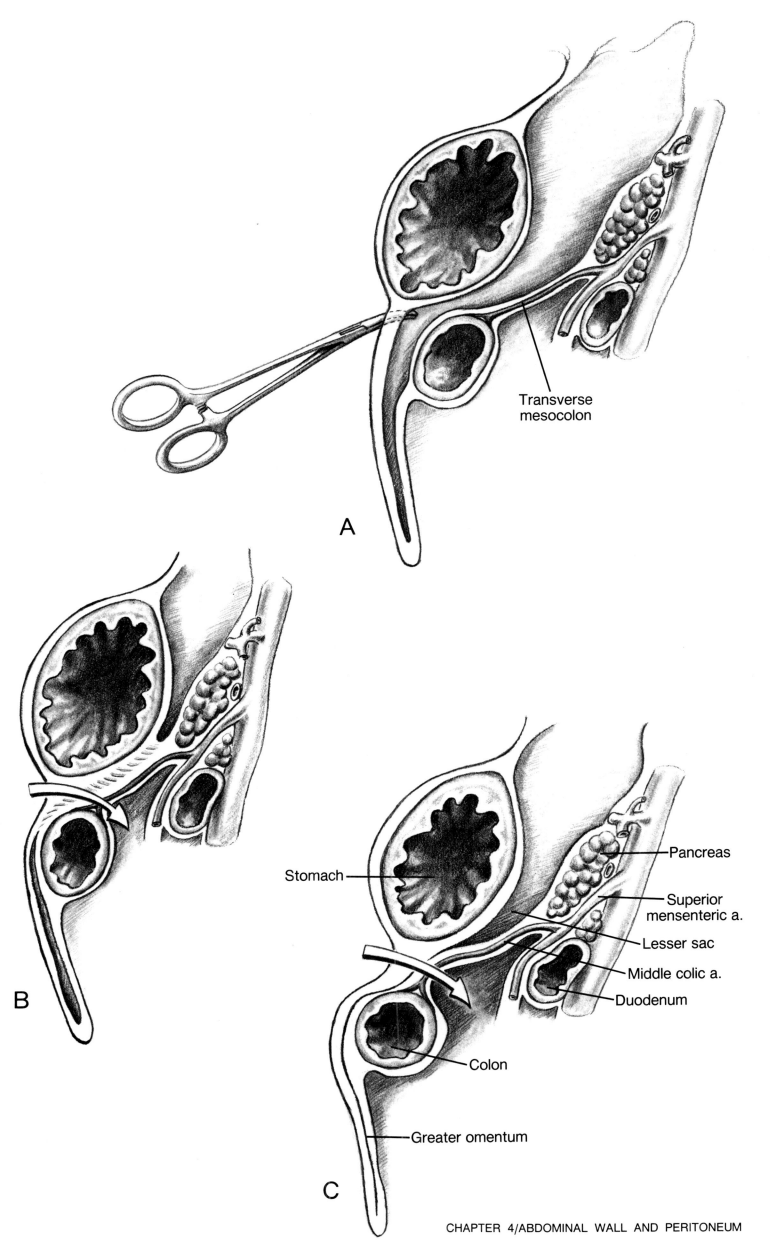

Transverse
mesocolon

A

B

C

Stomach

Pancreas

Superior
mensenteric a.

Lesser sac

Middle colic a.

Duodenum

Colon

Greater omentum

PLATE 4-7
The Peritoneal Cavity

A. The peritoneal cavity is divided into supracolic and infracolic compartments by the transverse mesocolon at the level of the first lumbar vertebra. The supracolic compartment is further divided into right (blue) and left (orange) compartments by a plane passing through the falciform ligament. The infracolic compartment is divided diagonally by the attachment of the mesentery of the small intestine into a right supramesenteric compartment (green) and a left inframesenteric compartment (pink). The pelvic cavity (purple) in the female is divided into anterior and posterior compartments by the uterus and the broad ligaments.

B. Diagram of the posterior abdominal wall with viscera removed. The peritoneal attachments of the organs are shown.

Remember:

The parietal peritoneum is sensitive to pain. The sensory innervation is from (1) spinal nerve branches of overlying muscles, (2) intercostal and lumbar nerve and (3) in the pelvis, the obturator nerve. Irritation of the diaphragm produces pain at the tip to the shoulder by way of the phrenic nerve (C_4).

The phrenocolic ligament forms a cranial limit to the general peritoneal cavity on the left; there is no such barrier on the right.

A

1. Supracolic compartment
2. Infracolic compartment

Right supracolic compartment
Left supracolic compartment
Right supramesenteric compartment
Left inframesenteric compartment
Pelvic compartment

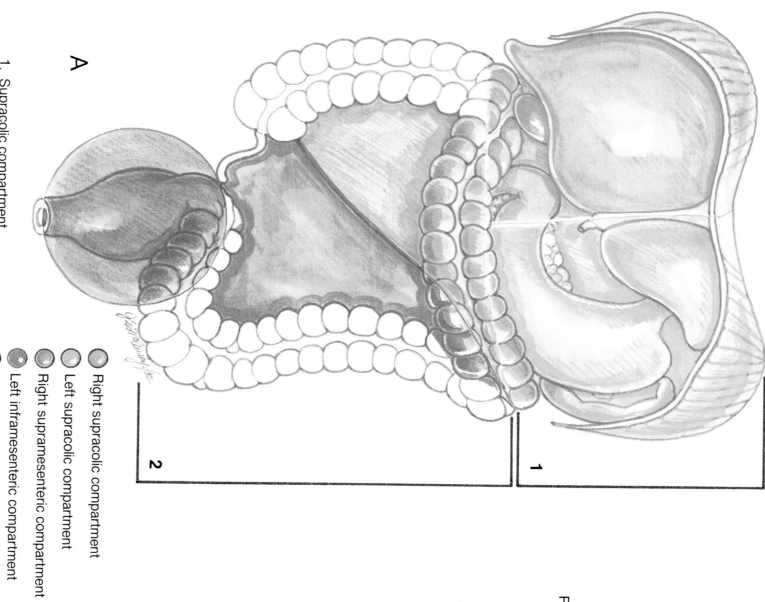

B

Right ureter
Right colon
Root of mesentery
Duodenum
Hepatic triad
Right triangular ligament
Coronary ligament
Bare area
Falciform ligament
Abdominal esophagus
Left triangular ligament
Transverse mesocolon
Phrenicocolic ligament
Jejunum
Left colon
Sigmoid mesocolon
Left ureter

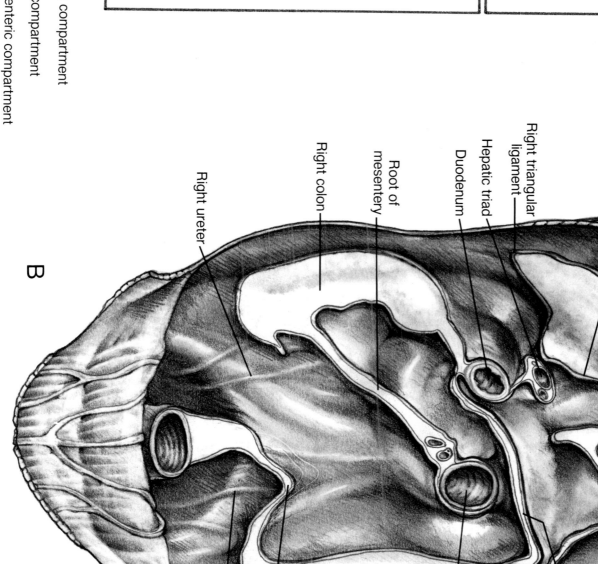

PLATE 4-8
Peritoneal Fossae

A. The most common paraduodenal fossae: (1) intermesocolic fossa; (2) superior duodenal fossa; (3) lateral fossa; (4) inferior duodenal fossa and (5) mesentericoparietal fossa.

B. Two peritoneal fossae in the ileocecal region. A loop of intestine may enter and become incarcerated in any of these fossae creating a peritoneal hernia. These hernias and their nomenclature are discussed in Chapter 14.

Table: Classification of Intraperitoneal Fossae and Apertures through Which Hernias May Occur

I Retroperitoneal
  Paraduodenal (Plates 4–8A, 14–19, 20)
  Paracecal (Plate 4–8B)

II Properitoneal
  Interparietal (Plate 14–9)
  Supravesical (Plates 14–10, 11)

III Endoperitoneal
  Mesenteric (Plate 14–21)
  Omental (Plate 14–22)
  Broad ligament (Plate 14–25)

IV Foraminal
  Epiploic (Plate 14–24)
  Sciatic (Plate 14–14)
  Obturator (Plate 14–13)

V Perineal (Plate 14–15)

Remember:

These fossae are not constant; rarely are all present in the same individual. Their presence predisposes to, but only occasionally results in, an actual hernia.

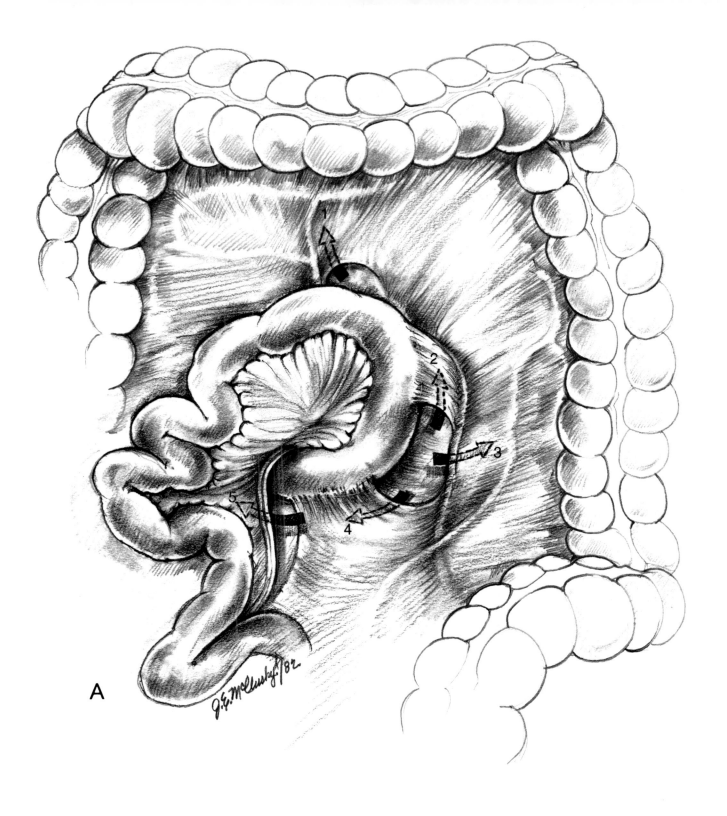

A

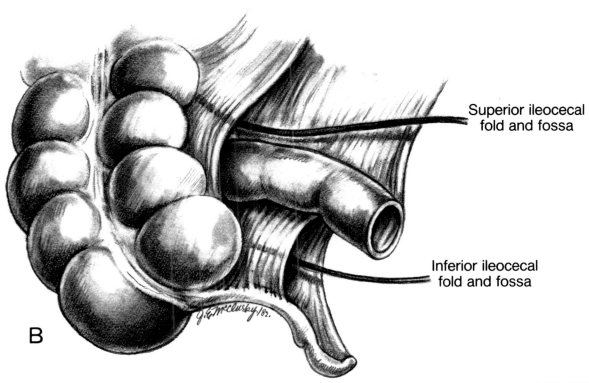

Superior ileocecal
fold and fossa

Inferior ileocecal
fold and fossa

B

PLATE 4-9
Anatomy of the Suprahepatic Spaces

Semidiagrammatic sagittal sections to illustrate the sites of suprahepatic (subdiaphragmatic) abscesses and fluid collections.

A. Abscess in the right anterior suprahepatic space.

B. Abscess in the right posterior suprahepatic space.

C. Abscess in the left posterior suprahepatic space.

D. Abscess in the left anterior suprahepatic space.

Part of the superior surface of the liver and the inferior surface of the diaphragm are in direct contact, the "bare area". Except for this area, the serous surfaces of the two organs are in apposition with a potential space between. The space is divided by the falciform ligament into right and left portions. These spaces may become the sites of intraperitoneal fluid collections and subphrenic abscesses.

Boundaries of the Right Suprahepatic Space:

Superior	Diaphragm
Inferior	Anterosuperior surface of right lobe and medial segment of left lobe of the liver
Medial	Falciform ligament
Posterior	Right anterior coronary and right triangular ligaments
Anteroinferior	Opens into general peritoneal cavity

Boundaries of the Left Supraheptic Space:

Superior	Diaphragm
Inferior	Lateral segment of left lobe of liver and fundus of stomach
Medial	Falciform ligament
Posterior	Left coronary and left triangular ligaments
Anterolateral	Opens into subhepatic space and general peritoneal cavity

Each of these spaces may be divided into anterior and posterior portions. In the absence of disease, the distinction is unimportant. A collection of fluid may form in the anterior (A), or the posterior (B), portions of the right hepatic space with pseudomembranes sealing off the corresponding posterior and anterior portions which are not involved.

The left space may be similarly divided by pathological pseudomembranes, limiting the lesion to the posterior (C) or anterior (D) portions only. Anterior lesions may extend into the subhepatic space.

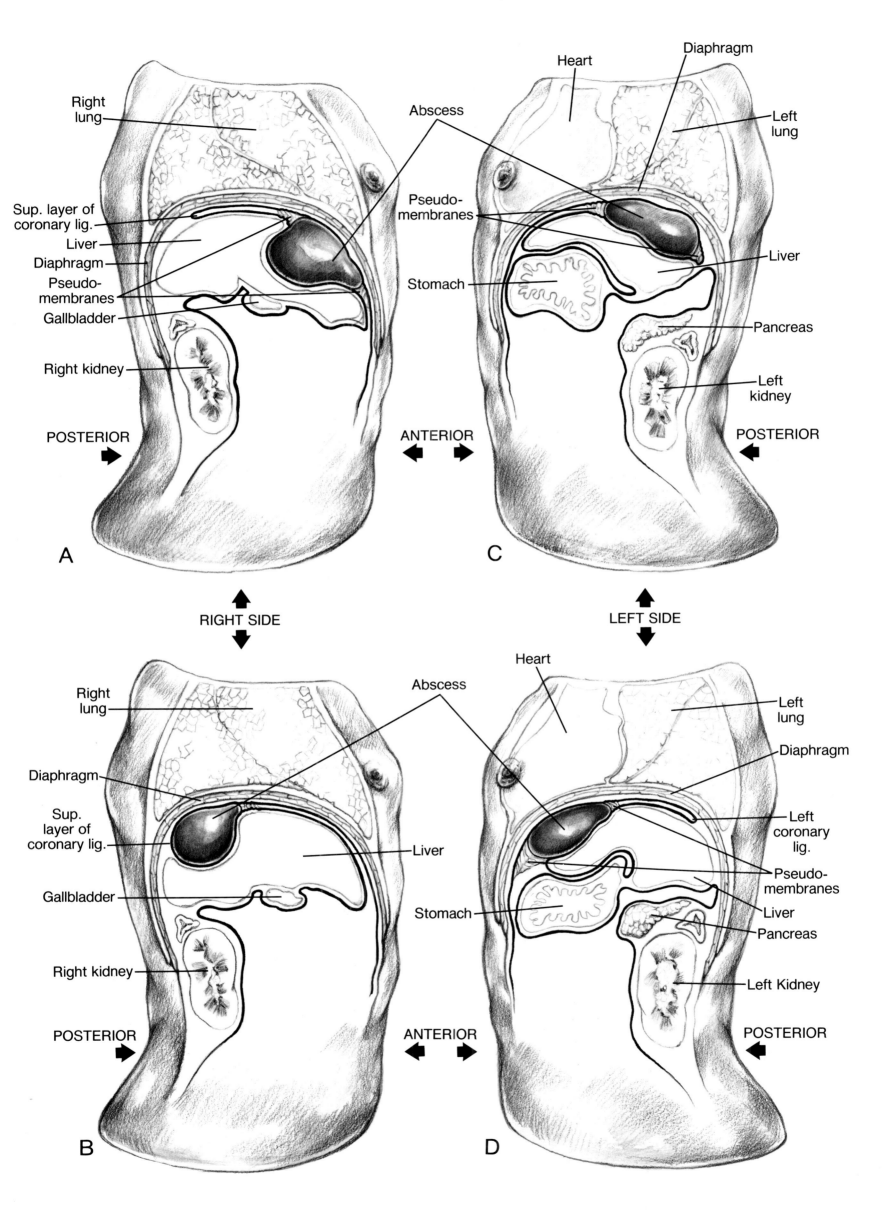

Right lung

Sup. layer of coronary lig.

Liver

Diaphragm

Pseudo-membranes

Gallbladder

Right kidney

POSTERIOR

A

Abscess

Pseudo-membranes

Heart

Diaphragm

Left lung

Liver

Stomach

Pancreas

Left kidney

ANTERIOR

POSTERIOR

C

RIGHT SIDE

LEFT SIDE

Right lung

Diaphragm

Sup. layer of coronary lig.

Gallbladder

Right kidney

POSTERIOR

B

Abscess

Liver

Heart

Left lung

Diaphragm

Left coronary lig.

Pseudo-membranes

Liver

Pancreas

Left Kidney

Stomach

ANTERIOR

POSTERIOR

D

CHAPTER 4/ABDOMINAL WALL AND PERITONEUM   107

PLATE 4-10
Examination of the Abdomen I

If the abdomen is to be opened, it should be explored even if the site of the lesion to be treated is known beforehand.

On the facing page is an example of an exploratory procedure. It is only an example. Any systematic procedure will suffice if it becomes habitual and automatic. The four criteria are: thoroughness, accuracy, gentleness and speed (acronym: TAGS).

Exploration of the abdomen is not without complications of its own. The cutting of folds and bands mistakenly thought to be bloodless can result in hemorrhage. Traction on the spleen occasionally leads to rupture. The failure to find or to recognize pathology that later becomes manifest must be considered to be the result of inadequate procedure.

Peritonitis is an ever present risk and its prevention should be uppermost in the surgeon's mind. Some strategies are listed below:

Strategy	Preventative Procedure
Prior to surgery	Antibiotics, hyperalimentation, cleansing enemas, respiratory toilet
At operation	Irrigation, antibiotics, closed suction drainage, delayed skin closure
After surgery	Antibiotics, hyperalimentation, respiratory toilet
Technique	Good surgery without "breaks"
Surgical anatomy	Understanding of the normal and pathological anatomy of the area is paramount.

PLATE 4-10
Examination of the Abdomen II

1) Inspect the abdomen for obvious pathology that may call for immediate treatment, or that may contraindicate further exploration.

2) Examine the greater omentum and the transverse colon.

3) Pull the colon downward; examine the supracolic compartment starting on the right. Inspect the right kidney and adrenal gland, the epiploic foramen and common bile duct, the gallbladder, the right lobe of the liver, the first and second portions of the duodenum, the pancreas, the left lobe segments of the liver, the pylorus, lesser curvature and fundus of the stomach, the abdominal esophagus, cardia and greater curvature of the stomach, the spleen and the left adrenal area.

4) Pull the colon upward; examine the infracolic compartment starting on the right. Inspect the cecum and appendix, the right colon, the right retroperitoneal space and lower pole of the right kidney, the third and fourth portions of the duodenum, the superior mesenteric vessels, the small intestine and its mesentery, the tail of the pancreas and the spleen, the left kidney, aorta and left retroperitoneal space, the left colon and the sigmoid colon.

5) Examine the pelvis. Inspect the sigmoid colon and rectum, the uterus, tubes and ovaries, the uterosacral ligaments, the pelvic wall, the inguinal and femoral regions and the iliac vessels.

Exception: The organ with the lesion for which the abdomen has been opened should be left to the last, in order that the operator's interest in it does not detract from careful examination of other organs.

PLATE 5-1
The Stomach and Greater Omentum

The liver has been removed to show the triangular, coronary, falciform and hepatoduodenal ligaments.

Remember:

1) For gastric resection, gently separate the posterior gastric surface from the stomach bed by incising the gastrocolic ligament after ligating the blood vessels. Separate the greater omentum from the transverse mesocolon which contains the middle colic artery.

2) Ligate the left triangular ligament before dividing it. This will avoid bleeding and possible bile leakage from small aberrant accessory bile ducts.

3) Ligate the falciform ligament before dividing it.

4) Either remove the greater omentum or preserve its blood supply by ligating the branches of the gastroepiploic vessels to the greater curvature. This will avoid postoperative fever from fat necrosis or infarction.

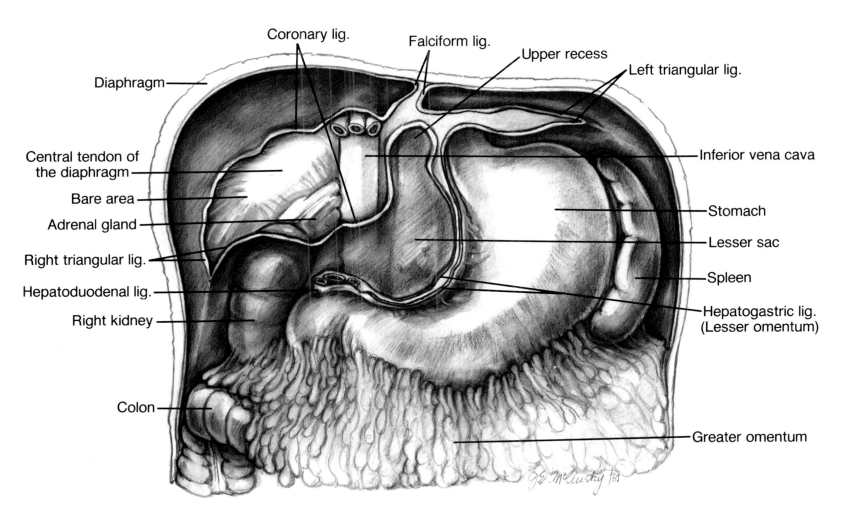

Coronary lig.

Falciform lig.

Upper recess

Left triangular lig.

Diaphragm

Central tendon of
the diaphragm

Bare area

Adrenal gland

Right triangular lig.

Hepatoduodenal lig.

Right kidney

Colon

Inferior vena cava

Stomach

Lesser sac

Spleen

Hepatogastric lig.
(Lesser omentum)

Greater omentum

PLATE 5-2
Relations of the Stomach

A. Diagram of the relations of the anterior surface of the stomach. (The length of the abdominal esophagus is exaggerated.)

B. Diagram of the relations of the posterior surface of the stomach (the stomach bed).

Remember:

1) The stomach varies in shape and position from one patient to another, and in the same patient at different times and in different positions.

2) The anterior surface is in contact with the liver, diaphragm and anterior abdominal wall.

3) The stomach bed is formed by the diaphragm, spleen, left kidney and left adrenal gland, pancreas and transverse mesocolon.

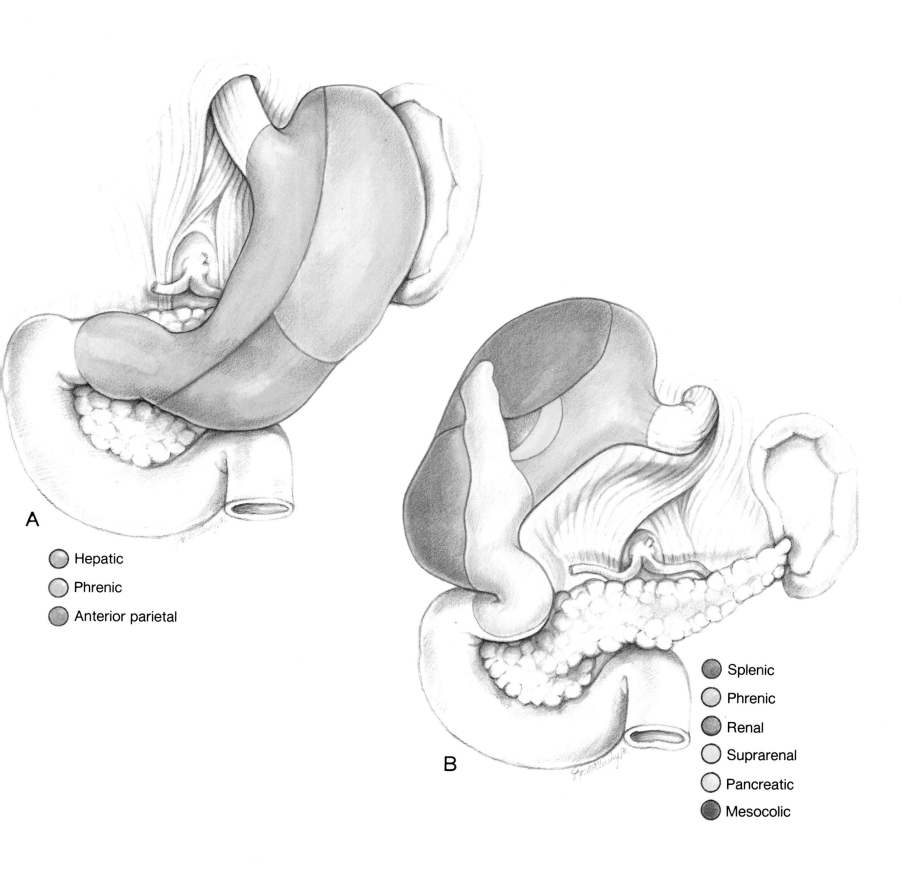

A

🔘 Hepatic

🔘 Phrenic

🔘 Anterior parietal

B

🔘 Splenic

🔘 Phrenic

🔘 Renal

🔘 Suprarenal

🔘 Pancreatic

🔘 Mesocolic

PLATE 5-3
Blood Supply of the Stomach I

A. The arterial supply to the stomach.

B. and C. The anterior and posterior relations of the branches of the gastroduodenal artery to the pylorus and the duodenum.

Extragastric ligation of the left and right gastric as well as the left and right epiploic arteries will not produce gastric necrosis due to the rich submucosal vascular plexus. The survival of the gastric remnants will depend on the ascending esophageal, the posterior gastric and short gastric arteries.

Remember:

1) The blood supply of the stomach is rich. The blood supply of the intestine is adequate. The blood supply of the colon is less adequate and the blood supply of the rectum is more adequate.

2) Extensive mobilization of the stomach can be accomplished by ligating three of the four main arteries.

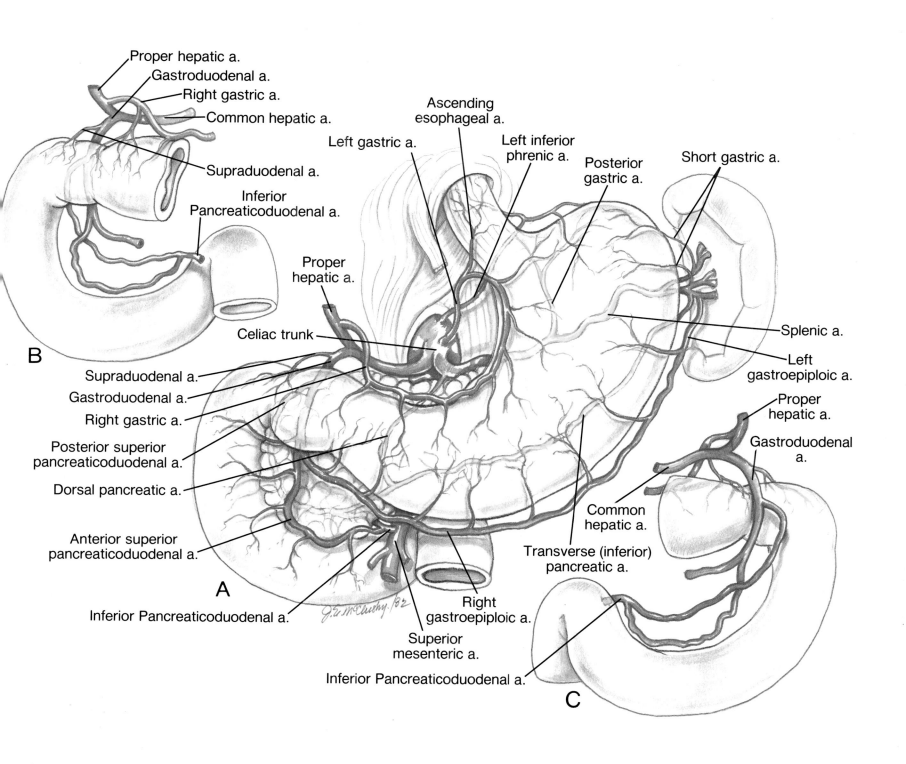

Proper hepatic a.
Gastroduodenal a.
Right gastric a.
Common hepatic a.
Supraduodenal a.
Inferior Pancreaticoduodenal a.

B

Ascending esophageal a.
Left gastric a.
Left inferior phrenic a.
Posterior gastric a.
Short gastric a.

Proper hepatic a.
Celiac trunk
Supraduodenal a.
Gastroduodenal a.
Right gastric a.
Posterior superior pancreaticoduodenal a.
Dorsal pancreatic a.
Anterior superior pancreaticoduodenal a.

A

Inferior Pancreaticoduodenal a.
Right gastroepiploic a.
Superior mesenteric a.
Inferior Pancreaticoduodenal a.

Splenic a.
Left gastroepiploic a.
Proper hepatic a.
Gastroduodenal a.
Common hepatic a.
Transverse (inferior) pancreatic a.

C

PLATE 5-4
Blood Supply of the Stomach II

A. Variations of the arteries of the proximal stomach, the distal esophagus and the diaphragm at the hiatus. With careful dissection from 3 to 12 cm of the normal esophagus can be mobilized (see also, Plate 3-9).

Remember:

If the spleen is removed, the ascending esophageal artery must be preserved since the short gastric arteries will be ligated.

B. The venous drainage of the stomach. The prepyloric vein (of Mayo), when present, indicates the site of the pyloric valve. Short gastric veins may enter a splenic vein or enter the substance of the spleen.

Remember:

1) At the abdominal esophagus the coronary vein (left gastric) anastomoses with the lower esophageal veins (porto-systemic anastomosis).

2) All the veins of the stomach drain directly or indirectly into the portal vein.

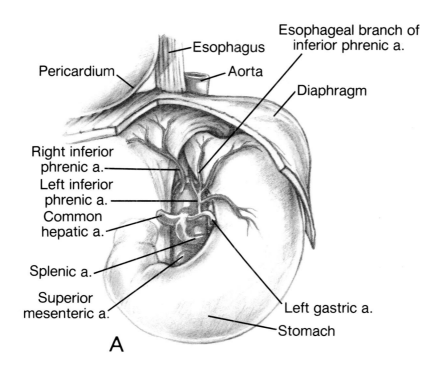

A

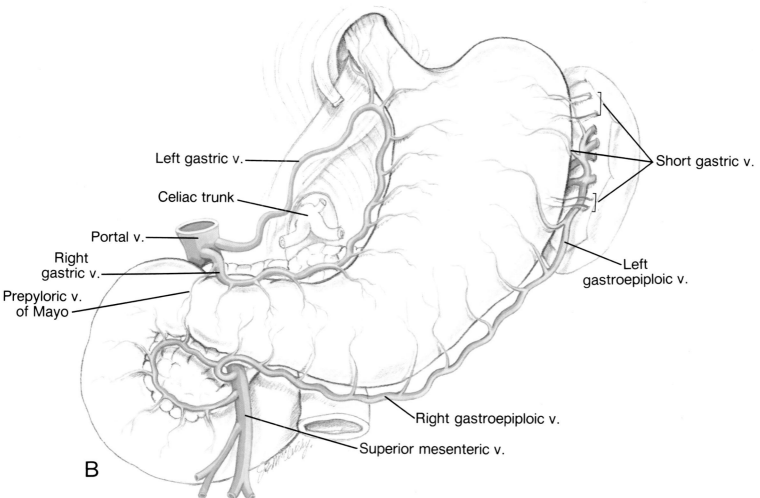

B

PLATE 5-5
Lymphatic Drainage of the Stomach

A. The lymphatic drainage and the major groups of lymph nodes of the stomach.

B. Diagram of lymphatic drainage of the four classic zones of the stomach. All drainage is ultimately to the celiac lymph nodes: the "vortex of the metastatic whorl."

Remember:

1) All the gastric lymph drains into the celiac nodes.

2) From the standpoint of lymphatic drainage and embryology, the ideal surgery for gastric carcinoma is total gastrectomy. The morbidity and mortality, however, dictate more conservative procedures such as radical subtotal, proximal or distal gastrectomy (see Plate 5–10).

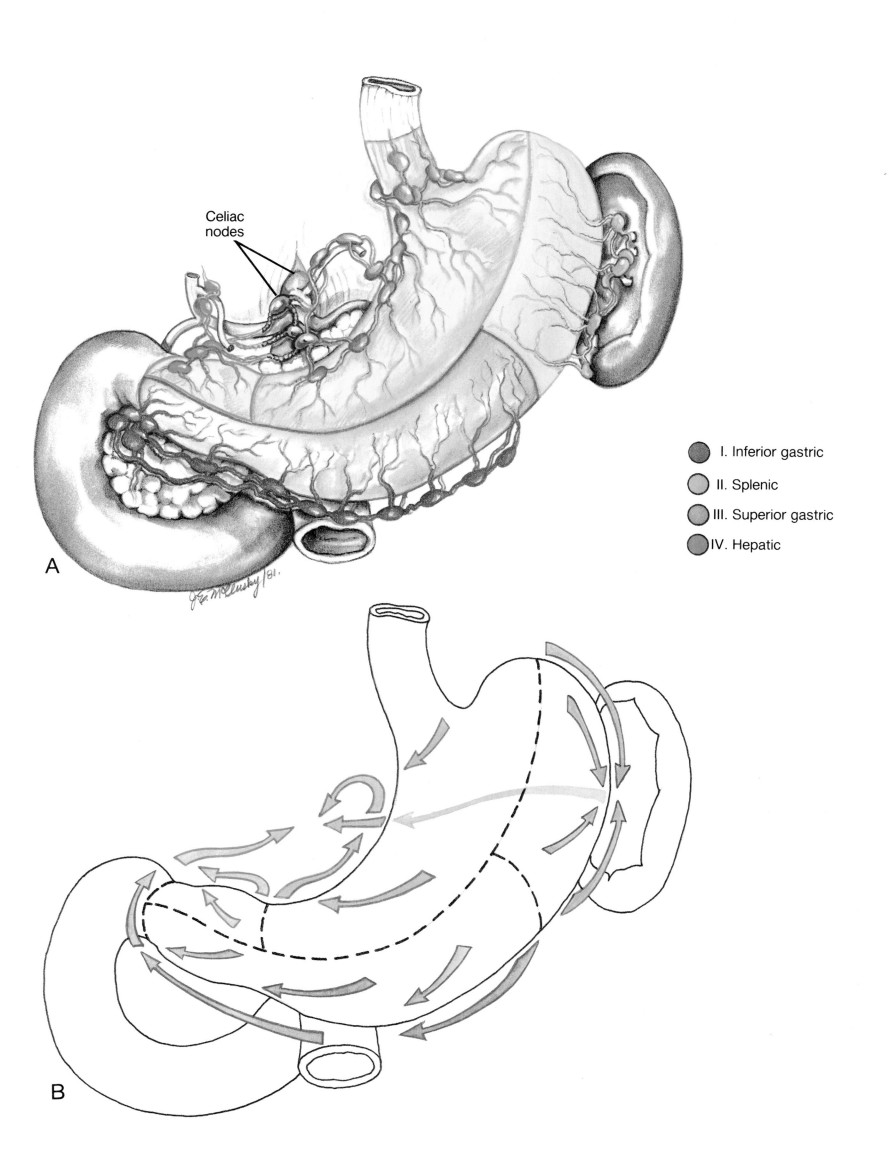

Celiac
nodes

I. Inferior gastric

II. Splenic

III. Superior gastric

IV. Hepatic

A

B

PLATE 5-6
Anatomy of the Vagus Nerves

A. Diagram of the vagus nerves, the esophageal plexus, and the distribution of the anterior vagal trunks below the diaphragm.

B. The posterior vagal trunk (broken lines) and the arteries from the aorta and the celiac trunk shown in anterior view.

Remember:

1) There is a constant anatomical pattern of the vagal trunks, divisions and branches below the diaphragm.

2) The surgeon should be familiar with the basic pattern and its variations, the "vagaries of the vagus" as it is distributed to the surface of the stomach.

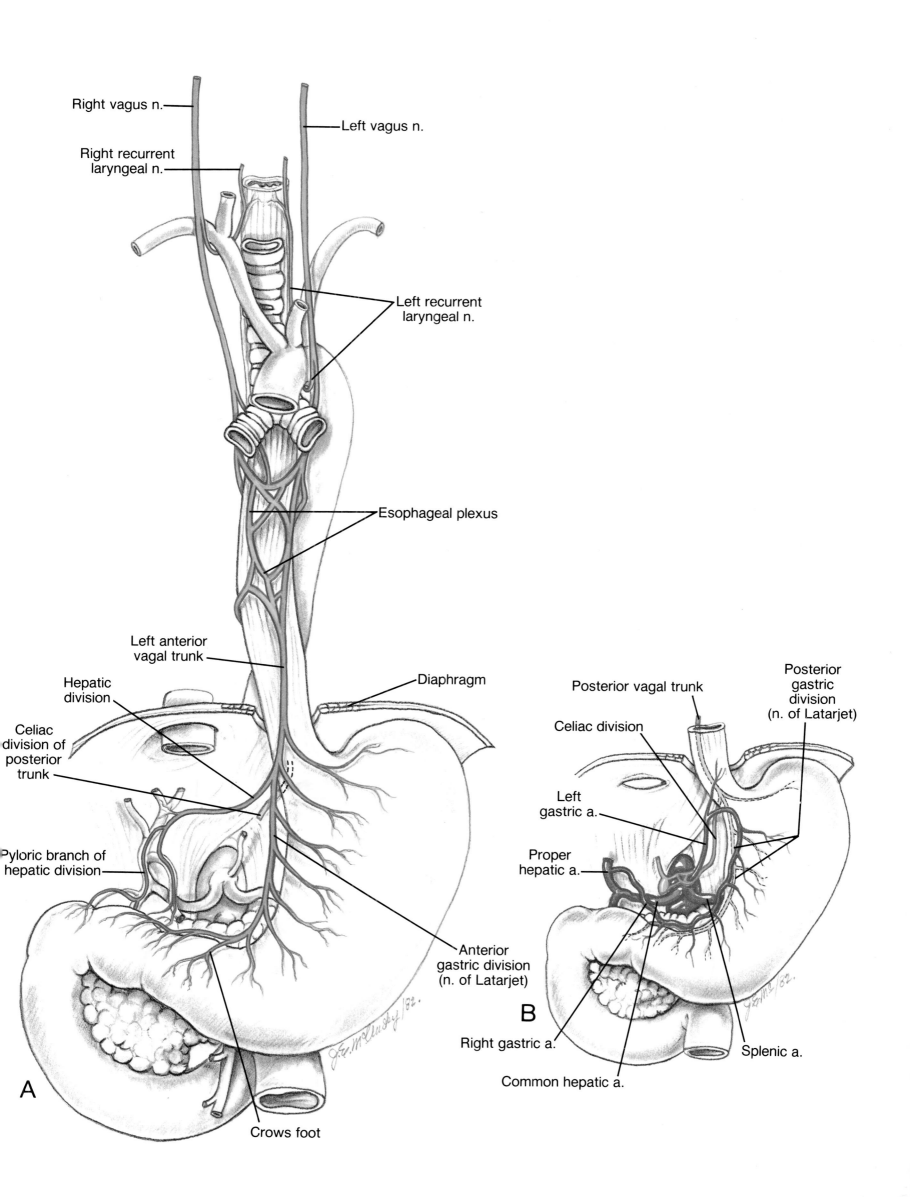

Right vagus n.

Right recurrent laryngeal n.

Left vagus n.

Left recurrent laryngeal n.

Esophageal plexus

Left anterior vagal trunk

Hepatic division

Diaphragm

Celiac division of posterior trunk

Pyloric branch of hepatic division

Anterior gastric division (n. of Latarjet)

Crows foot

A

Posterior vagal trunk

Posterior gastric division (n. of Latarjet)

Celiac division

Left gastric a.

Proper hepatic a.

Right gastric a.

Common hepatic a.

Splenic a.

B

PLATE 5-7
The Vagal Structures at the Diaphragm

A. Two vagal trunks pass through the diaphragm. This pattern was present in 88 of our 100 specimens. In the 88 specimens, 80 anterior trunks and 76 posterior trunks lay to the right of the midline. Only eight posterior and 12 anterior trunks lay to the left of the line.

B. Four vagal divisions at the diaphragm. The trunks have divided in the thorax. This pattern was present in seven of our 100 specimens.

C. More than four vagal structures at the diaphragm. The four major divisions have branched in the thorax. The vagal trunks are entirely in the thorax. This pattern was present in 2 of our 100 specimens.

D. More than four vagal structures at the diaphragm. The esophageal plexus is low; the vagal trunks are entirely within the abdomen. Three specimens had this configuration.

Remember:

1) The anterior trunk may be palpated at the front and slightly to the right. The posterior trunk may be felt as a cord-like structure, by the surgeon's finger, behind the esophagus, but closer to the aorta.

2) The anterior and posterior divisions may be found just below the gastroesophageal junction.

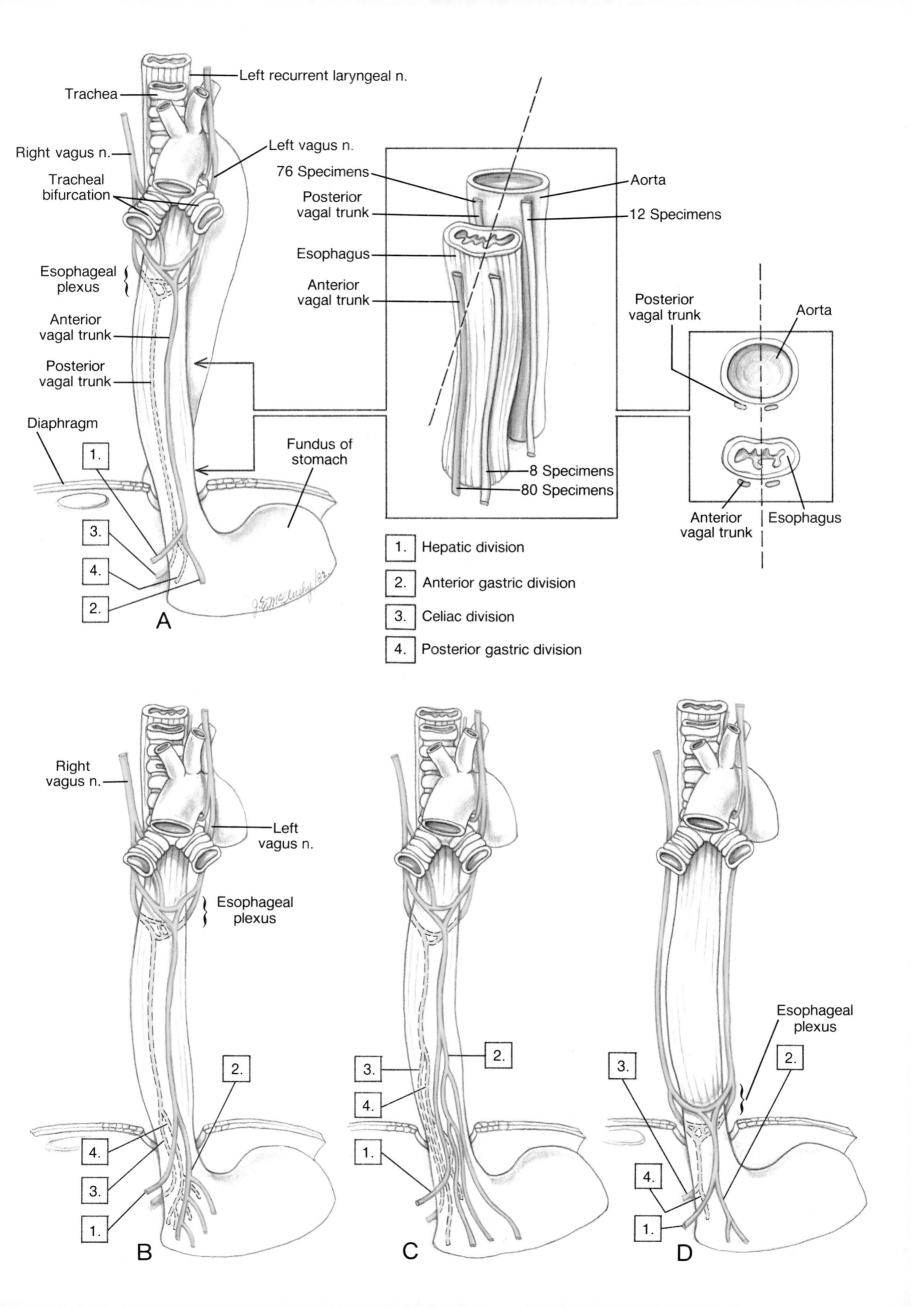

Left recurrent laryngeal n.

Trachea

Right vagus n.

Left vagus n.

Tracheal bifurcation

Esophageal plexus

Anterior vagal trunk

Posterior vagal trunk

Diaphragm

1.

3.

4.

2.

Fundus of stomach

A

76 Specimens

Aorta

Posterior vagal trunk

12 Specimens

Esophagus

Anterior vagal trunk

8 Specimens
80 Specimens

Posterior vagal trunk

Aorta

Anterior vagal trunk

Esophagus

1. Hepatic division

2. Anterior gastric division

3. Celiac division

4. Posterior gastric division

Right vagus n.

Left vagus n.

Esophageal plexus

2.

4.

3.

1.

B

3.

4.

2.

1.

C

3.

Esophageal plexus

2.

4.

1.

D

PLATE 5-8
Three Types of Abdominal Vagotomy

A. Truncal vagotomy. The anterior and posterior vagal trunks are cut just below the esophagus. The vagal structures proximal to the cut are in yellow; the structures distal to the cut are in red.

B. Selective vagotomy. The anterior and posterior gastric divisions (nerves of Latarjet) are cut; the hepatic and celiac divisions are spared.

C. Superselective or parietal cell vagotomy. The branches of the anterior and posterior gastric divisions are cut from proximal to distal, preserving the branches to the antrum (the crow's foot) and the pylorus. The celiac and hepatic divisions remain intact. The crow's foot, if present, is about 7 cm from the pylorus; the antrum begins a few centimeters cranial to it.

Remember:

1) The esophagus must be completely skeletonized, but too enthusiastic skeletonization can cause perforation.

2) Be careful to invaginate the lesser curvature to avoid postoperative necrosis.

3) Disappearance of the distal phalanx of the finger passed beneath the esophagus, together with the appearance of air bubbles, indicates pleural perforation by the fingertip.

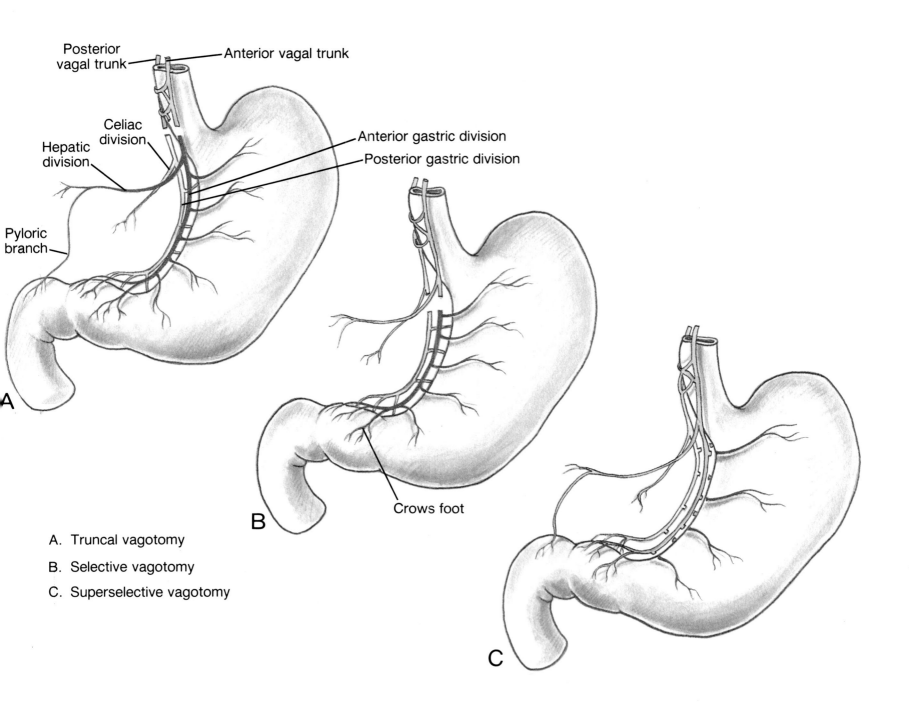

Posterior vagal trunk

Anterior vagal trunk

Celiac division

Hepatic division

Anterior gastric division

Posterior gastric division

Pyloric branch

A

Crows foot

B

A. Truncal vagotomy

B. Selective vagotomy

C. Superselective vagotomy

C

PLATE 5-9
Landmarks for Gastrectomy

A. Some arbitrary landmarks for 50% and 75% gastric resection and for antrectomy have been proposed.

50%: starting on the lesser curvature at the first descending branch of the left gastric artery, to the greater curvature at the midpoint of the left gastroepiploic artery.

75%: starting on the lesser curvature at the first branch of the left gastric artery, to a point on the greater curvature 2 cm below the spleen.

Antrectomy: starting at the incisura angularis or the midpoint of the lesser curvature and at the junction of the right and left epiploic arteries on the greater curvature. Neither point is obvious or constant, but such a resection will remove the antrum and its gastrin producing cells, together with a small cuff of distal gastric body. No satisfactory landmarks exist.

B. Proportionate numbers of parietal cells in the various parts of the stomach on a scale of 100.

Remember:

1) Do not devascularize more than 3 cm of the duodenum.

2) The gastroduodenal artery passes over (anterior to) the accessory pancreatic duct (of Santorini). If the artery must be ligated, the duct should be identified and protected. In 10% of subjects the accessory duct is the only drainage of all or part of the pancreas.

3) The distance between the pylorus and the papillae is shortened in patients with severe duodenitis or chronic ulcer disease.

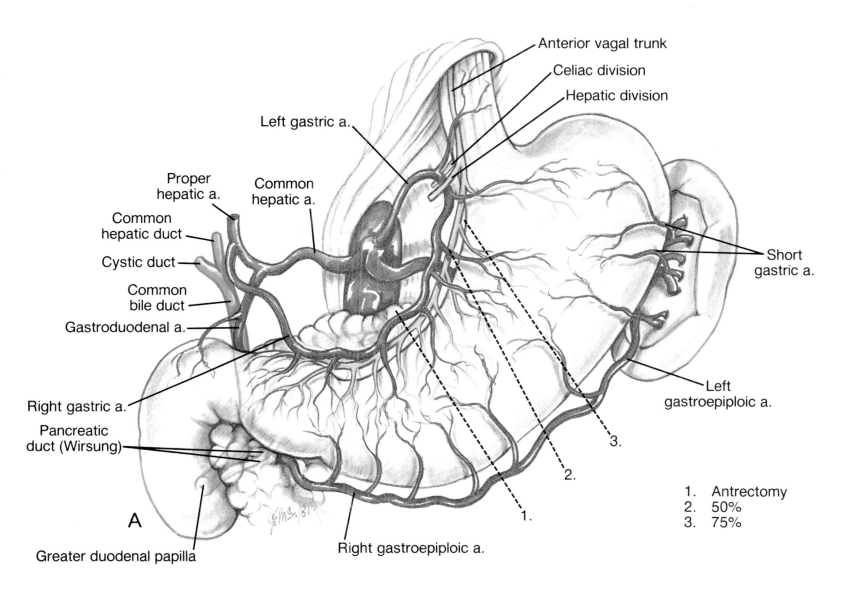

Anterior vagal trunk

Celiac division

Hepatic division

Left gastric a.

Proper hepatic a.

Common hepatic a.

Common hepatic duct

Cystic duct

Common bile duct

Gastroduodenal a.

Right gastric a.

Pancreatic duct (Wirsung)

Greater duodenal papilla

Short gastric a.

Left gastroepiploic a.

Right gastroepiploic a.

A

1. Antrectomy
2. 50%
3. 75%

1.
2.
3.

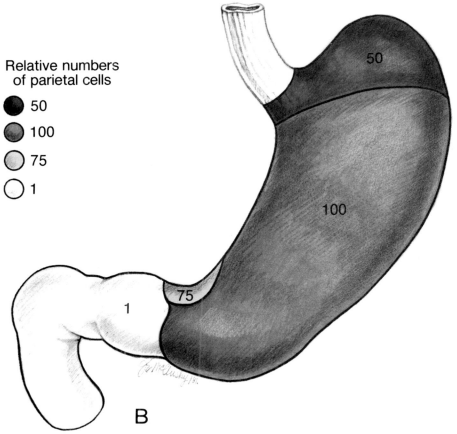

Relative numbers of parietal cells

● 50
● 100
○ 75
○ 1

50

100

75

1

B

PLATE 5-10
Theoretical Gastrectomy

Visalli and Grimes' proposal for *en bloc* resection of:

A. Structures related to the primitive dorsal epigastrium, having a common blood supply (left gastric and splenic arteries) and lymphatic drainage.

B. Structures related to the primitive ventral mesogastrium, supplied by the common hepatic artery. Note that the body and tail of the pancreas (from the dorsal anlage) lie in the proximal block while the head of the pancreas (from the ventral anlage) lies in the distal block.

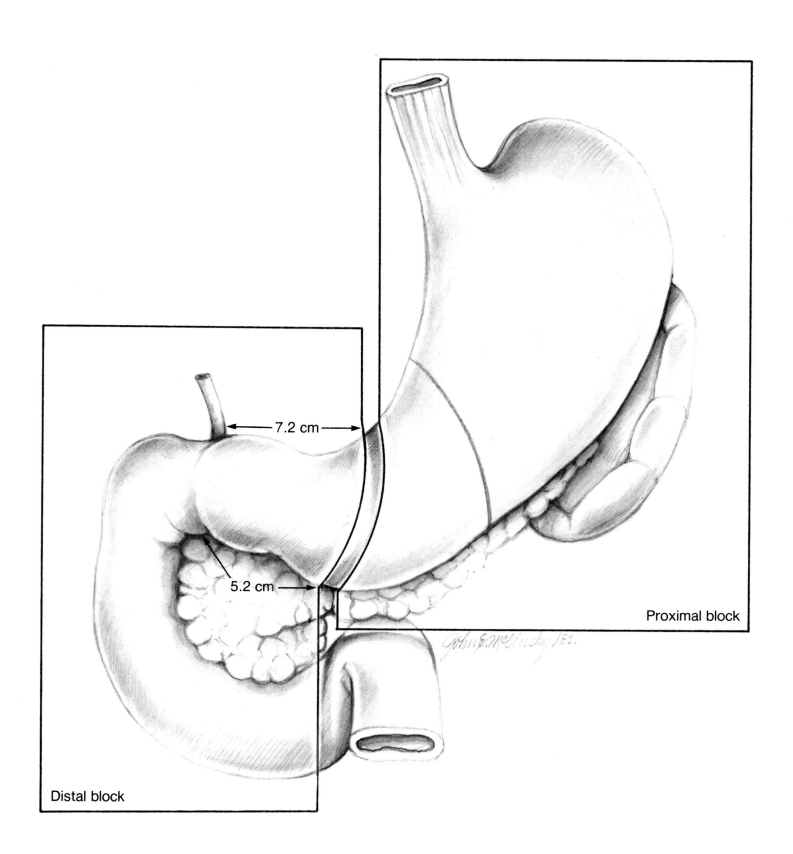

7.2 cm

5.2 cm

Proximal block

Distal block

PLATE 6-1
Development of the Pancreas

A. The appearance of dorsal and ventral pancreatic primordia at the end of the 4th week.

B. Rotation of the ventral primordium in the 5th and 6th weeks.

C and D. Fusion of the dorsal and ventral primordia. The pancreatic duct of the adult is formed distally by the duct of the dorsal primordium and proximally by the duct of the ventral primordium. The connecting duct appears only after fusion, at the end of the 6th week. The ventral primordium forms the uncinate process and part of the head of the pancreas; the dorsal primordium forms the remainder of the gland.

E. Final relationship of the two portions of the pancreas.

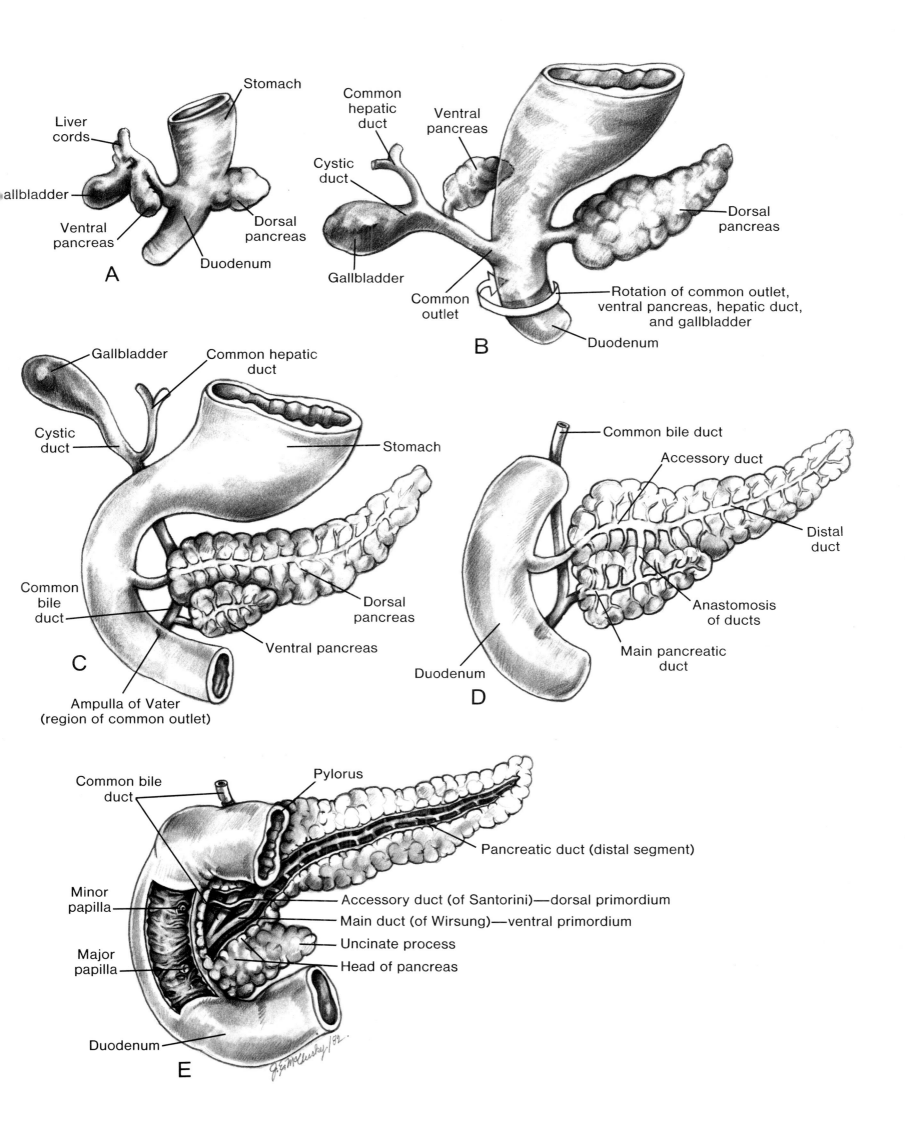

Liver cords

Stomach

Gallbladder

Ventral pancreas

Dorsal pancreas

Duodenum

A

Common hepatic duct

Ventral pancreas

Cystic duct

Dorsal pancreas

Gallbladder

Rotation of common outlet, ventral pancreas, hepatic duct, and gallbladder

Common outlet

Duodenum

B

Gallbladder

Common hepatic duct

Cystic duct

Stomach

Common bile duct

Dorsal pancreas

Ventral pancreas

C

Ampulla of Vater (region of common outlet)

Common bile duct

Accessory duct

Distal duct

Anastomosis of ducts

Main pancreatic duct

Duodenum

D

Common bile duct

Pylorus

Pancreatic duct (distal segment)

Minor papilla

Accessory duct (of Santorini)—dorsal primordium

Main duct (of Wirsung)—ventral primordium

Major papilla

Uncinate process

Head of pancreas

Duodenum

E

PLATE 6-2
Sites of Pancreatic Heterotopia

The distal stomach and the proximal duodenum are the most frequent sites of pancreatic heterotopia. Islets are usually present. At other sites, the pancreatic tissue is usually without islets.

The relative frequency of pancreatic heterotopia at various sites is indicated by the breadth of the arrows.

Remember:

1) In about 33% of cases of gastric pancreatic heterotopias, islets of Langerhans are present.

2) In most cases the accessory pancreatic tissue is functional.

3) In some systemic disorders, the heterotopic pancreas as well as the normal pancreas is affected.

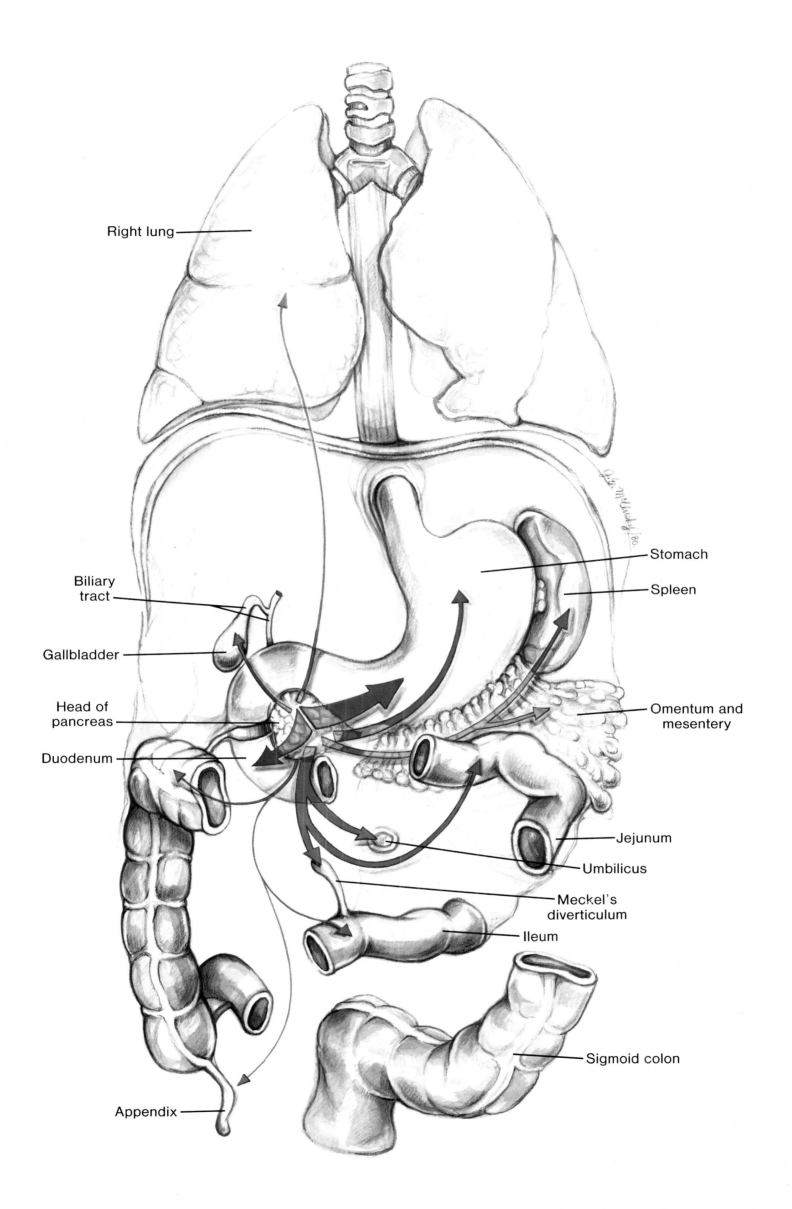

Right lung

Biliary
tract

Gallbladder

Head of
pancreas

Duodenum

Stomach

Spleen

Omentum and
mesentery

Jejunum

Umbilicus

Meckel's
diverticulum

Ileum

Sigmoid colon

Appendix

PLATE 6-3
Annular Pancreas and Other Variations

A. The ring of pancreatic tissue contains a large duct and may be heavily fixed to the duodenal musculature. The duodenum beneath the annulus is often stenosed. Thus, cutting the ring may not provide relief from symptoms of obstruction. There is also the danger of creating a pancreatic fistula or duodenal perforation. Duodenojejunostomy bypassing the annulus, is the accepted procedure.

Annular pancreas usually produces symptoms in the 1st year of life, but where the stenosis is mild or absent, it may remain silent for many years.

B. Occasionally a middle colic artery may arise from the superior mesenteric artery and pass through the head of the pancreas. It may supply twigs to the pancreas.

C–E. Common variations in the relation of the uncinate process to the superior mesenteric vessels. The uncinate process may be almost absent or it may completely envelop the superior mesenteric vessels and the portal vein. To avoid injury during pancreaticoduodenectomy, incise the neck of the pancreas at the front.

We have seen a case in which the inferior vena cava was enveloped by a tongue of pancreatic tissue from the posterior surface of the head.

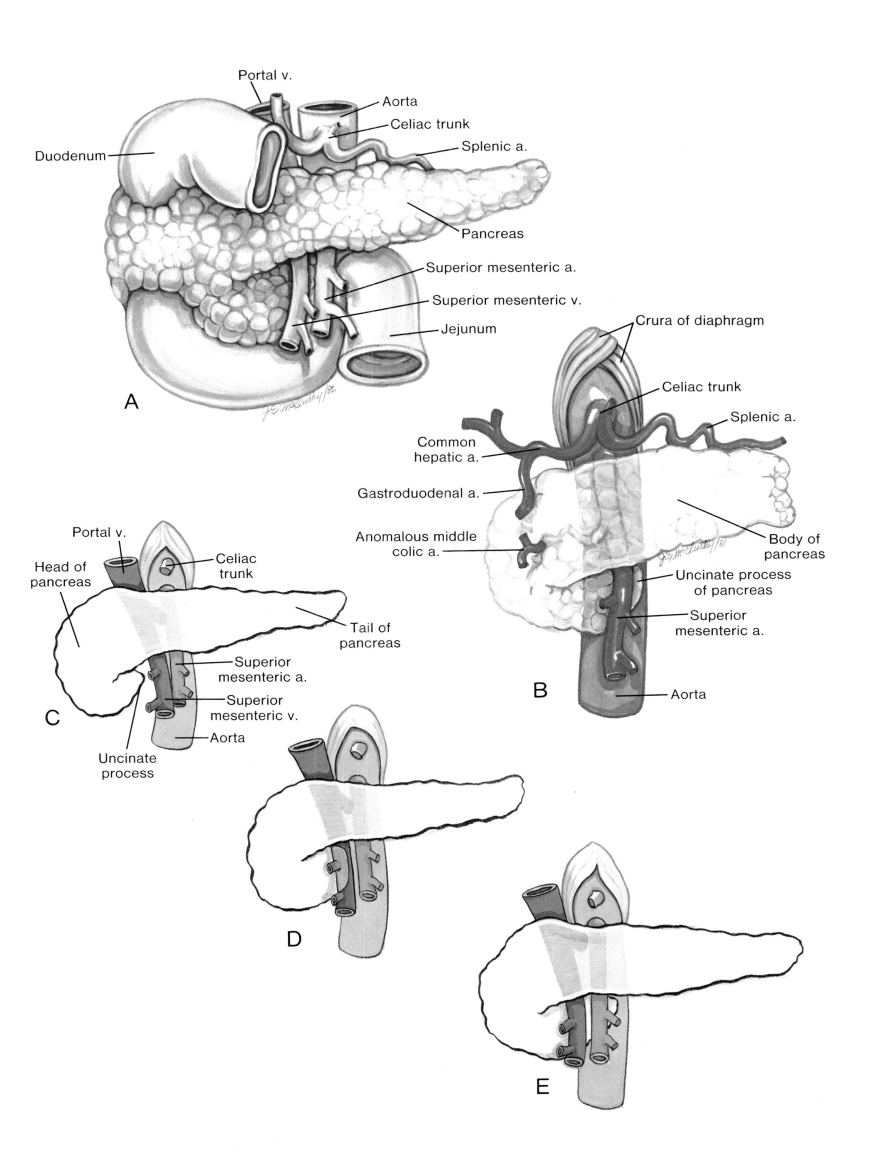

Portal v.

Aorta

Celiac trunk

Duodenum

Splenic a.

Pancreas

Superior mesenteric a.

Superior mesenteric v.

Jejunum

A

Crura of diaphragm

Celiac trunk

Splenic a.

Common
hepatic a.

Gastroduodenal a.

Body of
pancreas

Anomalous middle
colic a.

Uncinate process
of pancreas

Superior
mesenteric a.

Portal v.

Head of
pancreas

Celiac
trunk

Tail of
pancreas

Superior
mesenteric a.

Superior
mesenteric v.

Aorta

Uncinate
process

C

B

Aorta

D

E

PLATE 6-4
Types of Intestinal Atresias

A. Duodenal atresias. (1) Mucosal diaphragm. (2) Solid cord. (3) Segmental agenesis of the duodenum (rare). Note the dilated proximal segment and the undilated distal segment in all types. Forty percent of intestinal atresias are in the duodenum.

B. Similar atresias occur in the intestine. In segmental agenesis the mesentery also is usually absent.

Remember:

1) A mucosal diaphragm may perforate early in life producing a stenosis with symptoms of partial obstruction.

2) Restoration of the continuity of the intestinal tract requires some type of entero-enterostomy.

3) Duodenoduodenostomy after excision of the atretic or stenosed segment of the second part of the duodenum is preferred. Duodenojejunostomy or simple excision of the occluding diaphragm will relieve more distal obstruction.

4) Atresias of the first two types may be multiple. Do not forget the possibility of other, more distal, atresias or stenoses.

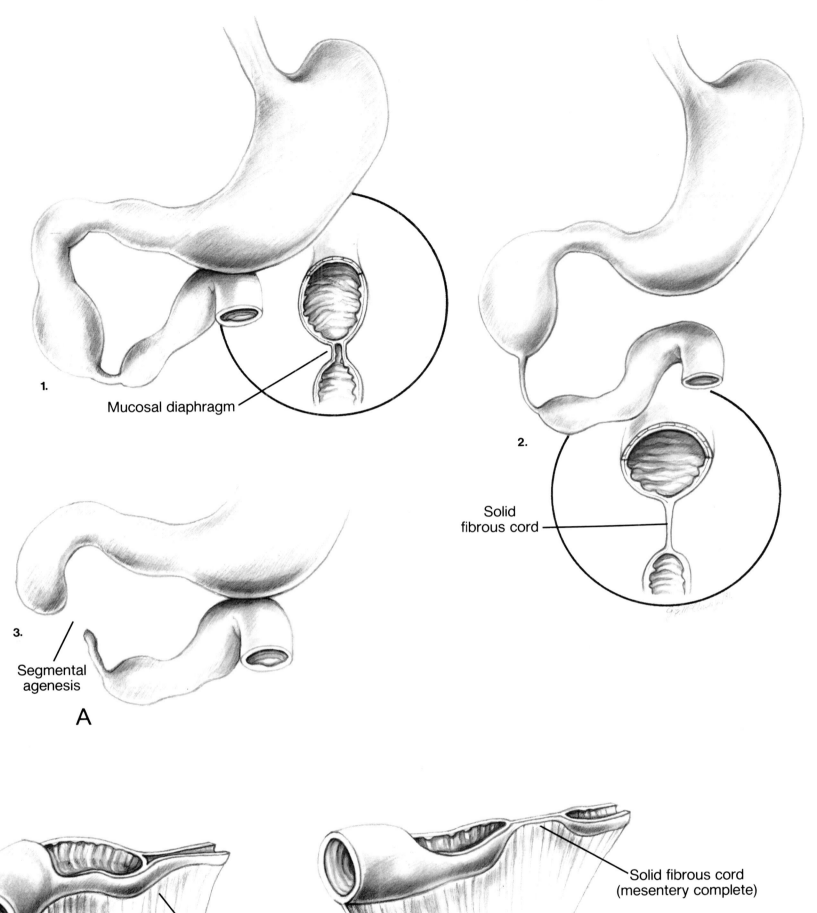

1. Mucosal diaphragm

2. Solid fibrous cord

3. Segmental agenesis

A

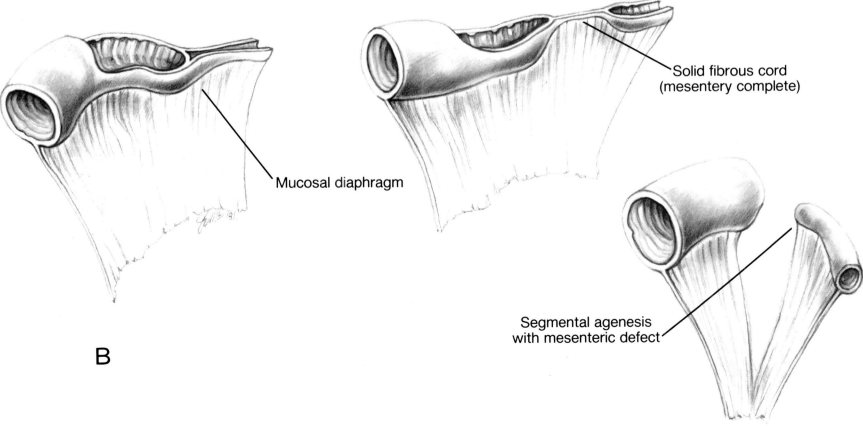

Mucosal diaphragm

Solid fibrous cord
(mesentery complete)

Segmental agenesis
with mesenteric defect

B

PLATE 6-5
Anterior View of the Duodenum and Pancreas

A. The stomach has been removed and the liver has been retracted upward to show the pancreas and duodenum. The body of the pancreas lies at the level of the first lumbar vertebra and the tail rises to the level of the 12th thoracic vertebra.

B. The regions of the pancreas. The division between the head and neck of the pancreas is marked anteriorly by the groove occupied by the gastroduodenal artery. The other boundaries are arbitrary.

C. Terminology of pancreatic resection. The site of distal resection varies with the location of the lesion. Although 85 and 95% resections are often effective, we believe that total resection is the ideal to be sought in pancreatic malignancy.

Remember:

A number of anatomical factors combine to make surgical removal of the pancreas difficult.

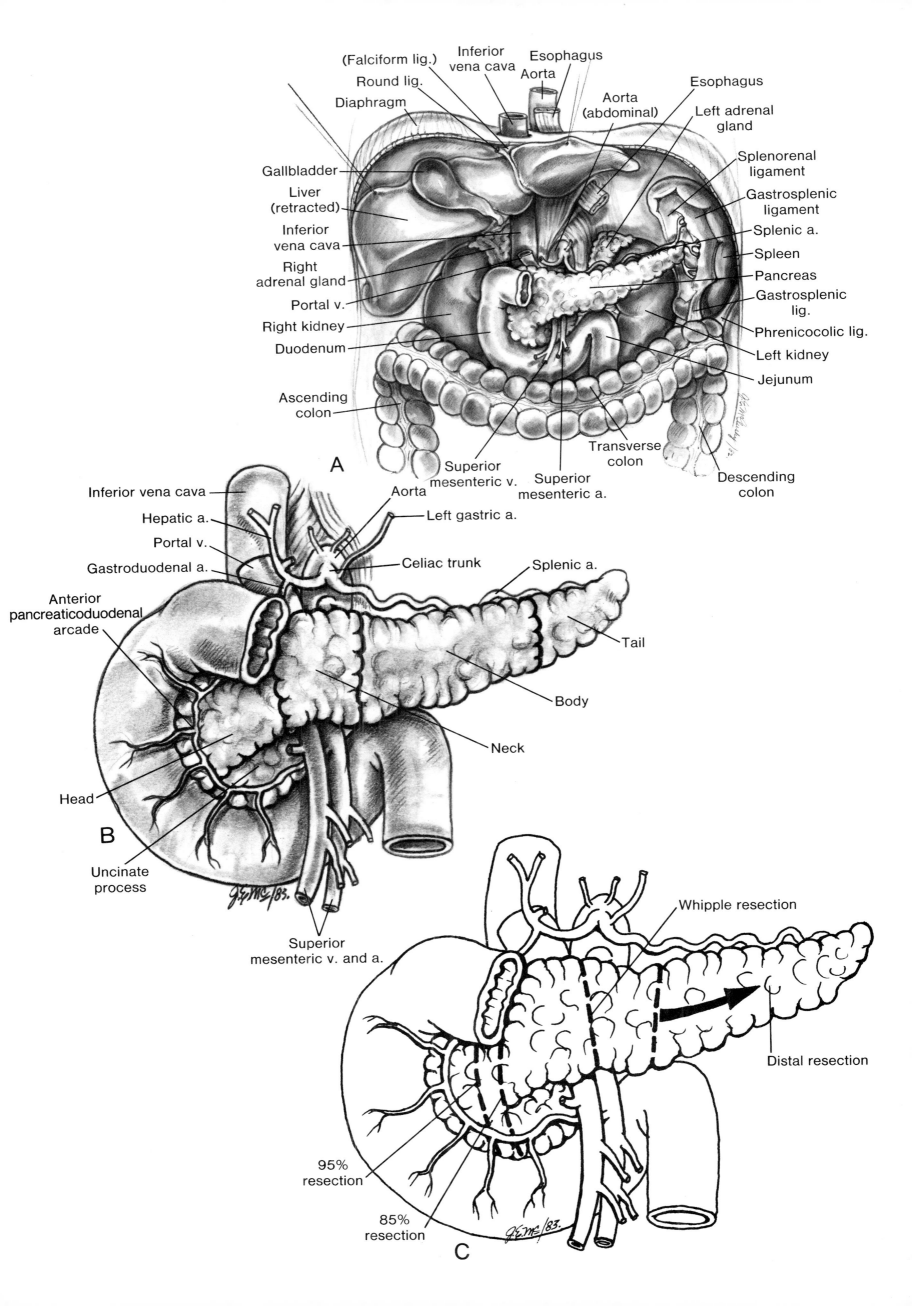

(Falciform lig.)

Inferior vena cava

Esophagus

Aorta

Diaphragm

Round lig.

Aorta (abdominal)

Esophagus

Left adrenal gland

Splenorenal ligament

Gastrosplenic ligament

Splenic a.

Spleen

Pancreas

Gastrosplenic lig.

Phrenicocolic lig.

Left kidney

Jejunum

Gallbladder

Liver (retracted)

Inferior vena cava

Right adrenal gland

Portal v.

Right kidney

Duodenum

Ascending colon

Superior mesenteric v.

Superior mesenteric a.

Transverse colon

Descending colon

A

Inferior vena cava

Aorta

Hepatic a.

Left gastric a.

Portal v.

Gastroduodenal a.

Celiac trunk

Splenic a.

Anterior pancreaticoduodenal arcade

Tail

Body

Neck

Head

Uncinate process

Superior mesenteric v. and a.

B

Whipple resection

Distal resection

95% resection

85% resection

C

PLATE 6-6
The Posterior Relations of the Pancreas

The pancreas is rendered transparent to show the relations of the posterior surface to the inferior vena cava, portal vein, superior mesenteric artery and vein, aorta and spleen.

The inferior mesenteric vein is shown here entering the splenic vein. In about 70% of subjects it enters the splenic or the superior mesenteric vein. In about 30% it enters at the junction of the two veins.

Remember:

1) Fixation by a tumor of duodenum or pancreas to underlying structures is a contraindication to pancreatic resection.

2) Kocherization or Jourdaniation (Jourdan described the procedure first in 1895) is mobilization of the second and proximal third parts of the duodenum.

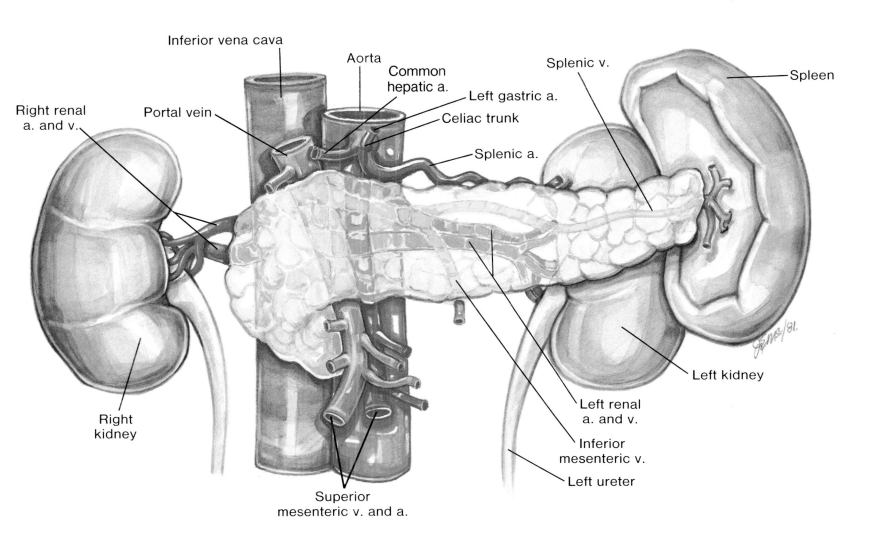

Inferior vena cava

Aorta

Common
hepatic a.

Left gastric a.

Splenic v.

Spleen

Right renal
a. and v.

Portal vein

Celiac trunk

Splenic a.

Left kidney

Right
kidney

Left renal
a. and v.

Inferior
mesenteric v.

Left ureter

Superior
mesenteric v. and a.

PLATE 6-7
Peritoneal Relations of the Duodenum and Pancreas

The stomach has been reflected upward to show the retroperitoneal pancreas. The transverse colon has been removed to show the relation of the pancreas to the transverse mesocolon and the root of the mesentery.

Remember:

1) With pancreatitis or pancreatic cancer, the pancreas and transverse mesocolon become adherent. Be gentle to avoid injury to the middle colic artery or to the colon. Prepare the colon before surgery; perforation is possible with the best of care.

2) The pancreas does not have a pancreatic capsule.

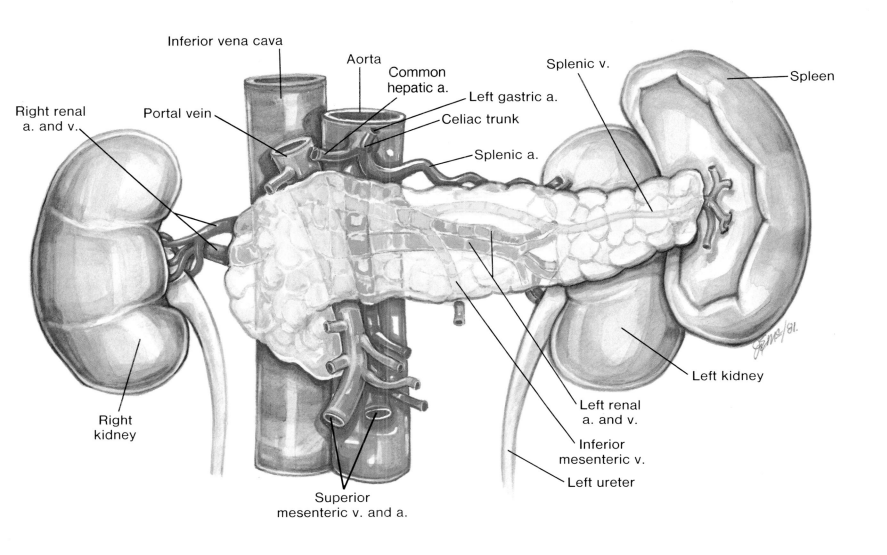

Inferior vena cava

Aorta

Common hepatic a.

Left gastric a.

Splenic v.

Spleen

Right renal a. and v.

Portal vein

Celiac trunk

Splenic a.

Right kidney

Left kidney

Superior mesenteric v. and a.

Left renal a. and v.

Inferior mesenteric v.

Left ureter

PLATE 6-7
Peritoneal Relations of the Duodenum and Pancreas

The stomach has been reflected upward to show the retroperitoneal pancreas. The transverse colon has been removed to show the relation of the pancreas to the transverse mesocolon and the root of the mesentery.

Remember:

1) With pancreatitis or pancreatic cancer, the pancreas and transverse mesocolon become adherent. Be gentle to avoid injury to the middle colic artery or to the colon. Prepare the colon before surgery; perforation is possible with the best of care.

2) The pancreas does not have a pancreatic capsule.

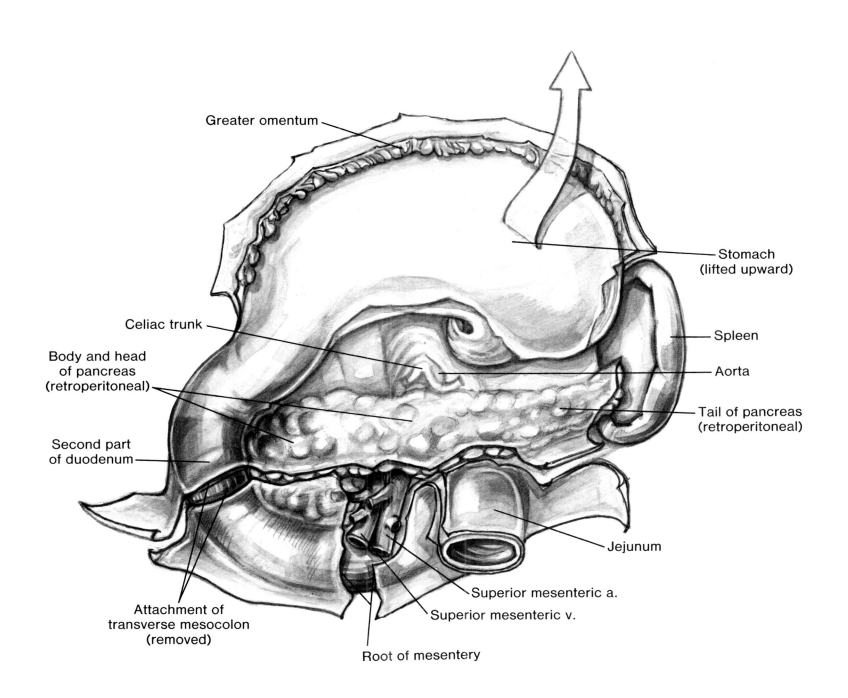

Greater omentum

Celiac trunk

Body and head
of pancreas
(retroperitoneal)

Second part
of duodenum

Attachment of
transverse mesocolon
(removed)

Root of mesentery

Superior mesenteric v.

Superior mesenteric a.

Jejunum

Tail of pancreas
(retroperitoneal)

Aorta

Spleen

Stomach
(lifted upward)

PLATE 6-8
The Pancreas and the Bile Ducts

Variations in the relation of the third part of the common bile duct to the posterior surface of the pancreas.

A and B. The common bile duct is partially covered by a fold of pancreatic tissue.

C. The duct is completely covered by pancreatic tissue.

D. The duct is uncovered, lying on the posterior surface of the pancreas.

E. The duct is partially covered (above and below) by two folds of pancreatic tissue.

In three fourths of patients, the configuration will be types A, B or C.

Remember:

1) The common bile duct, the head of the pancreas, and the duodenum form an inseparable embryological, anatomical and surgical unit demanding excision of the distal biliary tract during pancreatectomy.

2) We believe the anatomy of the pancreas, and the frequency of multicentric tumors demands total pancreatectomy. Total pancreatectomy avoids postoperative pancreatitis, has a better 5 year survival, and produces uncontrollable diabetes in only a few patients.

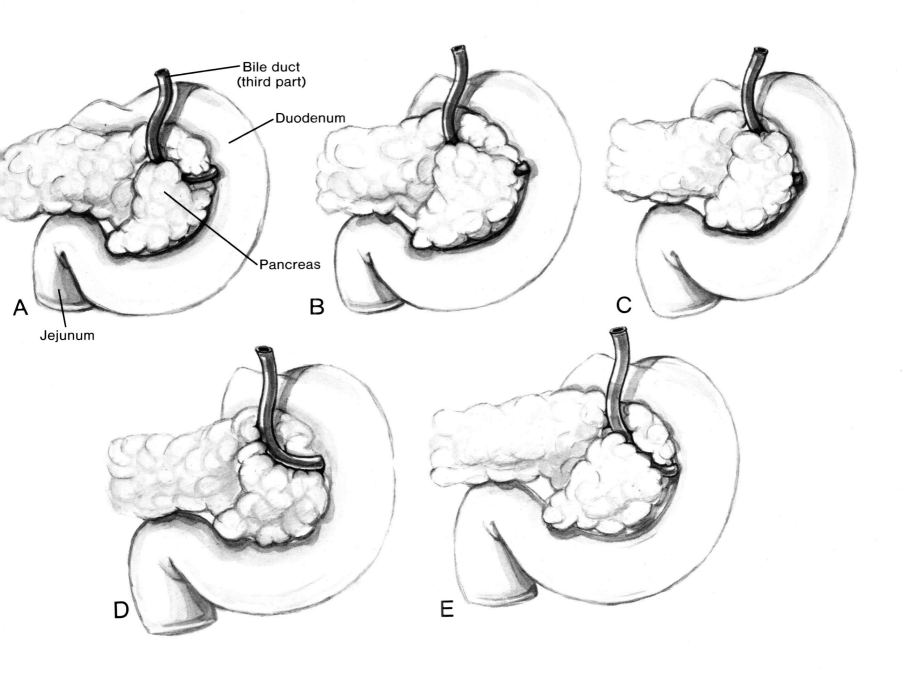

A

Bile duct
(third part)

Duodenum

Pancreas

Jejunum

B

C

D

E

PLATE 6-9
Variations of the Pancreatic Ducts

A. Both the main pancreatic duct (of Wirsung) and the smaller accessory pancreatic duct (of Santorini) open into the duodenum. This configuration is found in about 60% of subjects.

B. The accessory duct ends blindly before reaching the duodenal wall. It occurs in 30% of subjects.

C. The accessory duct drains most of the pancreas. The "main" duct is small or absent, draining only the head of the pancreas. This is "pancreas divisum" and represents incomplete fusion of the embryonic primordia. It occurs in about 10% of subjects.

D. Rare forms of the pancreatic ducts, including the presence of three ducts opening separately into the duodenum.

Remember:

1) The major duodenal papilla lies from 7 to 10 cm (extremes: 1.5 to 12 cm) below the pylorus. With duodenitis secondary to peptic ulcer disease at the cap or posterior bulbar area, the distance will be decreased.

2) The minor papilla is 2 cm cranial to the major papilla and the accessory duct is always *under* the gastroduodenal artery.

3) The best anatomical landmark for the papilla and duct of Santorini is the gastroduodenal artery which is located obliquely above and behind the duct.

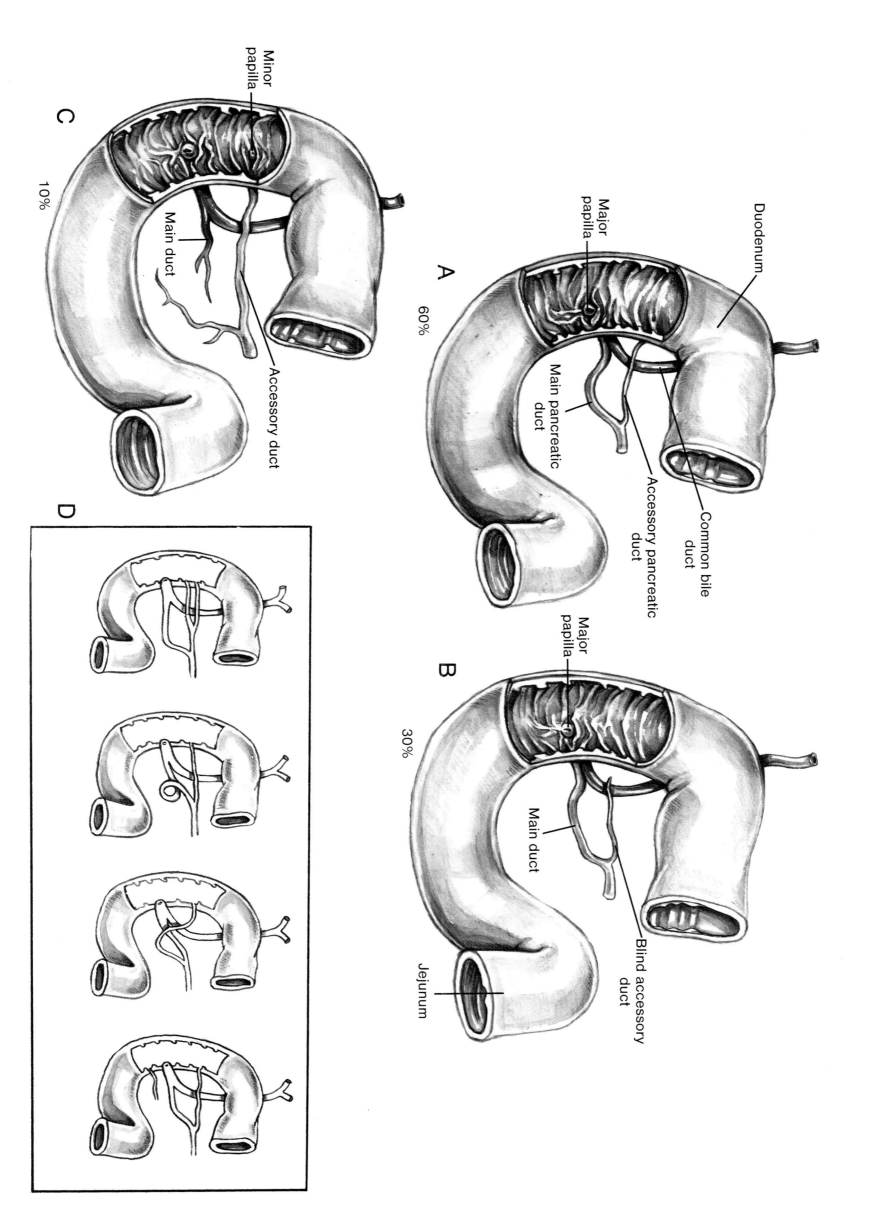

C

10%

Minor papilla

Main duct

Accessory duct

A

60%

Major papilla

Duodenum

Main pancreatic duct

Accessory pancreatic duct

Common bile duct

B

30%

Major papilla

Main duct

Blind accessory duct

Jejunum

D

PLATE 6-10
The Papilla of Vater and the Sphincter of Boyden

The structure and variations of the pancreatic and biliary ducts at their entrance into the duodenum and in the duodenal papilla of Vater.

A. The duodenal mucosa has been peeled away from the papilla to show the relation of its musculature to that of the duodenal wall.

B. The "T" formation of circular and longitudinal mucosal folds which aid in locating the duodenal papilla. The papilla is occasionally concealed by a circular fold of mucosa.

C and D. Diagrams of a long section of the duodenum showing the muscle fibers surrounding the biliary and pancreatic ducts at their junction within the duodenal wall. This complex of four small sphincters should be called the Sphincter of Boyden. Its total length is from 0.16 to 3.0 cm, depending upon the obliquity of its path through the duodenal wall.

E–G. Varying degrees of resorption of the ducts into the duodenum: Minimal resorption (E) leaves a long common channel, the ampulla (of Vater). Partial resorption (F) brings the ductal junction close to the tip of the papilla with no true ampulla. Complete resorption of the common channel (G) results in biliary and pancreatic ducts opening separately on the papilla.

Remember:

The common bile duct and the main pancreatic duct suddenly or gradually decrease in diameter as they enter the duodenal wall.

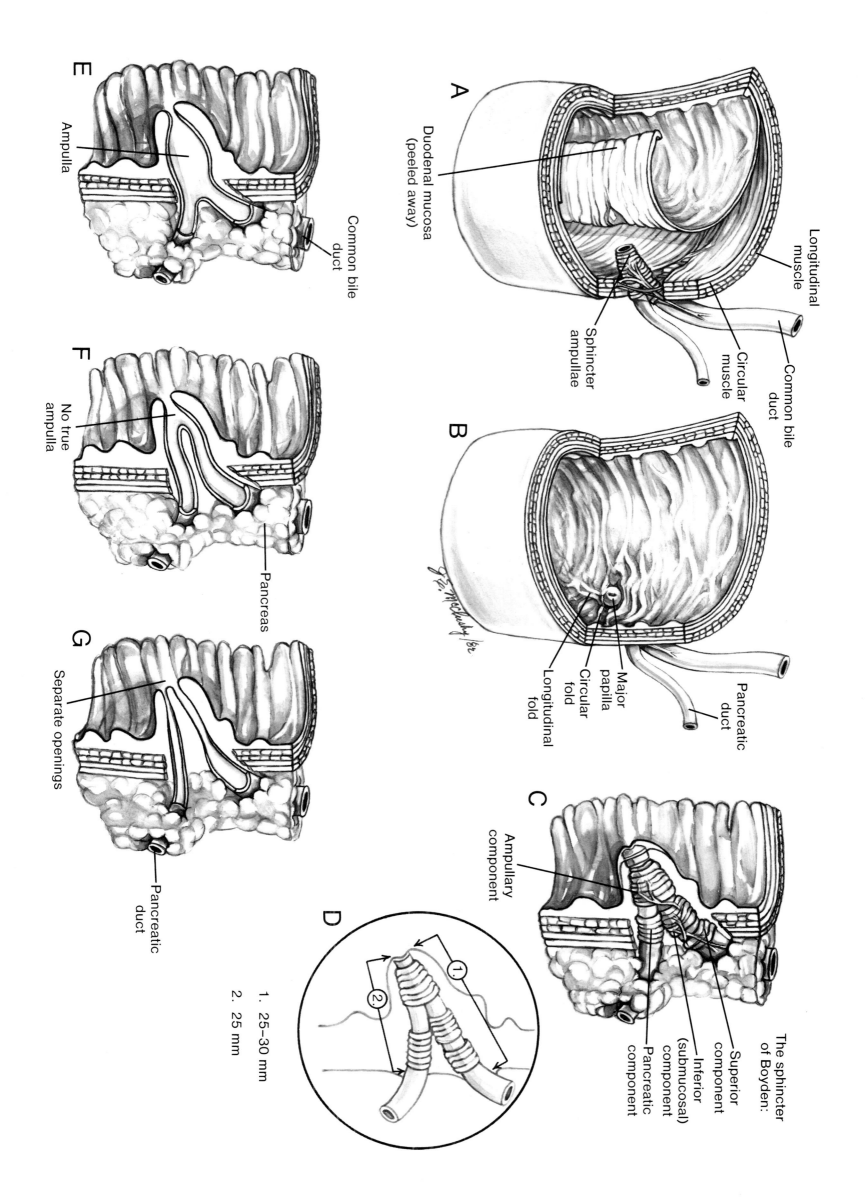

E

Ampulla

Common bile
duct

A

Duodenal mucosa
(peeled away)

Longitudinal
muscle

Common bile
duct

Sphincter
ampullae

Circular
muscle

F

No true
ampulla

Pancreas

B

Longitudinal
fold

Circular
fold

Major
papilla

Pancreatic
duct

G

Separate openings

Pancreatic
duct

C

Ampullary
component

The sphincter
of Boyden:

Superior
component

Inferior
(submucosal)
component

Pancreatic
component

D

1. 25–30 mm
2. 25 mm

PLATE 6-11
Arteries of the Pancreas and Duodenum

A. Arterial supply to the pancreas and duodenum, anterior view.

B. Arterial supply to the pancreas and duodenum, posterior view. For more details of the splenic vessels see Plates 7-3 and 7-4.

C. Diagrams of the three configurations of the blood supply to the distal pancreas:

Type I. The blood supply is from the splenic artery only.

Type II. The blood supply is from the splenic and transverse pancreatic arteries with anastomosis between them in the tail. This is the most common pattern.

Type III. The blood supply is from the splenic and transverse pancreatic arteries, having no distal anastomoses with each other. This configuration is susceptible to infarction from emboli in the transverse artery.

Remember:

1) The head of the pancreas is attached to the medial surface of the second and third parts of the duodenum. Blood vessels from the pancreas continue onto the duodenum. It is this vascular relationship that makes resection of the head of the pancreas, while sparing the duodenum, very difficult.

2) The blood supply is greatest to the head of the pancreas, less to the body and tail, and least to the neck.

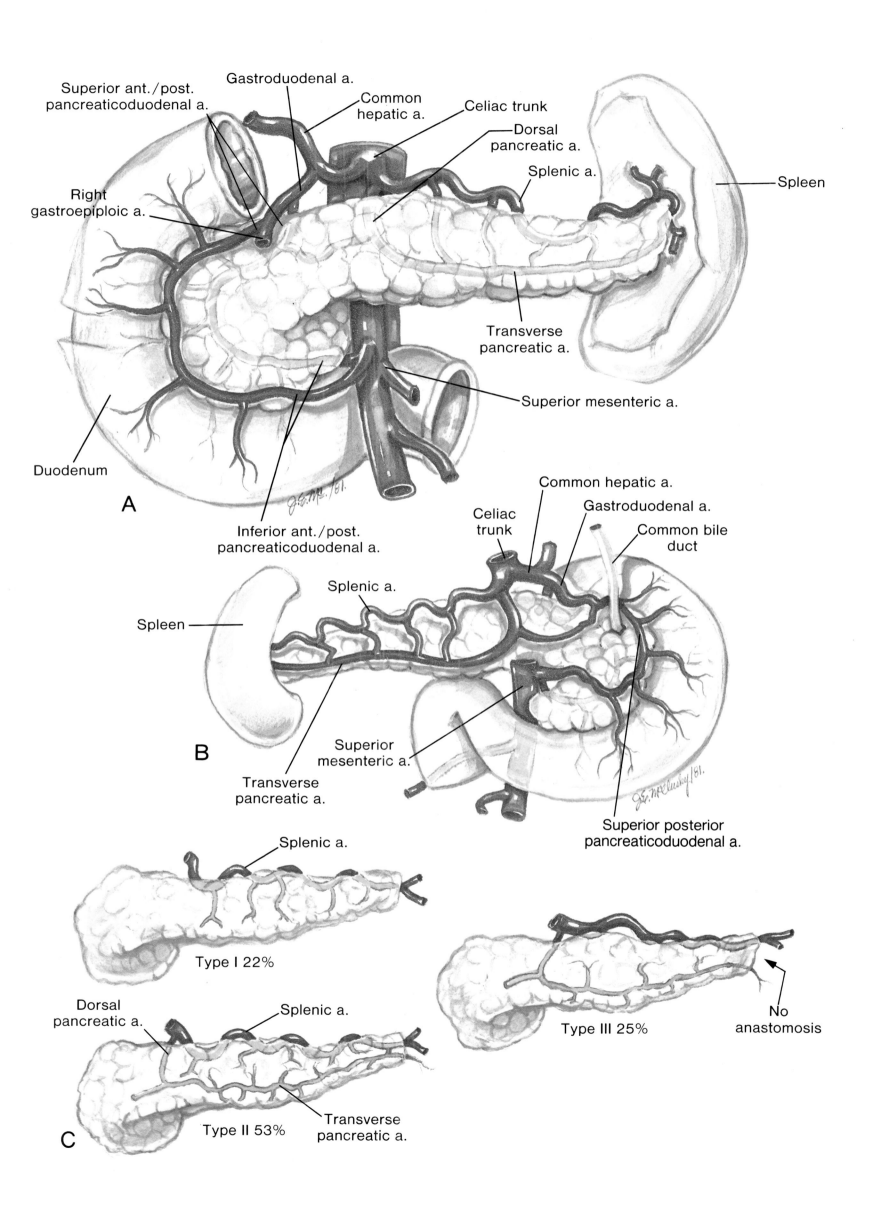

Superior ant./post. pancreaticoduodenal a.

Gastroduodenal a.

Common hepatic a.

Celiac trunk

Dorsal pancreatic a.

Splenic a.

Spleen

Right gastroepiploic a.

Transverse pancreatic a.

Superior mesenteric a.

Duodenum

A

Inferior ant./post. pancreaticoduodenal a.

Common hepatic a.

Celiac trunk

Gastroduodenal a.

Common bile duct

Splenic a.

Spleen

B

Superior mesenteric a.

Transverse pancreatic a.

Superior posterior pancreaticoduodenal a.

Splenic a.

Type I 22%

Dorsal pancreatic a.

Splenic a.

Type III 25%

No anastomosis

Type II 53%

Transverse pancreatic a.

C

PLATE 6-12
Veins of the Pancreas and Duodenum

A. The veins of the pancreas and duodenum, anterior view.

B. The veins of the pancreas and duodenum, posterior view. See also Plate 7-3.

Remember:

1) Be slow and careful during pancreatic mobilization, avoiding traction on the head of the pancreas. Isolate gently and ligate all small veins to avoid avulsion.

2) The veins lie parallel with, and superficial to, the arteries.

3) The arterial and venous pancreatic network lies posterior to the ducts.

4) The splenic vein, receiving short veins from the pancreas, readily disseminates cancer cells.

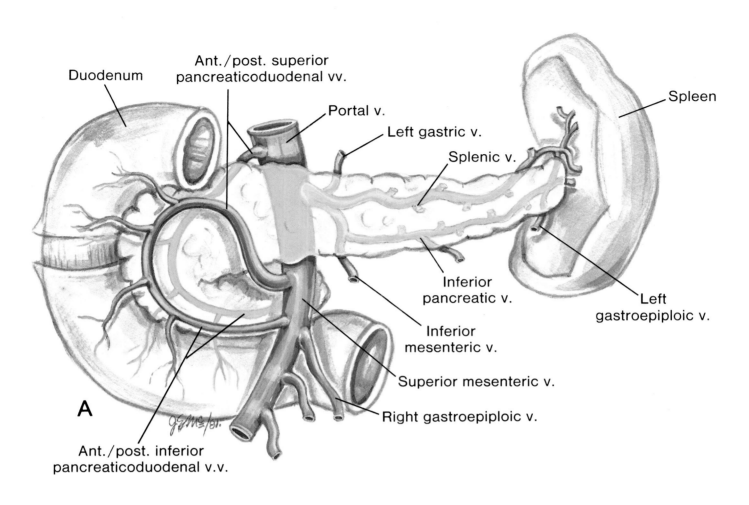

Duodenum

Ant./post. superior
pancreaticoduodenal vv.

Portal v.

Left gastric v.

Splenic v.

Spleen

Inferior
pancreatic v.

Inferior
mesenteric v.

Superior mesenteric v.

Right gastroepiploic v.

Left
gastroepiploic v.

Ant./post. inferior
pancreaticoduodenal v.v.

A

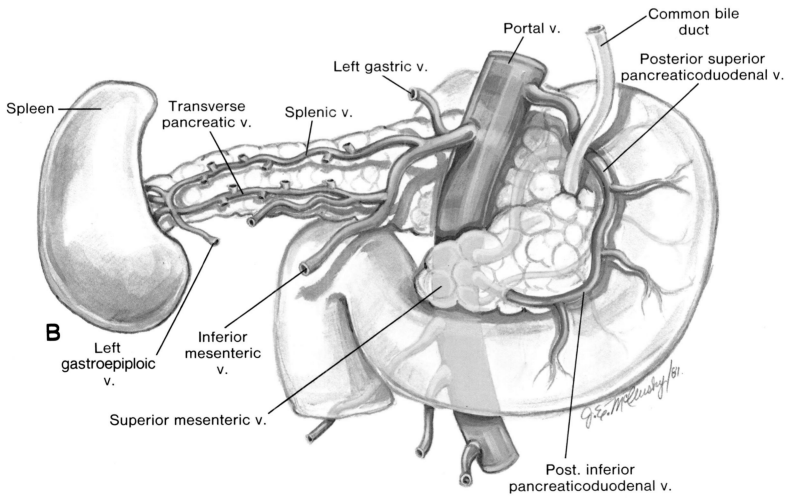

Spleen

Transverse
pancreatic v.

Splenic v.

Left gastric v.

Portal v.

Common bile
duct

Posterior superior
pancreaticoduodenal v.

Left
gastroepiploic
v.

Inferior
mesenteric
v.

Superior mesenteric v.

Post. inferior
pancreaticoduodenal v.

B

PLATE 6-13
Lymph Drainage of the Duodenum, Pancreas and Spleen

Drainage is to the nearest group of nodes. The rich network of lymphatics favors nodal metastasis.

Remember:

1) Seventy-two percent of pancreatic tumors occur in the head, 25% in the body and 3% in the tail.

2) Ninety percent of pancreatic carcinoma arises from the ducts and 10% from the acini.

3) Multicentric malignant foci are not rare in pancreatic carcinoma.

4) Ninety percent of pancreatic carcinoma has already spread to the lymph nodes at the time of surgery; 80% has spread to the liver.

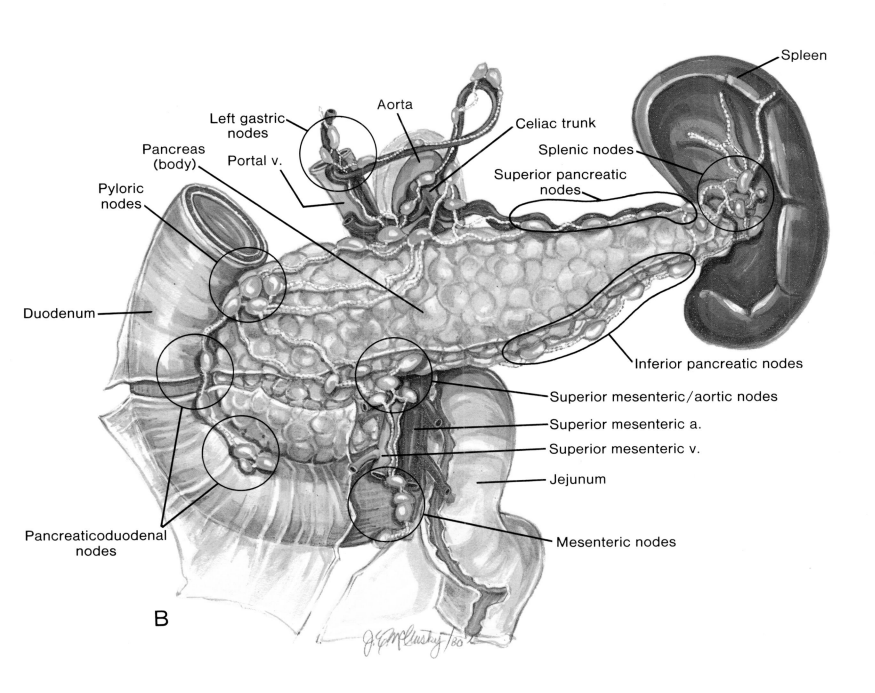

Spleen

Aorta

Left gastric nodes

Celiac trunk

Pancreas (body)

Splenic nodes

Portal v.

Superior pancreatic nodes

Pyloric nodes

Duodenum

Inferior pancreatic nodes

Superior mesenteric/aortic nodes

Superior mesenteric a.

Superior mesenteric v.

Jejunum

Pancreaticoduodenal nodes

Mesenteric nodes

B

PLATE 6-14
Vascular Compression of the Duodenum I

The third part of the duodenum crosses the spine at the level of L_3 and lies in the angle formed by the aorta and the superior mesenteric artery. In this vascular angle lie the left renal vein, the uncinate process of the pancreas and the third part of the duodenum.

The superior mesenteric artery, crossing the duodenum, may produce obstruction by compression. Occasionally compression is from the middle colic artery (Plate 6-15) or, very rarely, from the right colic artery.

A. Left lateral view showing the vascular angle.

B. Anterior view showing the artery crossing the duodenum.

C. Diagram of the mesenteric and vascular relations of the aortomesenteric arterial angle.

Remember:

1) Very few patients with duodenal compression are fat, although they may have a history of recent weight loss. Anorexia in women is common.

2) Immobilization in the supine position or use of a total body cast may produce vascular compression within a short time.

3) Cineradiography provides the best basis for diagnosis; it is the characteristic *activity* of the duodenum rather than its static appearance that will reveal the obstruction.

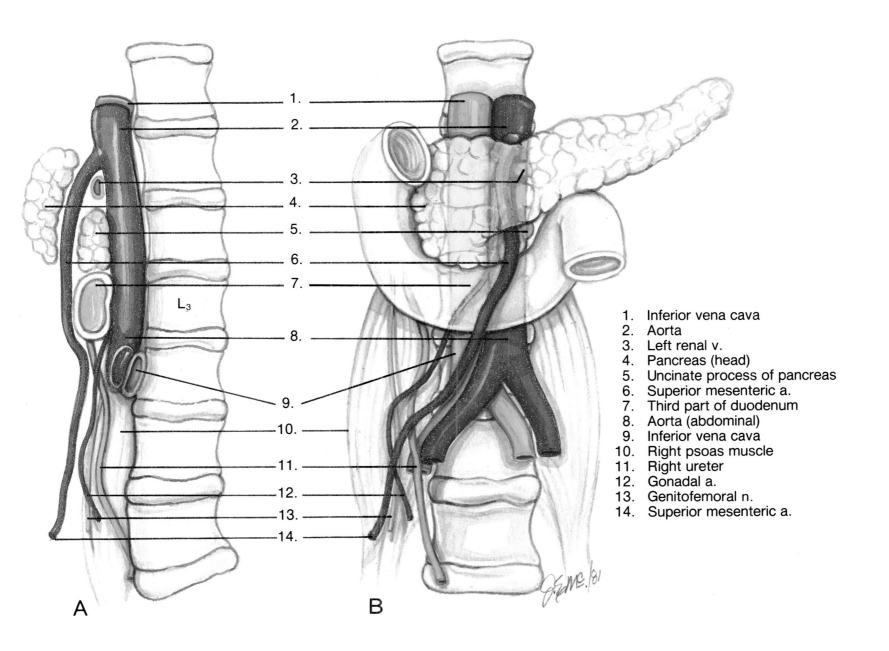

1. Inferior vena cava
2. Aorta
3. Left renal v.
4. Pancreas (head)
5. Uncinate process of pancreas
6. Superior mesenteric a.
7. Third part of duodenum
8. Aorta (abdominal)
9. Inferior vena cava
10. Right psoas muscle
11. Right ureter
12. Gonadal a.
13. Genitofemoral n.
14. Superior mesenteric a.

A

B

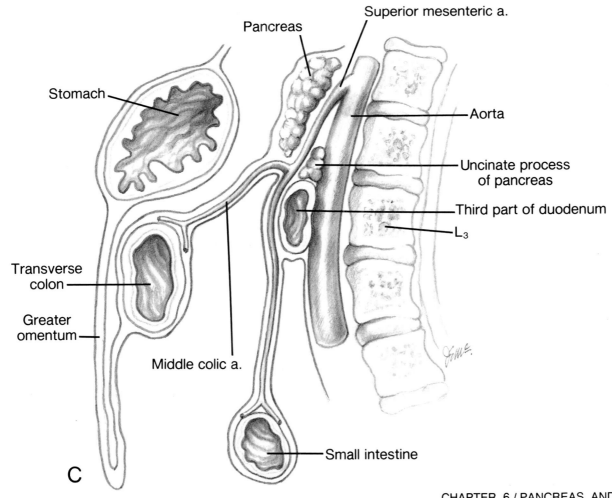

C

PLATE 6-15
Vascular Compression of the Duodenum II

A. The colon in its normal position: the middle colic artery as well as the superior mesenteric artery crosses the duodenum, occasionally producing compression.

B. The colon and its mesentery reflected upward showing the middle colic artery with no obvious relation to the duodenum. This may lead the surgeon to forget the possible role of this artery in duodenal compression.

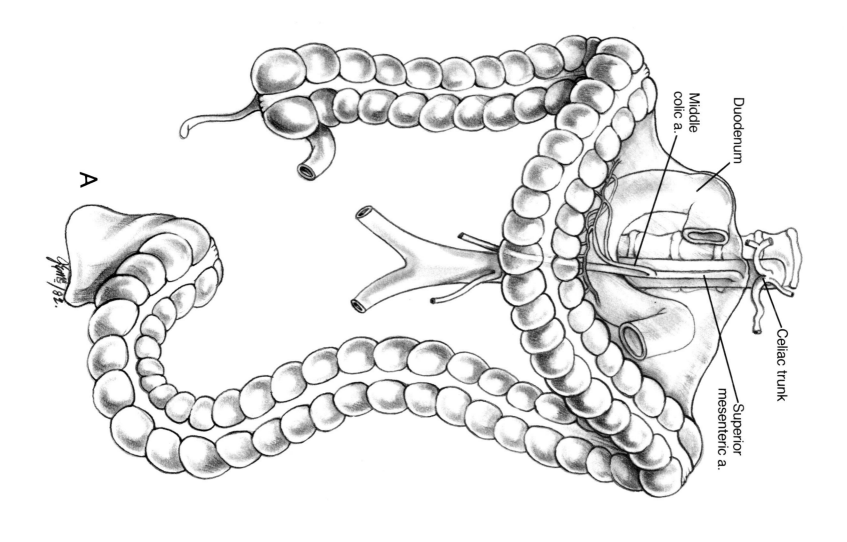

A

Middle colic a.

Duodenum

Celiac trunk

Superior mesenteric a.

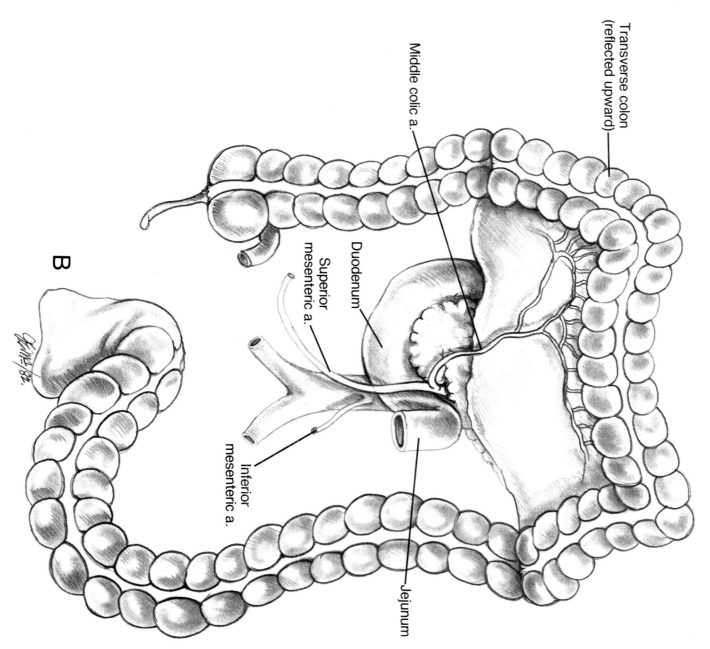

B

Transverse colon (reflected upward)

Middle colic a.

Duodenum

Superior mesenteric a.

Inferior mesenteric a.

Jejunum

PLATE 6-16
Vascular Compression of the Duodenum III

A. A duodenum lying high in the vascular angle formed by the superior mesenteric artery and the aorta is more susceptible to compression.

B. A duodenum lying in the vascular angle at a lower level is less likely to be compressed.

C. Relief of vascular compression of the duodenum is obtained by section of the suspensory muscle (ligament of Treitz), permitting the breadth of two fingers to pass easily into the angle above the duodenum. If the duodenum does not come down far enough to relieve the symptoms of compression, duodenojejunostomy will be necessary.

Exposure of the duodenum:

1) Mobilize the second and proximal third portions of the duodenum by the Jourdan (Kocher) maneuver.

2) Incise the gastrocolic omentum and reflect the right colon to expose the duodenum distal to the superior mesenteric vessels.

3) Incise the suspensory muscle. Avoid the inferior mesenteric artery.

Remember:

When cutting the suspensory muscle, avoid injury to the inferior mesenteric vein lying to the left of the duodenojejunal flexure.

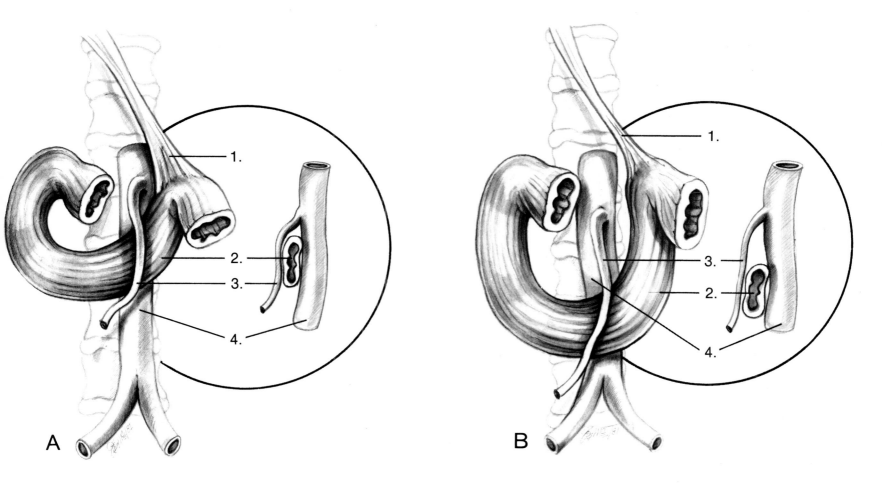

A

B

1. Suspensory lig.
2. Duodenum
3. Superior mesenteric a.
4. Aorta

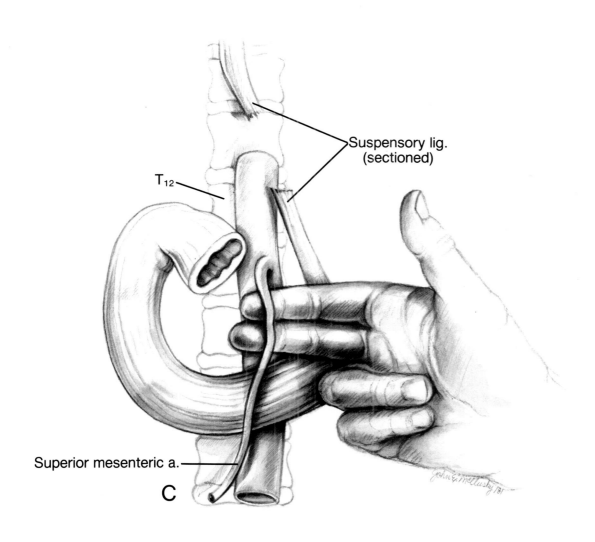

Suspensory lig.
(sectioned)

T$_{12}$

Superior mesenteric a.

C

PLATE 6-17
The Suspensory Muscle of the Duodenum (Ligament of Treitz)

A. The muscle attaches to the jejunal flexure only.

B. The muscle attaches to the flexure and the third and fourth portions of the duodenum.

C. The muscle attaches to the third and fourth portions of the duodenum.

D. Multiple attachments of the suspensory muscle are occasionally found.

Remember:

Be careful to isolate, cut and ligate all attachments of the ligament of Treitz to the duodenum during surgical treatment of superior mesenteric artery syndrome.

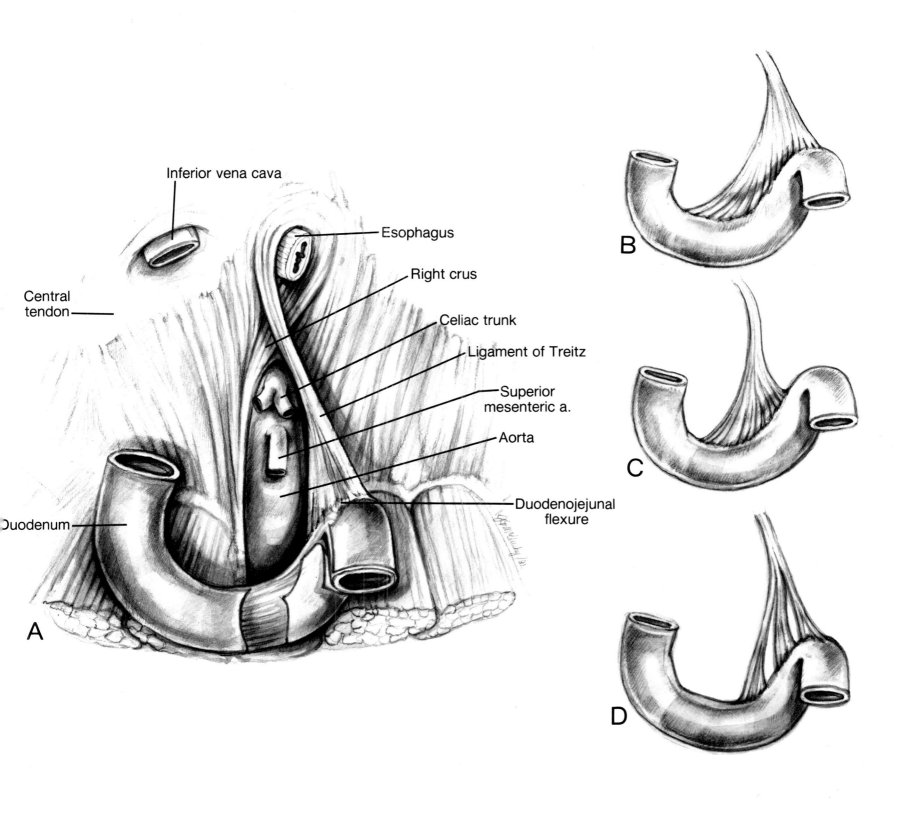

Inferior vena cava

Central tendon

Duodenum

Esophagus

Right crus

Celiac trunk

Ligament of Treitz

Superior mesenteric a.

Aorta

Duodenojejunal flexure

A

B

C

D

PLATE 6-18
Differential Diagnosis of Pancreatic Disease in the Operating Room

Pathology	Pancreas	Gallbladder/Common Bile Duct
Carcinoma of the Pancreas	Discrete mass in head (67%), less often in body or tail.	With CA of head, common duct is dilated, thin-walled and bluish.
	Pancreas distal to tumor is pale, indurated and rounder; the tail may be retracted from the splenic hilum.	With distal CA common duct is not involved.
	Distal duct is dilated and palpable ventrally.	Gallbladder is usually distended.
Carcinoma of the Ampulla	Marble-like structure projecting from medial wall of duodenum.	Same as above.
	If main duct is obstructed (20–25%), then pancreas is as above.	
Chronic Pancreatitis	If the main duct is obstructed the appearance is as with cancer.	If jaundice is present, then the gallbladder and common bile duct are distended, thick-walled, edematous and pale; gastrohepatic ligament is inflamed.
Penetrating Duodenal Ulcer	Localized induration in the head of the pancreas, without obstruction of the pancreatic duct.	No jaundice.
	No other pancreatic changes.	No dilation of gallbladder or common bile duct.
Impacted Stone	Stone in the head of the pancreas without projecting into the lumen of the duodenum, induration around the stone.	Gallstones in 93% cases.
	No pancreatic changes.	Gallbladder and common bile duct are rarely distended.

PLATE 6-19
Complications of Pancreatic Diagnostic Procedures

Procedure	Complications
1) Arteriography	Hemorrhage
2) Percutaneous transhepatic cholangiography	Hemorrhage Bile peritonitis Cholangitis
3) Transpancreatic or transduodenal pancreatography	Pancreatitis
4) Endoscopic retrograde cholangiopancreatography (ERCP)	Transient hyperamylasemia and hyperamylasuria Pancreatitis Drug reactions Pancreatic sepsis and pseudocyst abscess Cholangitis Instrumental injury

PLATE 6-20
Complications of Pancreatic Resection

Procedure	Complications
1) Pancreatoenteric Anastomosis (least secure anastomosis)	Leakage or disruption with: a) Abscess or peritonitis b) Ileus c) Pancreatic fistula d) Wound infection and dehiscence e) Bleeding from erosion of large vessels f) Ductal fibrosis, obstruction and pancreatitis
2) Biliary-Enteric Anastomosis (most secure anastomosis)	Leakage or disruption with: a) Abscess or bile peritonitis b) Biliary obstruction c) Biliary fistula d) Obstruction at the anastomotic site e) Ascending or descending cholangitis
3) Inadequate Gastric Resection	Gastrojejunal ulceration (anastomotic ulcer)
4) General	Operating room hemorrhage from major vessels: a) Portal vein b) Hepatic artery, normal or aberrant c) Superior mesenteric artery or vein d) Splenic artery or vein e) Inferior vena cava f) Renal arteries or veins g) Middle colic artery Acute postoperative pancreatitis with: a) Ductal obstruction b) Direct injury to pancreas with leakage from pancreatic parenchyma c) Interference with blood supply or drainage

PLATE 6-21
Complications of Surgical Procedures for Chronic Pancreatitis

Procedure	Complications
1) Internal drainage of pancreatic cyst	
cysto gastrostomy	Hemorrhage Pancreatitic necrosis
cysto duodenostomy	Injury to common bile duct Injury to pancreatic duct Hemorrhage
cysto jejunostomy (Roux-en-Y preferred)	Hemorrhage Reflux from too short defunctionalized limb or too small stoma

Comment: The site selected for internal drainage depends upon the location of the cyst. The lowest portion of the cyst must be able to drain by gravity into the anastomotic viscus chosen. Thus the operation must be planned to satisfy the need of the particular patient.

2) External drainage of pancreatic cyst	Complications minimal Peritonitis

Comment: External drainage is outdated and is unpleasant for the patient. We have had to use it only twice. In a poor risk patient with multiple problems, external drainage of a pancreatic cyst should not be considered a sign of timidity but rather evidence of mature surgical judgment.

3) Excision of cyst	Duodenal fistula Hemorrhage Recurrence of cyst Injury to common bile duct

Comment: Because the cyst is usually fixed firmly to surrounding organs, excision is not often recommended. It is the ideal operation where the cyst is in the body or tail and can be removed by itself. Only about 13% are of this type. The mortality following excision is 8.7%.

4) Sphincterotomy and sphincteroplasty	Operating room complications:
	    Duodenal perforation
	    Acute pancreatitis
	    Postoperative hemorrhage
	    Postoperative fibrosis and stenosis of ampulla
	    Incomplete division of sphincter
	Endoscopic complications
	    Injury to bile duct
	    Acute pancreatitis

5) Pancreaticoduodenostomy and pancreaticojejunostomy (Puestow procedure)	Anastomotic leak Hemorrhage Inadequate stoma Injury to ducts with leakage and obstruction Pancreatic necrosis from injury to vessel

PLATE 7-1
Splenic Anomalies

The spleen appears as a bulge in the mesoderm of the left side of dorsal mesogastrium early in the 6th week. There is no embryological or phylogenetic evidence that the spleen has a bilateral origin.

Accessory spleens are not rare. Most (75%) are found at the hilus, but they may occur at other sites, the chief of which is the tail of the pancreas. An accessory spleen with the gonad is rare but striking. It is associated with absence of limbs (ectromelia) and reduced size of the mandible (micrognathia).

Most other splenic anomalies are associated with cardiac malformations or more or less severe situs anomalies.

Table: Anomalies of the Spleen and Associated Malformations

Splenic Anomaly	Associated Malformations
Accessory spleen	None
Absence of spleen (asplenia syndrome)	Partial situs inversus Severe cardiac anomalies Mesenteric defects Spina bifida
Right-sided spleen	Kartagener's triad: (Total situs inversus, bronchiectasis, malformed paranasal sinuses)
Multiple spleens (polysplenia syndrome)	Partial situs inversus Severe cardiac anomalies
Splenogonadal fusion	Ectromelia (absence of limbs) Micrognathia (small mandible)

Remember:

1) Accessory spleens are found in 14 to 30% of patients, but in patients with hematologic disorders, the incidence is greater.

2) Accessory spleens are rarely found in more than one site.

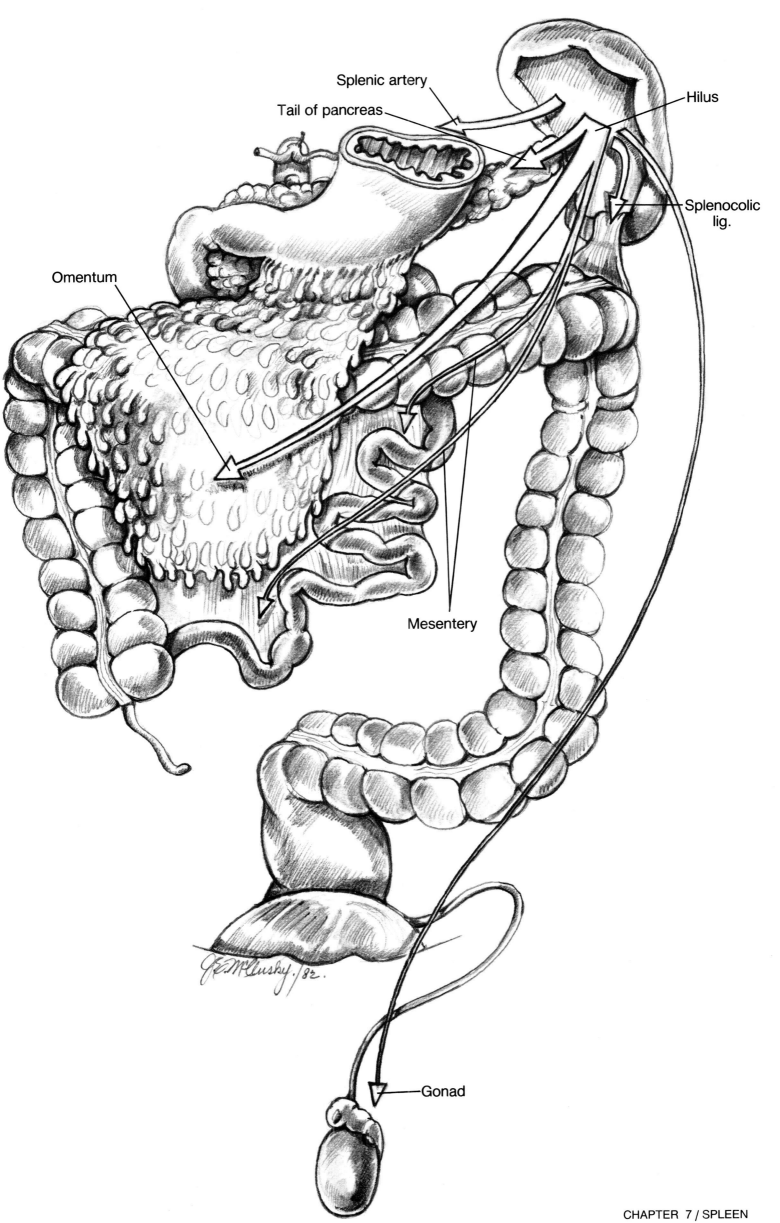

Splenic artery

Tail of pancreas

Hilus

Omentum

Splenocolic lig.

Mesentery

Gonad

PLATE 7-2
Peritoneal Reflections of the Spleen

A. The splenic pedicle consists of the splenorenal and gastrosplenic ligaments and the presplenic fold.

B. If the presplenic fold is absent, the pedicle is formed by two ligaments only.

Remember:

1) The splenorenal ligament is a double layer of peritoneum extending from the left kidney to the spleen, containing the splenic artery and vein as well as the tail of the pancreas.

2) The gastrosplenic ligament is a double layer of peritoneum extending from the greater curvature of the stomach to the spleen and contains the short gastric vessels above and the left gastroepiploic vessels below. Ligate, transfix and suture the area of the greater curvature to avoid future bleeding.

3) The splenic pedicle is the splenic portion of the splenorenal and gastrosplenic ligaments.

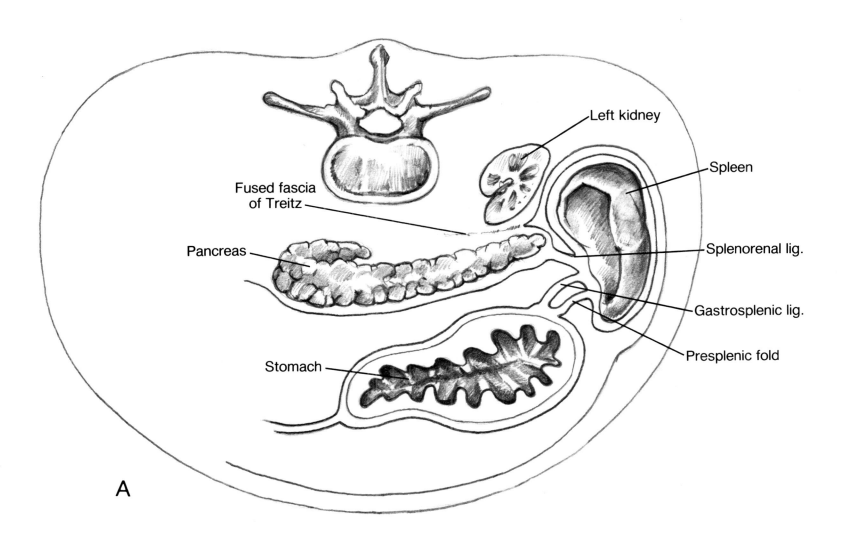

A

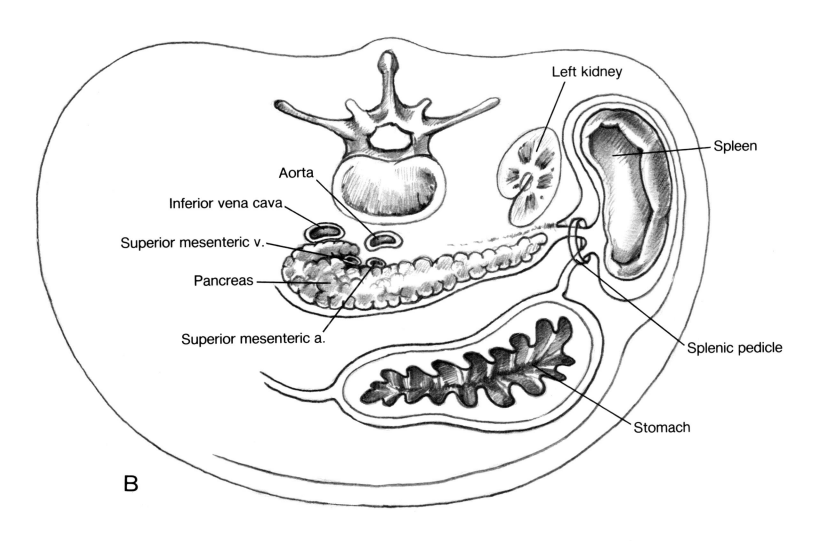

B

PLATE 7-3
The Splenic Artery and Vein

Variations of the relations of the splenic artery and vein.

A. The splenic artery lies anterior to the splenic vein.

B. The splenic artery lies posterior to the splenic vein.

C. The splenic artery lies anterior to the vein proximally and posterior to the vein distally.

Most, but not all, short gastric veins enter the spleen. The left gastric vein may enter the portal vein (A) (67%) or the splenic vein (B) (33%). The inferior mesenteric vein may enter the superior mesenteric vein (B) (33%), the splenic vein (C) (33%), or at the junction of the superior mesenteric and splenic veins (A) (33%).

Remember:

1) If the splenic artery is injured it may be ligated. If the splenic vein is injured, a splenectomy will usually be necessary.

2) If the spleen is to be removed, doubly ligate the splenic artery and vein, separately or as a unit, distal to the origin of the gastroepiploic vessels. This will avoid postoperative bleeding.

3) The splenic vein contributes about 30% of the portal blood.

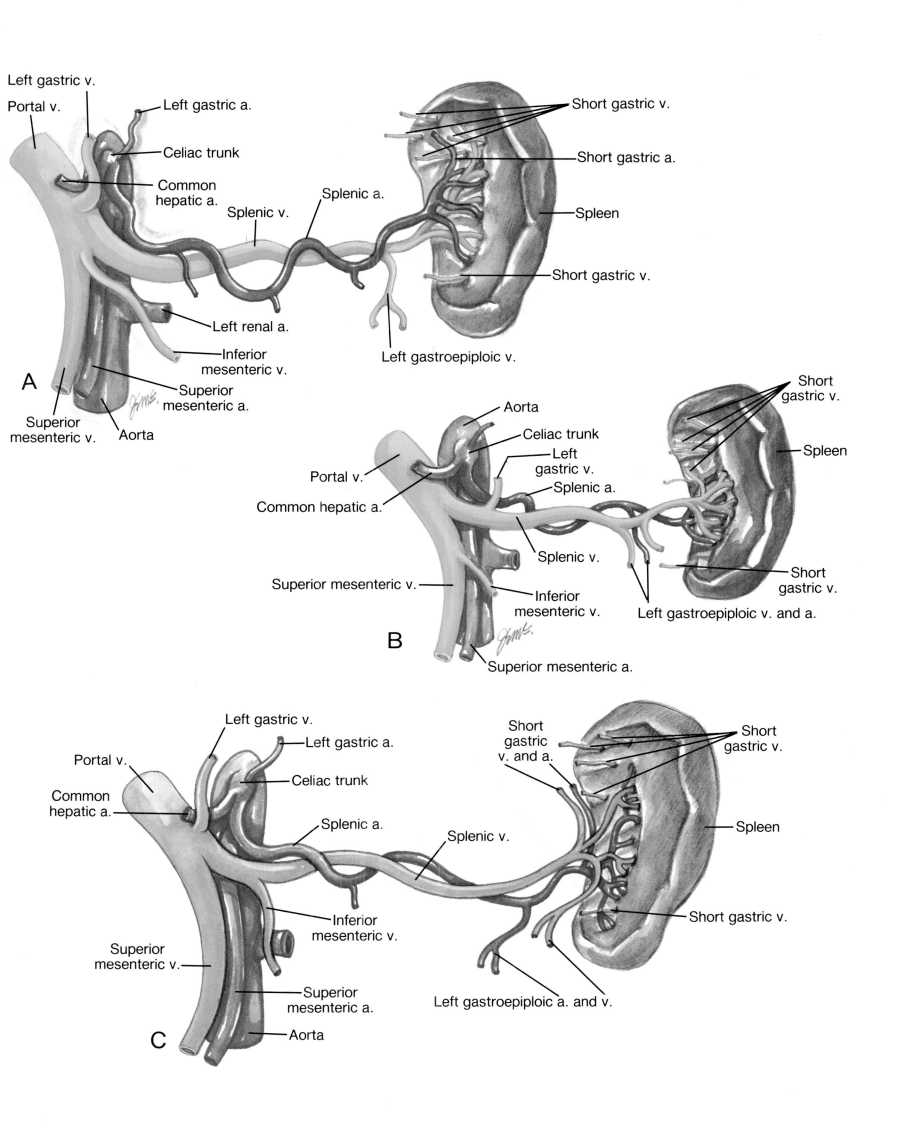

PLATE 7-4
Arterial Supply of the Spleen and Pancreas

The splenic artery emerges from behind the body of the pancreas to cross the tail of the pancreas.

A. Two terminal splenic branches and two polar arteries are present. The left gastroepiploic artery arises directly from the splenic artery.

B. Two terminal branches of the splenic artery are present. The left gastroepiploic artery arises from the inferior terminal branch which also receives the transverse pancreatic artery. The right gastroepiploic artery arises from the gastroduodenal artery.

C. A small transverse pancreatic artery anastomoses with the splenic artery. The left gastroepiploic artery arises from the inferior terminal branch of the splenic artery.

D. Only the distal portion of the transverse pancreatic artery is present. It (as the caudal pancreatic artery) joins the inferior terminal branch of the splenic artery at the hilum.

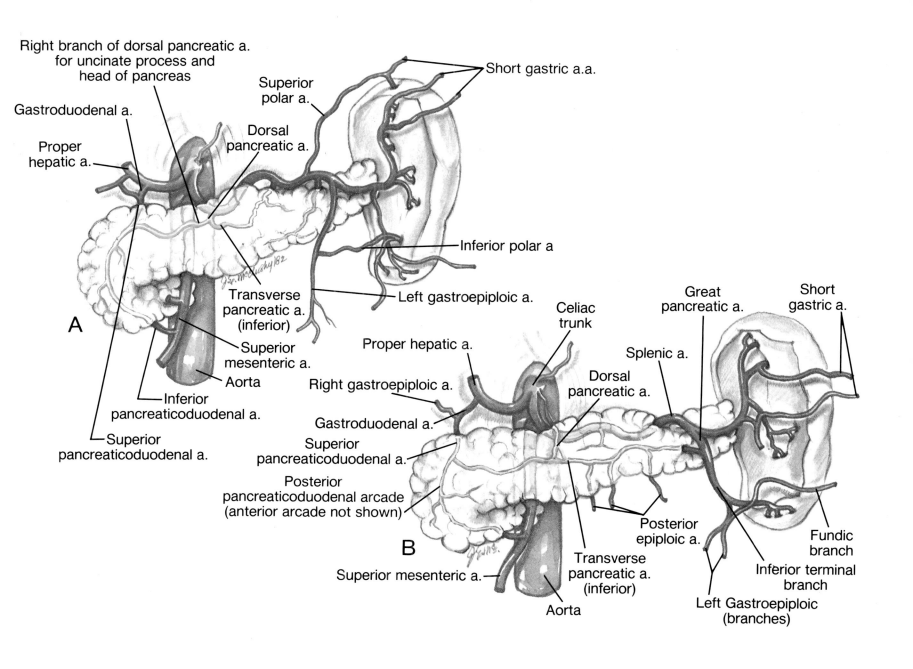

Right branch of dorsal pancreatic a. for uncinate process and head of pancreas

Short gastric a.a.

Superior polar a.

Dorsal pancreatic a.

Gastroduodenal a.

Proper hepatic a.

Inferior polar a

Transverse pancreatic a. (inferior)

Left gastroepiploic a.

Superior mesenteric a.

Aorta

Inferior pancreaticoduodenal a.

Superior pancreaticoduodenal a.

A

Celiac trunk

Great pancreatic a.

Short gastric a.

Proper hepatic a.

Splenic a.

Right gastroepiploic a.

Dorsal pancreatic a.

Gastroduodenal a.

Superior pancreaticoduodenal a.

Posterior pancreaticoduodenal arcade (anterior arcade not shown)

Posterior epiploic a.

Fundic branch

Superior mesenteric a.

Transverse pancreatic a. (inferior)

Inferior terminal branch

Left Gastroepiploic (branches)

Aorta

B

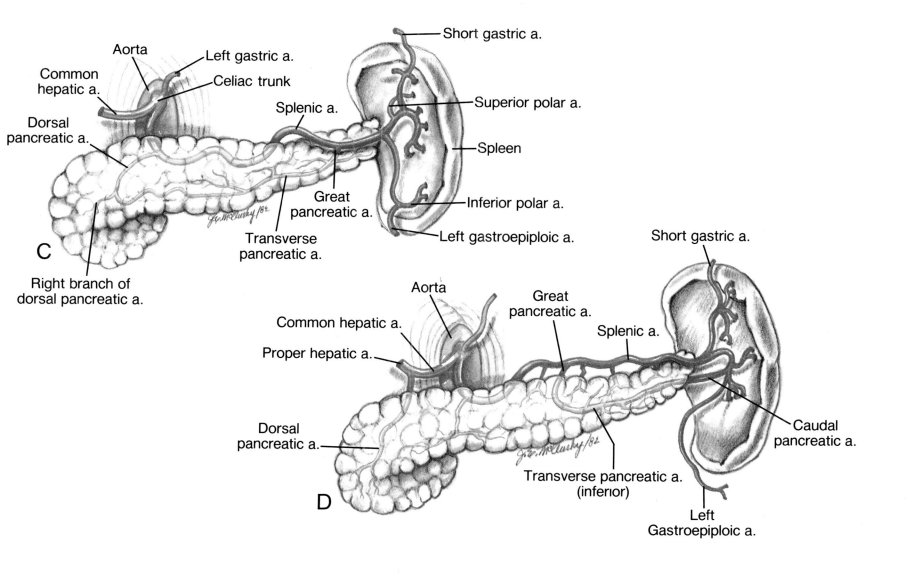

Aorta

Left gastric a.

Short gastric a.

Common hepatic a.

Celiac trunk

Dorsal pancreatic a.

Splenic a.

Superior polar a.

Spleen

Great pancreatic a.

Inferior polar a.

Transverse pancreatic a.

Left gastroepiploic a.

C

Right branch of dorsal pancreatic a.

Aorta

Great pancreatic a.

Short gastric a.

Common hepatic a.

Splenic a.

Proper hepatic a.

Caudal pancreatic a.

Dorsal pancreatic a.

Transverse pancreatic a. (inferior)

Left Gastroepiploic a.

D

PLATE 7-5
Relations of the Spleen and Pancreas: Lymphatic Drainage

A. Relation of the spleen to the tail of the pancreas. (1) is found in 8%, (2) in 50% and (3) in 42%. In about one third of subjects the two organs are in contact.

B. Lymphatic drainage of the spleen as well as that of the tail of the pancreas is to lymph nodes at the hilus of the spleen. Drainage of the parts of the pancreas is to left gastric, pancreaticoduodenal and mesenteric nodes.

Remember:

1) The surgery of the spleen, total or segmental, requires anatomical mobilization of the organ by division and ligation of the splenic ligaments.

2) The anatomical entities responsible for bleeding are the (a) short gastric vessels, (b) splenic pedicle and (c) left gastroepiploic vessels.

3) Transfix ligatures of the short gastric vessels.

4) Ligate splenic artery and vein distal to the origin of the left gastroepiploic vessels.

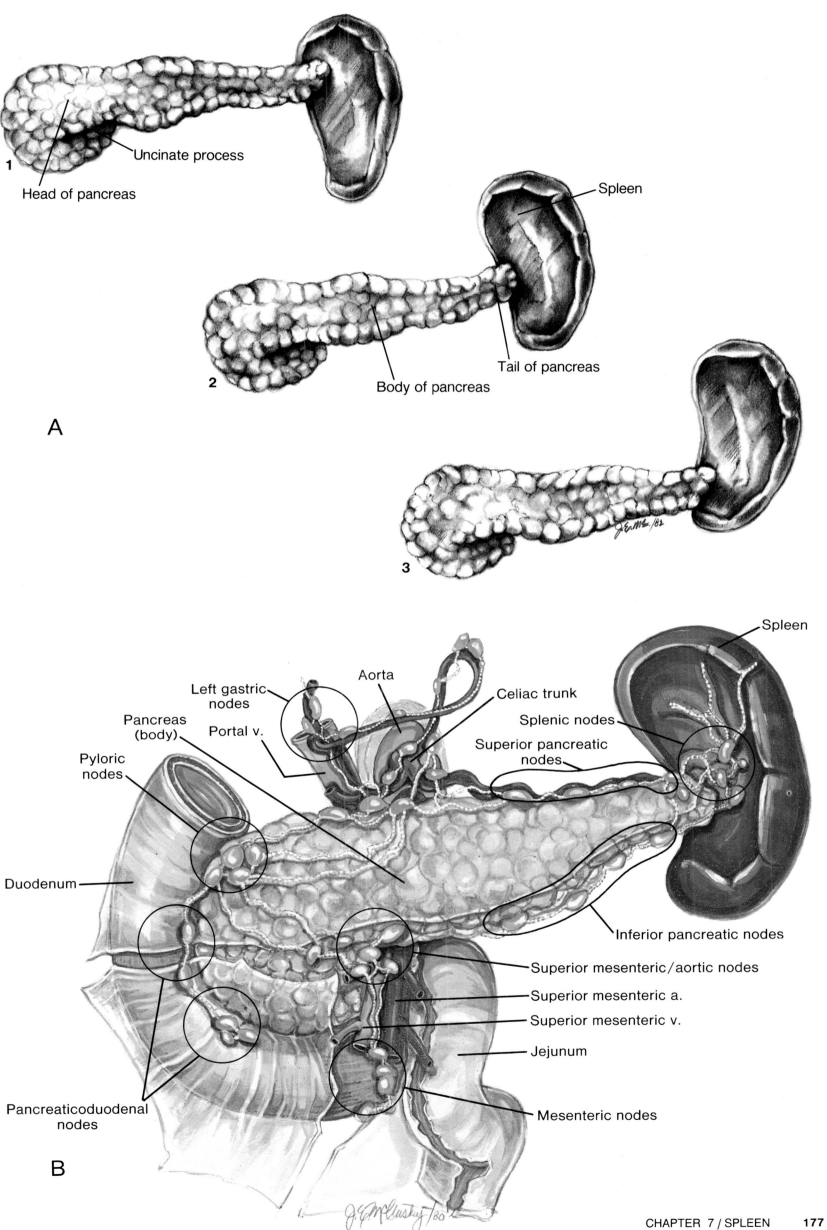

A

1

Head of pancreas

Uncinate process

2

Body of pancreas

Tail of pancreas

Spleen

3

B

Left gastric
nodes

Aorta

Celiac trunk

Pancreas
(body)

Portal v.

Splenic nodes

Pyloric
nodes

Superior pancreatic
nodes

Spleen

Duodenum

Inferior pancreatic nodes

Superior mesenteric/aortic nodes

Superior mesenteric a.

Superior mesenteric v.

Jejunum

Pancreaticoduodenal
nodes

Mesenteric nodes

PLATE 7-6
Segments of the Spleen

A and B. The splenic artery usually divides into two or three major terminal branches before entering the spleen.

C and D. Segmental anatomy of the spleen. One or two avascular planes may be found between the areas served by terminal branches.

In 84% of spleens there are superior, middle and inferior segments. These segments are the basis for partial (segmental) splenectomy, which will avoid postsplenectomy sepsis.

Remember:

1) The splenic artery must be dissected carefully at the hilus. The branch or branches to the segments to be resected, should be ligated with through and through parenchymal sutures to prevent bleeding. Gelfoam or Avitene should be used as necessary.

2) Save the spleen if possible.

3) Avoid capsular avulsion and traction of the spleen.

4) Isolate the splenic artery.

5) Do not attempt to isolate the splenic vein. It is fragile.

6) The two prerequisites for successful splenic surgery are mobilization and good hemostasis.

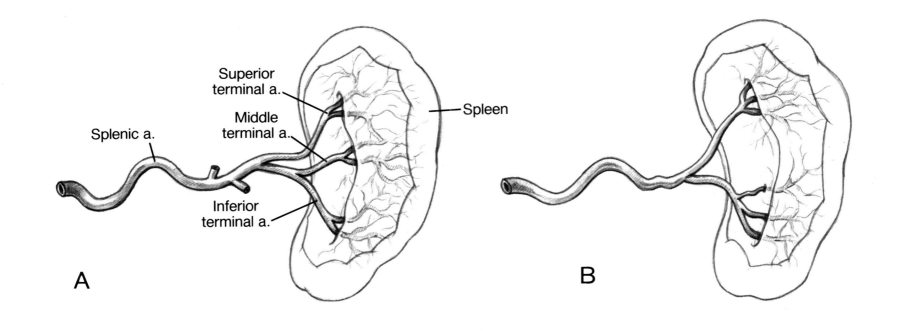

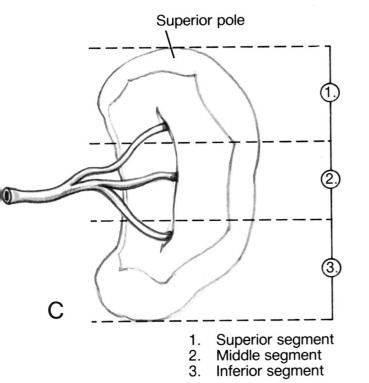

1. Superior segment
2. Middle segment
3. Inferior segment

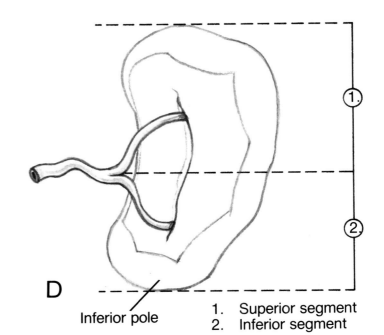

1. Superior segment
2. Inferior segment

PLATE 8-1
Peritoneal Reflections and Projections of the Liver

A. Peritoneal reflections of the liver, stomach and spleen. The liver has been removed to show the bare area and the cut edges of the two layers of the coronary ligament. The right leaf of the falciform ligament forms the anterior layer of the coronary ligament.

B. Anterior erect projection of the liver.

C. Posterior erect projection of the liver.

D. Left lateral supine projection of the liver.

Remember:

1) The rib levels of the liver, lung and pleura (from Lockhart, Hamilton and Fyfe)

	Lateral Sternal Line	Mid Axillary Line	Vertebral Spines
Liver (superior border)	5	6	8
Lung (inferior border)	6	8	10
Pleura (inferior border)	7	10	12

2) The hepatogastric ligament contains the following structures: (a) left gastric artery and vein; (b) hepatic division of left vagus nerve; (c) lymph nodules; (d) occasionally both vagal trunks; (e) occasionally branches of the right gastric artery and vein; (f) left hepatic artery if it arises from the left gastric artery.

3) The anterior and posterior layers of the coronary ligament are almost in apposition on the left.

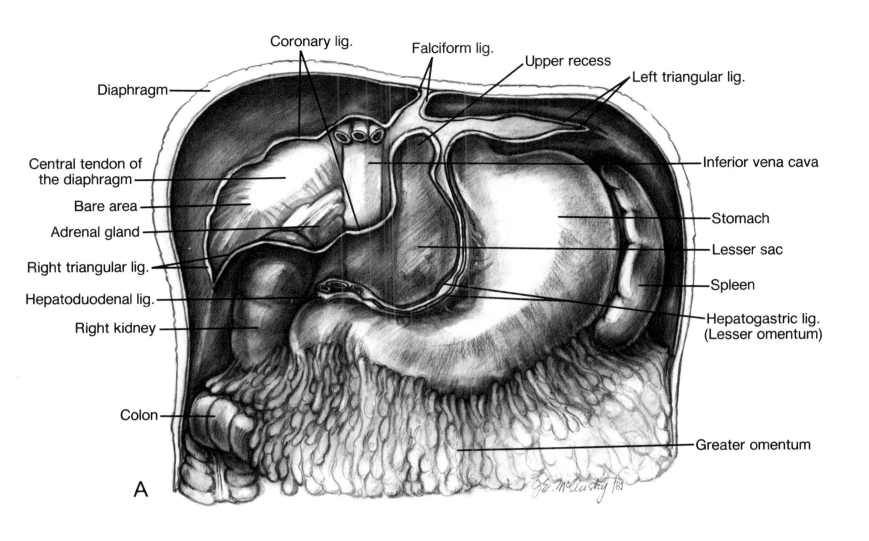

Coronary lig.
Falciform lig.
Upper recess
Left triangular lig.
Diaphragm
Central tendon of the diaphragm
Bare area
Adrenal gland
Right triangular lig.
Hepatoduodenal lig.
Right kidney
Colon
Inferior vena cava
Stomach
Lesser sac
Spleen
Hepatogastric lig. (Lesser omentum)
Greater omentum

A

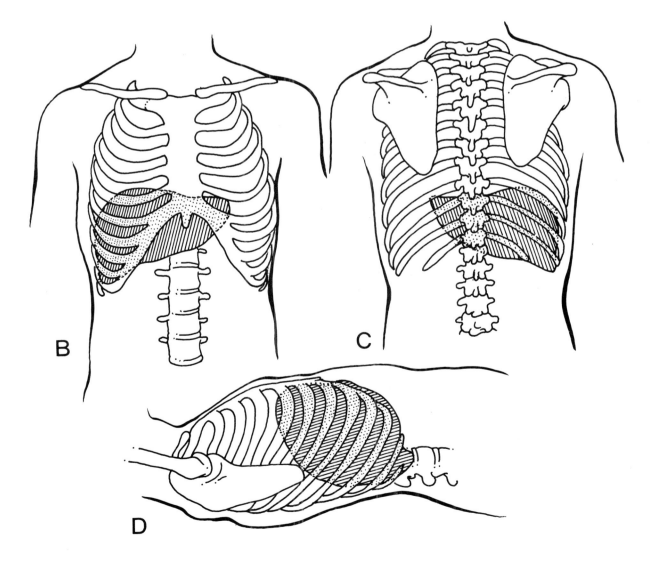

B

C

D

PLATE 8-2
The Three Surfaces of the Liver

A. Anterior surface. The sharp anterior edge is that which is palpated at physical examination, while the blunt rounded posterior margin is seen as the "edge" in a plain abdominal x-ray.

B. Visceral surface of the liver.

C. Posterior surface of the liver.

Remember:

The liver shows almost no external indication of its lobation. Only the division between medial and lateral segments of the left lobe is clearly marked by the falciform ligament. The fissure between anterior and posterior segments of the right lobe is rarely distinguishable.

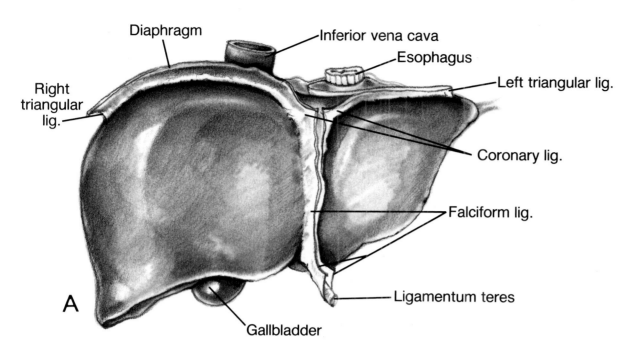

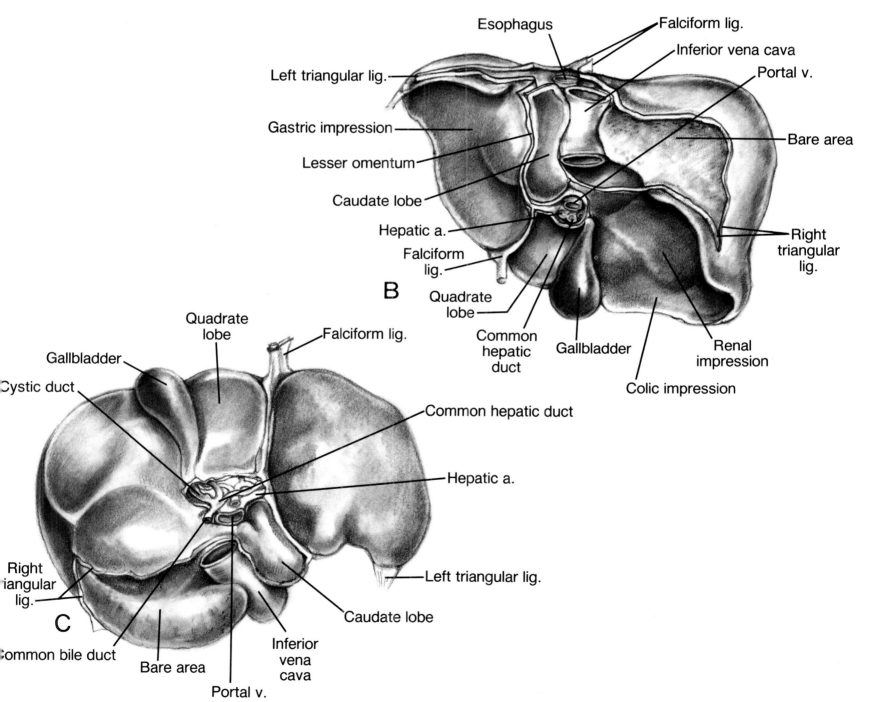

PLATE 8-3
The Lobulation of the Liver

A. Posterior surface. The broken line (line of Rex) marks the division into right and left lobes (from the inferior vena cava to the gallbladder).

B. The "H" monogram of the liver (Hepar).

C. Anterior surface. The broken line marks the division into the right and left lobes.

D. Anterior surface. The two lobes, four segments, and eight areas are indicated.

Remember:

1) The interlobar fissure between right and left lobes is not indicated on the hepatic surface. For practical purposes it is on the line from the inferior vena cava to the gallbladder.

2) The right and left lobes have approximately the same mass, though a different shape. The blood vessels to each lobe have approximately the same diameter.

3) The quadrate "lobe" lies between the gallbladder and the falciform ligament. It belongs to the medial segment of the left lobe.

4) The caudate "lobe" receives vessels from the left and right; the lobar dividing line passes through it.

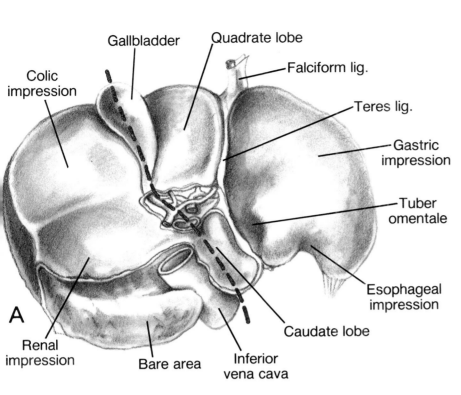

Colic
impression

Gallbladder

Quadrate lobe

Falciform lig.

Teres lig.

Gastric
impression

Tuber
omentale

Esophageal
impression

Caudate lobe

Renal
impression

Bare area

Inferior
vena cava

A

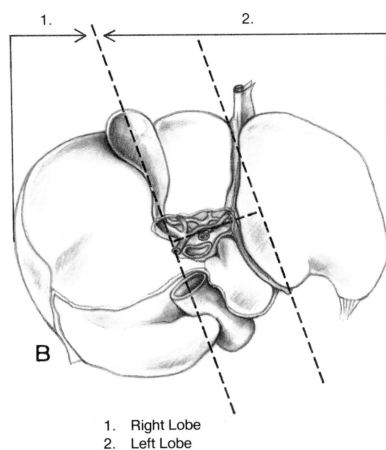

B

1. Right Lobe
2. Left Lobe

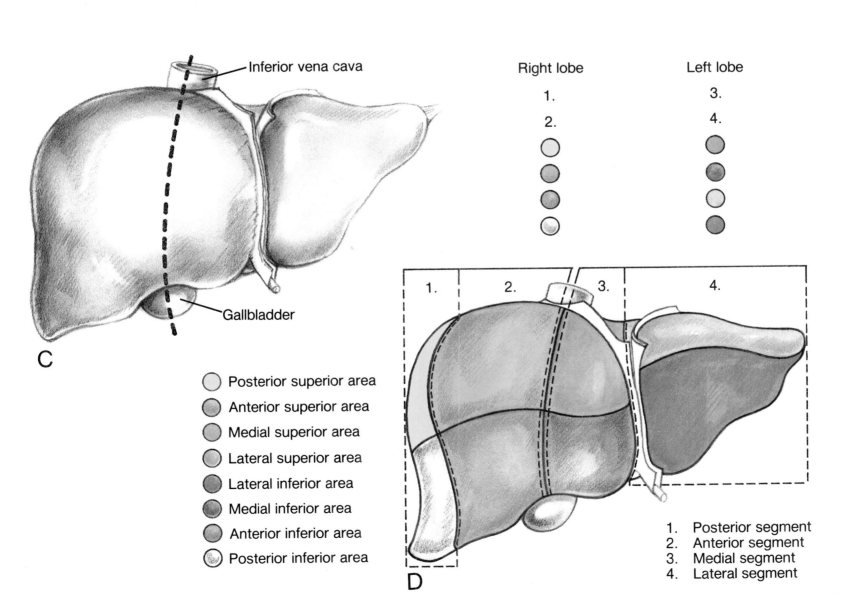

Inferior vena cava

Gallbladder

C

Right lobe
1.
2.

Left lobe
3.
4.

Posterior superior area
Anterior superior area
Medial superior area
Lateral superior area
Lateral inferior area
Medial inferior area
Anterior inferior area
Posterior inferior area

D

1. Posterior segment
2. Anterior segment
3. Medial segment
4. Lateral segment

PLATE 8-4
Intrahepatic Blood Vessels

The intrahepatic distribution of blood vessels. The broken line indicates the plane of division between right and left lobes.

A. Distribution of the hepatic artery. Translobar and subcapsular collateral circulation makes it possible to ligate the left or right hepatic artery, but such ligation should be avoided if possible.

B. Distribution of the hepatic veins. The middle and left hepatic veins usually form a common trunk before they emerge from the liver. The extrahepatic veins are from 0.5 to 1.5 cm in length. The hepatic veins, unlike the other hepatic blood vessels, lie *between* the lobes rather than within them.

C. Distribution of the portal veins. Portal veins may be ligated but atrophy of the affected segment usually follows.

Remember:

1) The hepatic artery supplies 25% of hepatic blood; the portal vein supplies 75%.

2) After ligation of the right or left hepatic artery, hepatic bile ducts, or portal vein, the affected lobe becomes atrophic; the unligated lobe becomes hypertrophic.

3) Hepatic artery ligation is tolerated by most patients.

4) Hepatic arteries appear to be end arteries in cadavers, but *in vivo* arteriograms show arterial anastomoses between right and left hepatic lobes.

5) Anastomoses between portal veins are few, but the lobar portal vein may be ligated.

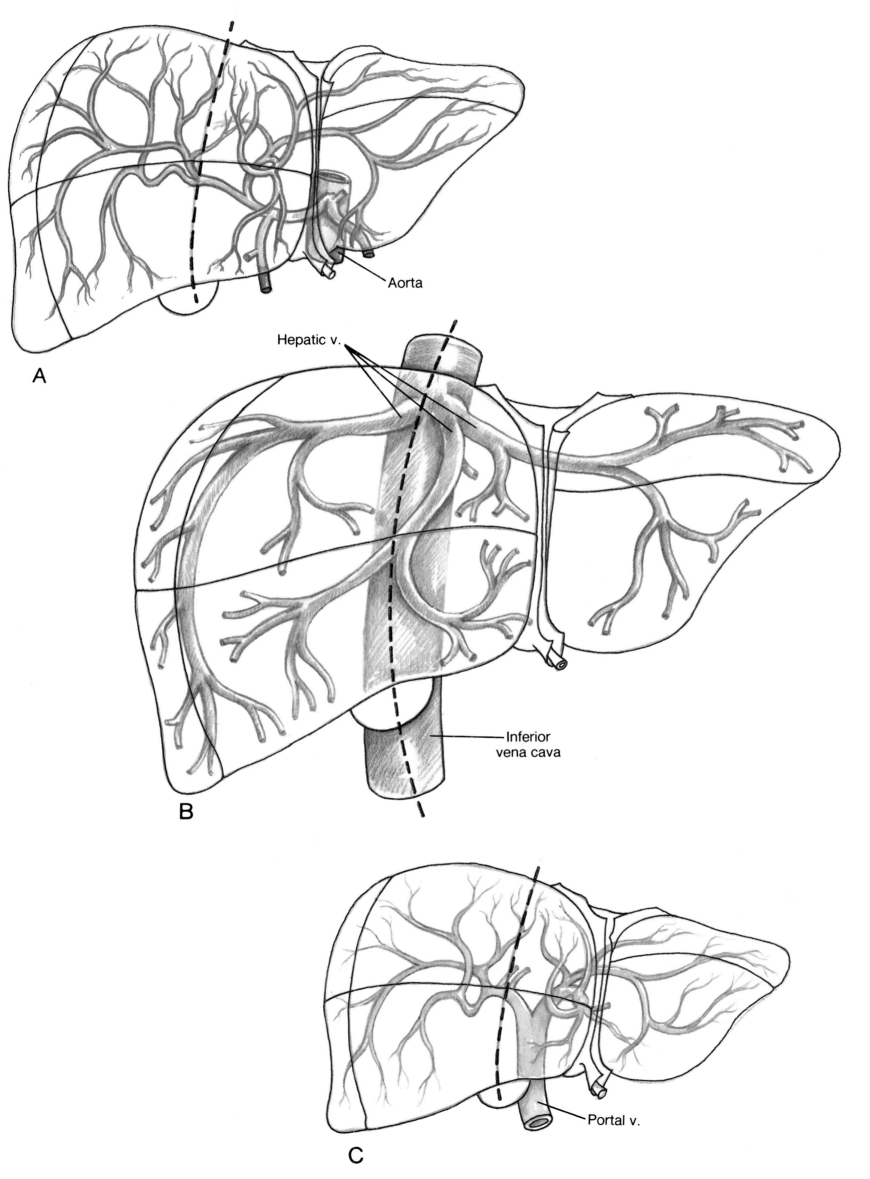

A

Hepatic v.

Inferior
vena cava

B

Aorta

Portal v.

C

PLATE 8-5
Intrahepatic and Extrahepatic Bile Ducts

A. Distribution of the intrahepatic bile ducts. Injury to the bile ducts must be repaired. If repair is impossible, ligate the duct and resect the affected segment.

B. The extrahepatic bile ducts and the gallbladder on the visceral surface of the liver.

C. Variations of intrahepatic segmental ducts. (1) Usual pattern. (2) Anomalous origin of the right anterior duct from the left hepatic duct. (3) Anomalous origin of the right posterior duct from the left hepatic duct. In (2) and (3), the aberrant ducts cross the interlobar line. They may complicate surgical procedures.

Remember:

1) The biliary tract has many variations, both intrahepatic and extrahepatic. Before you cut or ligate be sure to identify the right and left hepatic ducts, the common hepatic duct and the cystic duct.

2) Ligation of an extrahepatic bile duct results in atrophy of the corresponding lobe.

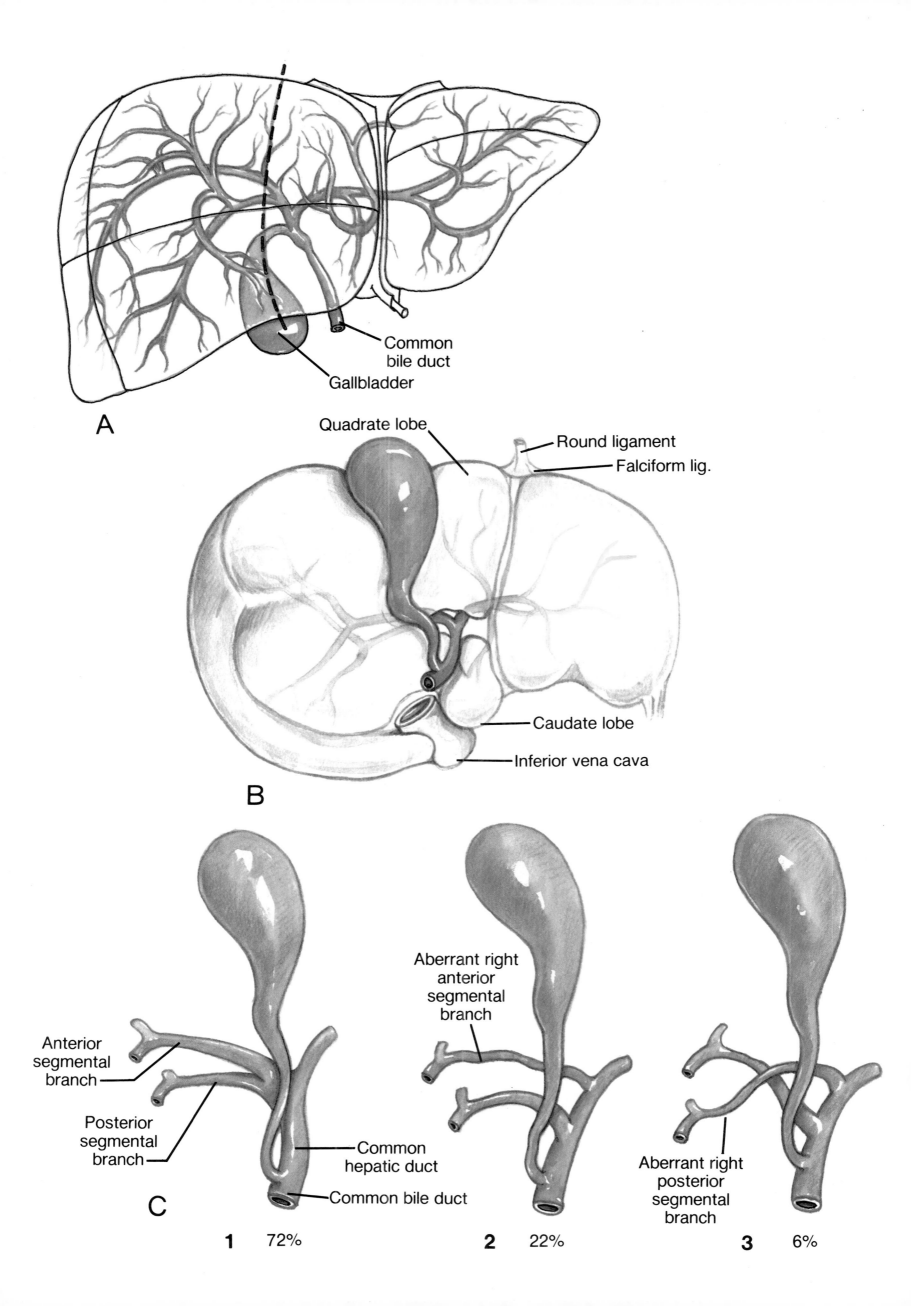

Common
bile duct

Gallbladder

A

Quadrate lobe

Round ligament

Falciform lig.

Caudate lobe

Inferior vena cava

B

Anterior
segmental
branch

Posterior
segmental
branch

Aberrant right
anterior
segmental
branch

Common
hepatic duct

Common bile duct

Aberrant right
posterior
segmental
branch

C

1 72%   **2** 22%   **3** 6%

PLATE 8-6
The Anatomy and Terminology of Liver Resection

Areas to be resected are shaded:

A. Right lobectomy

B. Right trisegmentectomy

C. Left lobectomy

D. Left lateral segmentectomy

E. Left trisegmentectomy

Remember:

1) The line of resection for a right lobectomy must be placed just to the right of the interlobar plane, and for a left lobectomy, just to the left of it (from inferior vena cava to gallbladder).

2) Resection of 10 to 20% of the liver is compatible with life.

3) Regeneration of the liver takes place by hypertrophy of the remaining hepatic tissue within 4 to 6 months.

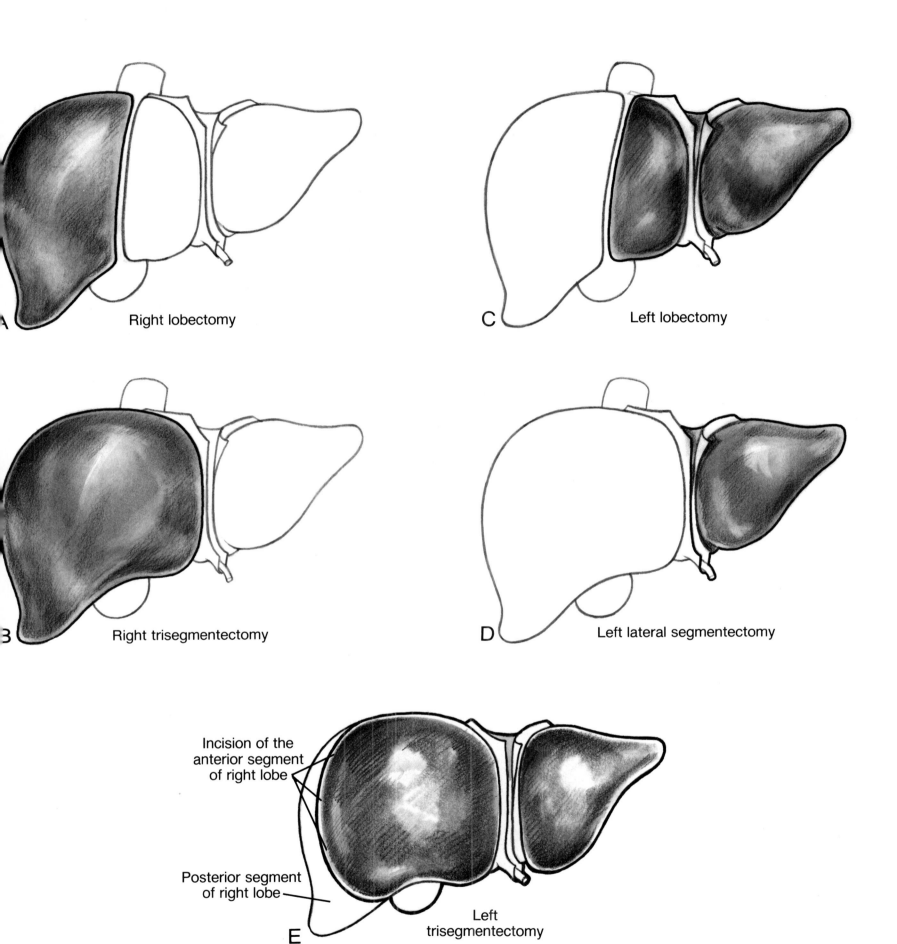

A   Right lobectomy

B   Right trisegmentectomy

C   Left lobectomy

D   Left lateral segmentectomy

Incision of the
anterior segment
of right lobe

Posterior segment
of right lobe

E   Left
trisegmentectomy

PLATE 8-7
Lymphatic Drainage of the Liver

Diagram of lymphatic drainage of the liver. See Plate 3-10 for transdiaphragmatic drainage to nodes in the thorax.

Remember:

1) The lymphatics of the liver are not well known.

2) 25 to 50% of the lymph reaching the thoracic duct comes from the liver.

3) 25 to 50% of patients dying of cancer have liver metastasis.

4) Metastasis to the liver may occur by (a) portal circulation, (b) arterial hepatic circulation, (c) lymphatic vessels or (d) direct extension.

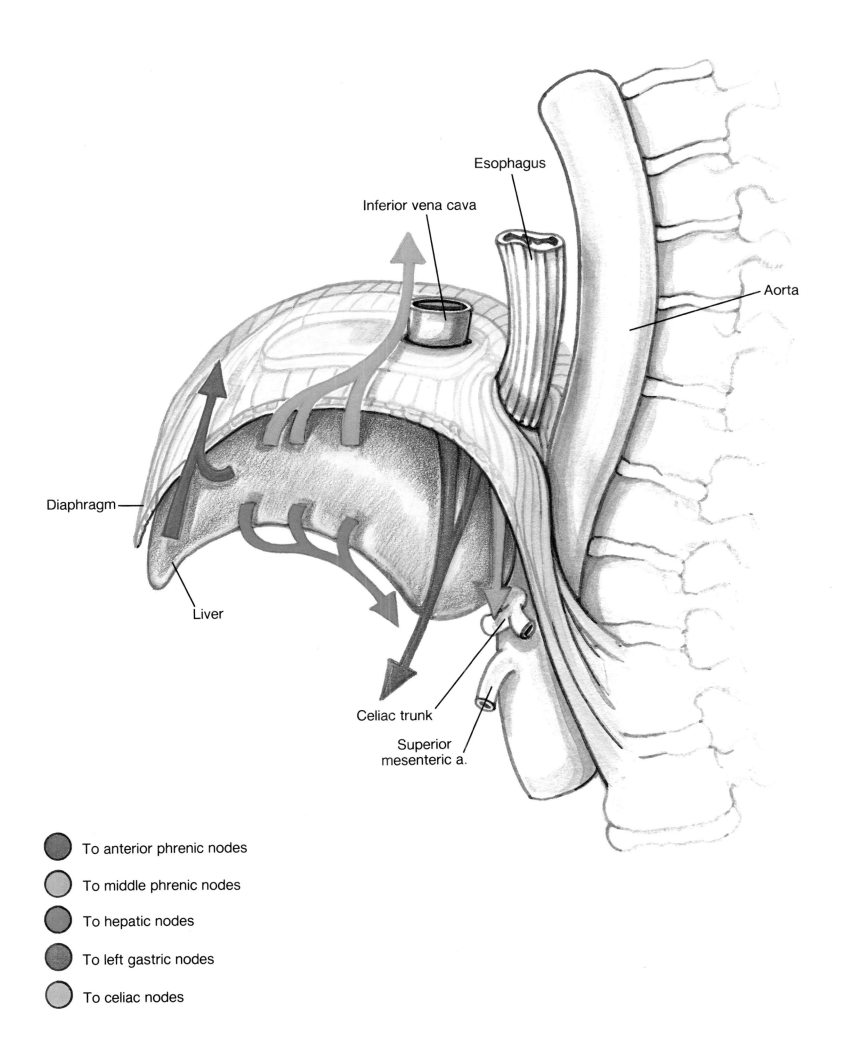

Esophagus

Inferior vena cava

Aorta

Diaphragm

Liver

Celiac trunk

Superior
mesenteric a.

To anterior phrenic nodes

To middle phrenic nodes

To hepatic nodes

To left gastric nodes

To celiac nodes

PLATE 8-8
The Hepatic Triad and Celiac Trunk

The relations of the biliary tract (green), the hepatic artery (red), and the portal vein (blue), at the hepatic porta. The branches of the celiac trunk (red) and the inferior vena cava (violet) also are shown.

Remember:

1) The cystic artery may be single or double, short or long, anterior or posterior to the right or left hepatic duct, common hepatic duct or common bile duct.

2) The gallbladder is drained by numerous small veins entering the quadrate lobe. There is no cystic vein as such.

3) The length of the common hepatic duct and the common bile duct depends upon the point at which the cystic duct joins the common hepatic duct.

4) The mnemonic for the relations of structures of the triad is "Don't Act Vain" (DAV): Duct, above; Artery, middle; Vein, beneath.

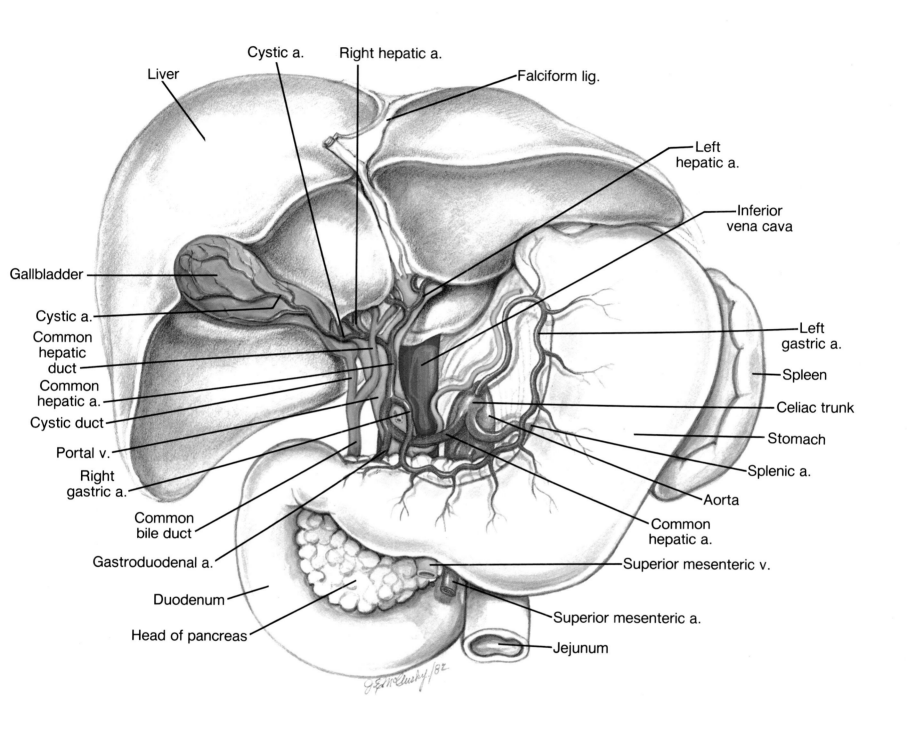

Liver

Cystic a.

Right hepatic a.

Falciform lig.

Left hepatic a.

Inferior vena cava

Gallbladder

Cystic a.

Common hepatic duct

Common hepatic a.

Cystic duct

Portal v.

Right gastric a.

Common bile duct

Gastroduodenal a.

Duodenum

Head of pancreas

Left gastric a.

Spleen

Celiac trunk

Stomach

Splenic a.

Aorta

Common hepatic a.

Superior mesenteric v.

Superior mesenteric a.

Jejunum

PLATE 8-9
The Cystic and Common Hepatic Ducts

A. Diagram of structures at the hepatic porta. The left lobe and part of the right lobe of the liver have been removed. Note the relationship of the anatomical entities of the hepatic triad to the inferior vena cava.

B. Variations at the junction of the cystic duct with common hepatic duct. (1–3) Possible configurations of the junction of the cystic duct with common hepatic duct. (4) Sessile gallbladder. "Absence" of the cystic duct. (5) Short cystic duct. (6) "Absence" of the common hepatic duct. The cystic duct enters the duodenum with the common bile duct. (7) "Phrygian cap" deformity of the fundus of the gallbladder. (8) Hartmann's pouch deformity of the neck of the gallbladder.

Remember:

1) This is an area of variations and anomalies. Variant ducts are found in 18 percent of patients. Most will be asymptomatic and hence give no warning of their presence.

2) To be safe, dissect the gallbladder from above downward during cholecystectomy.

3) The cystic duct should be ligated close to the common bile duct to avoid the "cystic remnant" syndrome.

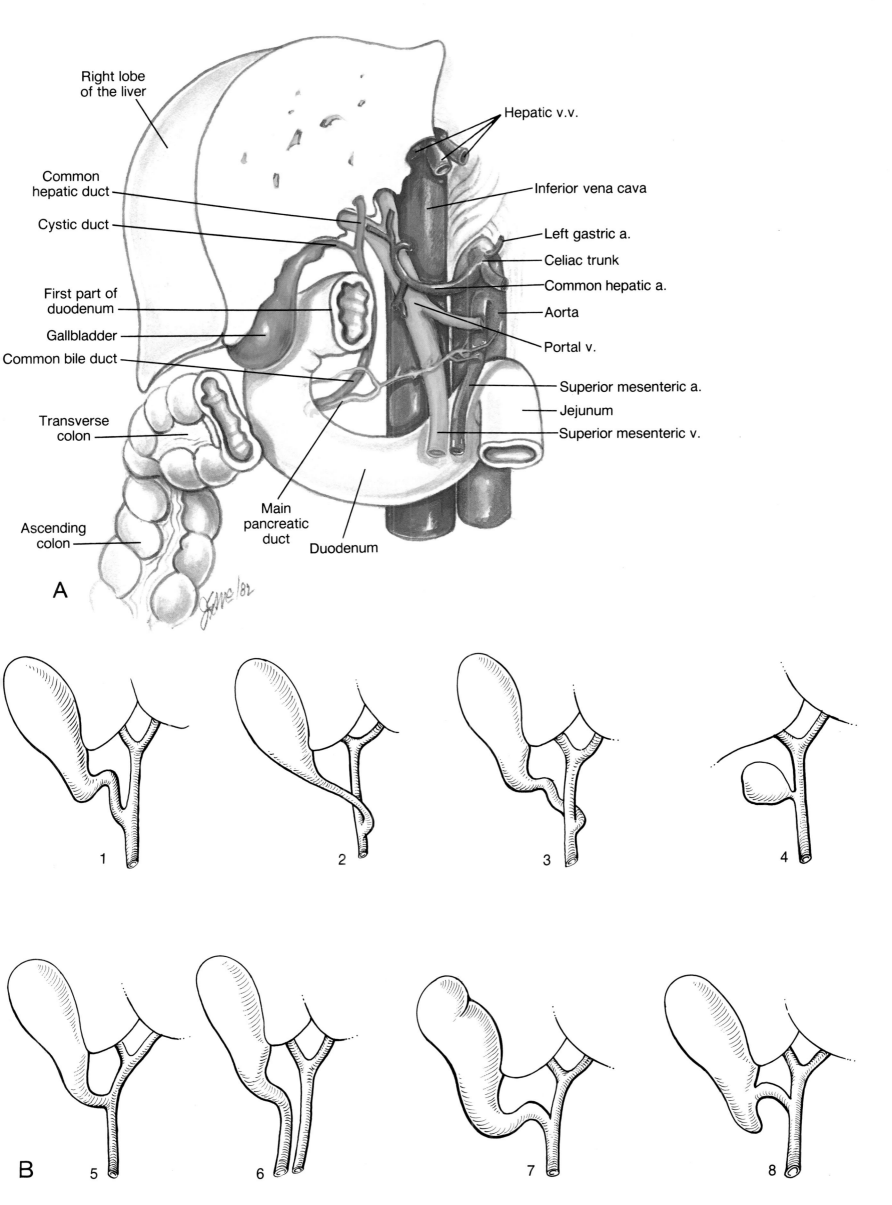

Right lobe
of the liver

Common
hepatic duct

Cystic duct

First part of
duodenum

Gallbladder

Common bile duct

Transverse
colon

Ascending
colon

A

Main
pancreatic
duct

Duodenum

Hepatic v.v.

Inferior vena cava

Left gastric a.

Celiac trunk

Common hepatic a.

Aorta

Portal v.

Superior mesenteric a.

Jejunum

Superior mesenteric v.

B

1

2

3

4

5

6

7

8

PLATE 8-10
The Hepatocystic Triangle and the Triangle of Calot

A. The hepatocystic triangle is defined laterally by the cystic duct and gallbladder, medially by the common hepatic duct and superiorly by the margin of the right lobe of the liver. It is larger than the triangle of Calot (1891), which is bounded superiorly by the cystic artery. Within the larger triangle are a number of structures that must be identified before they may be ligated or cut. These include: right hepatic artery, aberrant right hepatic artery, right hepatic duct, cystic artery and accessory bile ducts.

B. The pattern found in about 75% of subjects. The cystic artery (shaded) arises from the right hepatic artery and passes posterior to the common hepatic duct.

C. In about 20%, the artery arises from the common or left hepatic artery and passes anterior to the duct.

D. In about 2.5%, the cystic artery arises from the gastroduodenal artery.

E and F. Rarely a "recurrent" cystic artery reaches the gallbladder at the body or fundus.

Remember:

The frequency of structures found in the hepatocystic triangle: (a) cystic artery 90%, (b) right hepatic artery 82%, (c) all aberrant arteries 95% and (d) all aberrant ducts 91%.

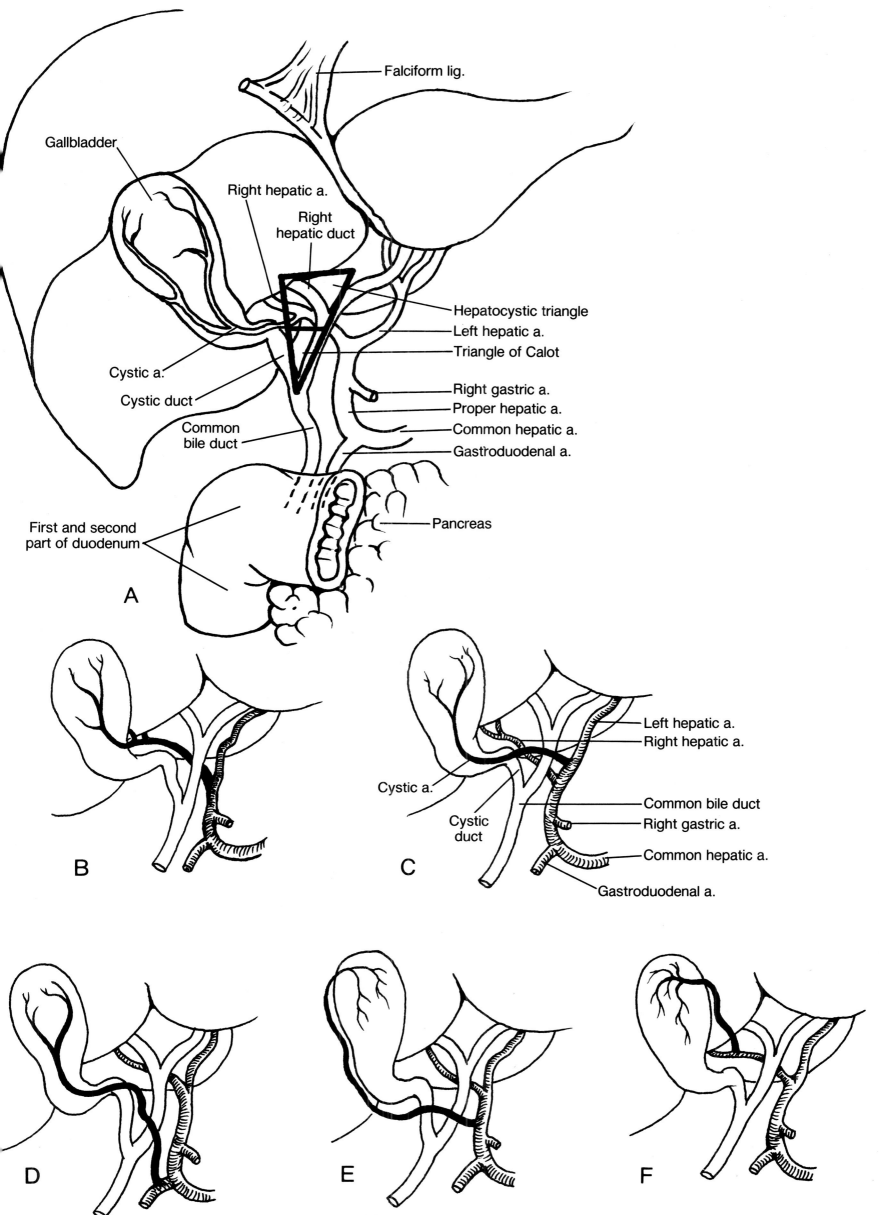

Falciform lig.

Gallbladder

Right hepatic a.

Right hepatic duct

Hepatocystic triangle

Left hepatic a.

Triangle of Calot

Right gastric a.

Proper hepatic a.

Common hepatic a.

Gastroduodenal a.

Cystic a.

Cystic duct

Common bile duct

Pancreas

First and second part of duodenum

A

B

C

Left hepatic a.

Right hepatic a.

Cystic a.

Cystic duct

Common bile duct

Right gastric a.

Common hepatic a.

Gastroduodenal a.

D

E

F

PLATE 8-11
Variations in the Arteries of the Liver

A. The usual configuration. The common hepatic artery arises from the celiac trunk and divides into right and left hepatic arteries.

B. A right hepatic artery arises from the superior mesenteric artery. This is an "accessory" aberrant hepatic artery; normal right and left hepatic arteries are present. It may give rise to the gastroduodenal artery and even to the dorsal pancreatic artery.

C. The only hepatic artery arises from the superior mesenteric artery. This is a "replacing" aberrant artery.

D. A left hepatic artery arises from the superior mesenteric artery. This is a "replacing" aberrant artery.

E. An aberrant left "replacing" hepatic artery arises from the gastroduodenal artery.

Remember:

The blood supply to the liver is unpredictable. An arteriogram prior to surgery is a great comfort.

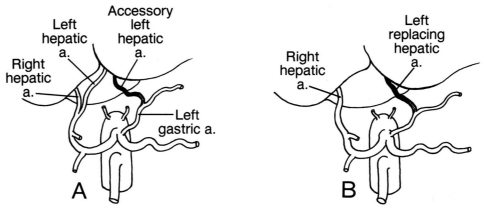

A. *Accessory* left hepatic artery (shaded) from the left gastric artery.
B. *Replacing* left hepatic artery (shaded).

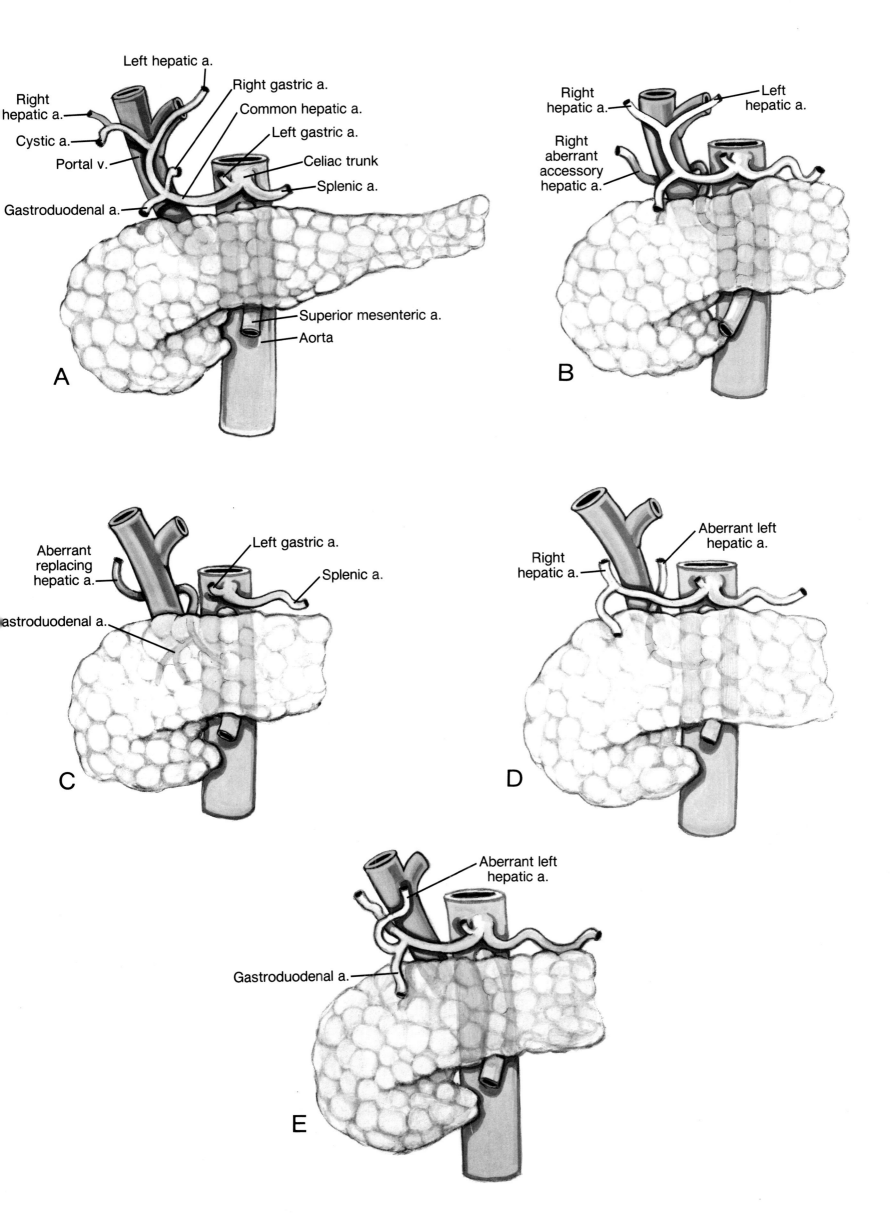

A

Left hepatic a.
Right hepatic a.
Cystic a.
Portal v.
Gastroduodenal a.
Right gastric a.
Common hepatic a.
Left gastric a.
Celiac trunk
Splenic a.
Superior mesenteric a.
Aorta

B

Right hepatic a.
Left hepatic a.
Right aberrant accessory hepatic a.

C

Aberrant replacing hepatic a.
Gastroduodenal a.
Left gastric a.
Splenic a.

D

Right hepatic a.
Aberrant left hepatic a.

E

Aberrant left hepatic a.
Gastroduodenal a.

PLATE 8-12
Portosystemic Shunts

A. The anatomy of the portal venous system. Portal blood enters the systemic circulation through the sinusoids of the liver and the hepatic veins. In addition, normal anastomoses between portal and systemic veins occur in several other locations in the body.

B to F. If venous flow through the hepatic sinusoids is impeded, portal venous pressure will rise and varices will form at these locations. Relief may be obtained by creating a portosystemic shunt.

Table: Sites of Normal Portosystemic Anastomoses

Region	Hepatic Portal Veins	Systemic Veins
Umbilical	Veins of falciform ligament	Epigastric veins
Lower esophagus	Gastric and esophageal veins	Hemiazygos vein
Bare area of liver	Veins of liver	Phrenic veins
Abdomen, posterior to hepatic flexure of colon	Veins of peritoneum and colon	Tributaries of renal veins
Rectum	Superior rectal vein	Middle and inferior rectal veins

Remember:

Portal vein obstruction permits more blood to pass from portal to systemic veins at the normal anastomoses.

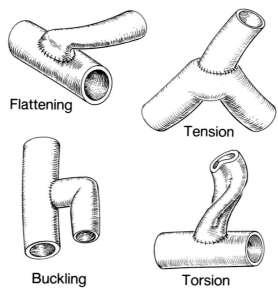

Flattening

Tension

Buckling

Torsion

Possible vascular deformities resulting from incorrectly constructed shunts.

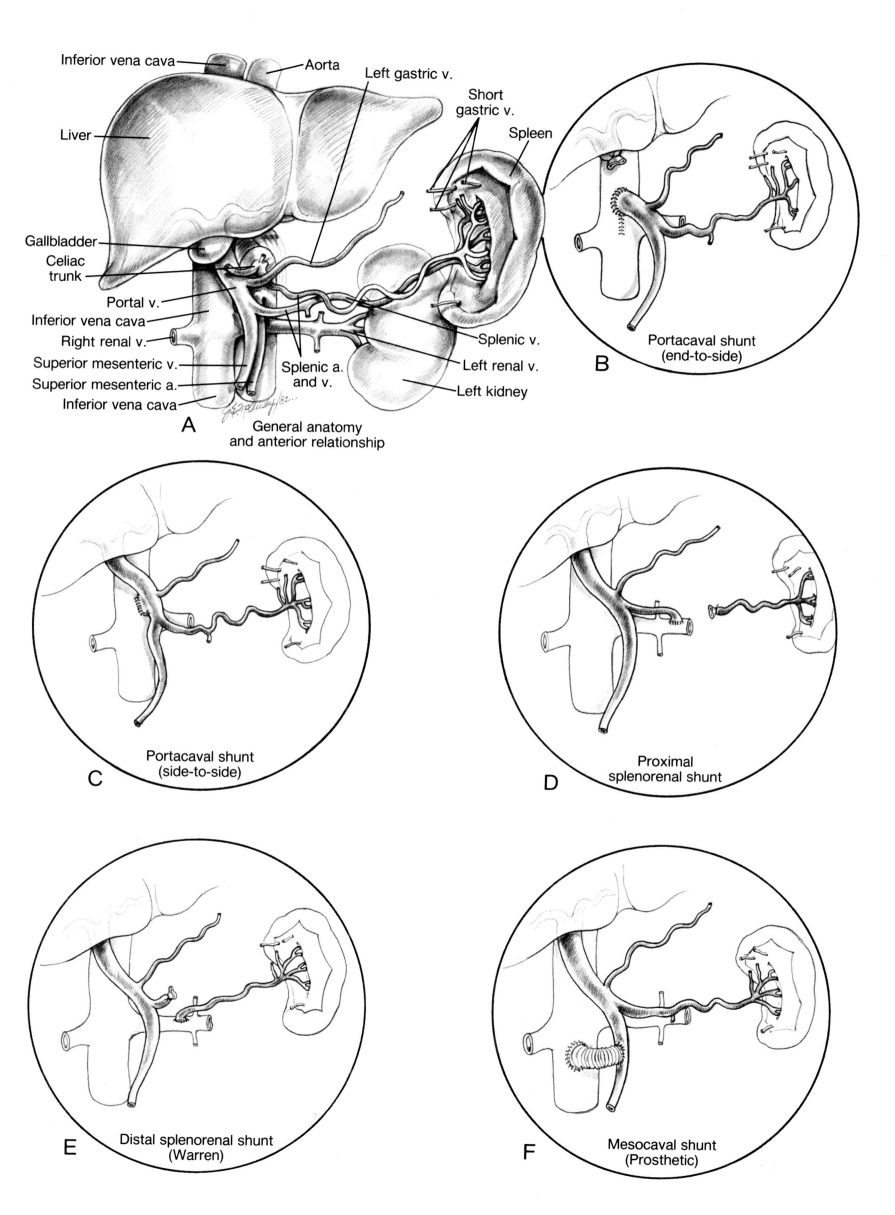

Inferior vena cava — Aorta

Left gastric v.

Short gastric v.

Spleen

Liver

Gallbladder

Celiac trunk

Portal v.

Inferior vena cava

Right renal v.

Superior mesenteric v.

Superior mesenteric a.

Inferior vena cava

Splenic a. and v.

Splenic v.

Left renal v.

Left kidney

A General anatomy and anterior relationship

B Portacaval shunt (end-to-side)

C Portacaval shunt (side-to-side)

D Proximal splenorenal shunt

E Distal splenorenal shunt (Warren)

F Mesocaval shunt (Prosthetic)

PLATE 9-1
Rotation of the Intestines I

A. The intestines grow in length faster than the embryonic body so that the midgut buckles ventrally through the umbilical ring into the extraembryonic celom of the umbilical cord during the 6th week. At the apex of the herniated loop is the attachment of the vitelline duct served by the vitelline artery, the proximal portion of which will become the superior mesenteric artery.

B. The initial twist is 90 degrees counterclockwise, bringing the cranial limb of the gut to the right of the caudal limb. Continued elongation of the cranial limb forms some six intestinal loops, whereas the caudal limb, the future colon, remains shorter and straighter. The cecum is indicated by a small swelling a short distance caudal to the site of the vitelline duct.

C. In the 10th week, the herniated intestines return, rather suddenly, to the abdominal cavity, undergoing a further 180 degree counterclockwise rotation.

D. The long cranial limb returns first, passing under the superior mesenteric artery. The shorter caudal limb returns last, the distal part lying in front of the superior mesenteric artery.

E. The cecum, at birth, is under the liver. Subsequent postnatal growth will bring it down into the right lower quadrant.

Table: Synopsis of Anomalies of Intestinal Rotation

Condition	Incidence	Symptoms
Nonrotation	Common; more frequent in males	Asymptomatic, or may result in volvulus
Mixed rotation	Common	Volvulus often present in first few days of life; twisted barium column in duodenum; signs of duodenal obstruction
Reversed rotation	Rare; more frequent in males	Ileocecal volvulus eventually develops; attacks become progressive
Hyperrotation	Rare	Asymptomatic

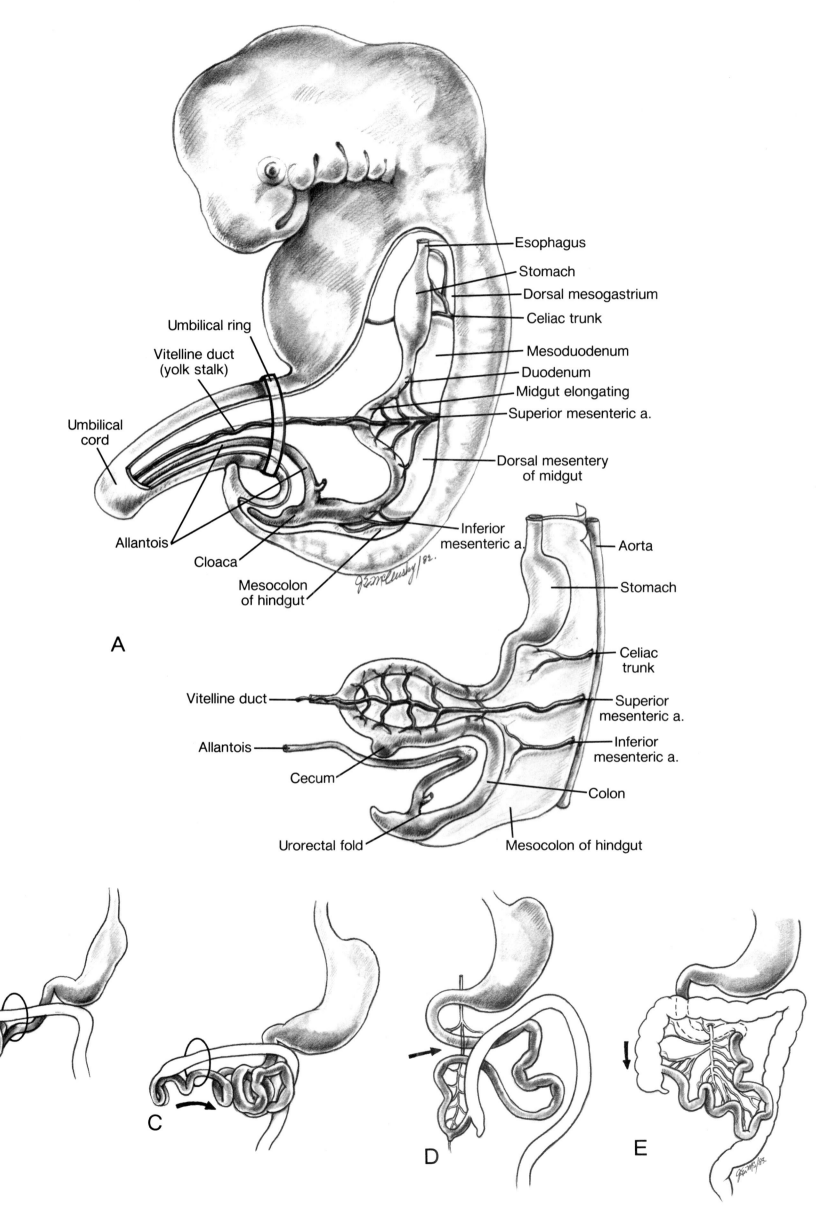

Esophagus

Stomach

Dorsal mesogastrium

Celiac trunk

Mesoduodenum

Duodenum

Midgut elongating

Superior mesenteric a.

Dorsal mesentery
of midgut

Umbilical ring

Vitelline duct
(yolk stalk)

Umbilical
cord

Allantois

Cloaca

Mesocolon
of hindgut

Inferior
mesenteric a.

A

Aorta

Stomach

Celiac
trunk

Superior
mesenteric a.

Inferior
mesenteric a.

Colon

Mesocolon of hindgut

Vitelline duct

Allantois

Cecum

Urorectal fold

B

C

D

E

PLATE 9-2
Rotation of the Intestines II

The last stage of intestinal development is fixation of the ascending, transverse and descending colon. There are varying degrees of fixation of the ascending and descending colon.

A. The right colon may be completely retroperitoneal, filling the right paracolic gutter and covered by peritoneum containing branches of the second lumbar artery (Jackson's veil). This covering predisposes to obstruction.

B. The term "mobile cecum" describes a right colon with a mesentery. Such a mesentery predisposes to volvulus of the colon. A similar situation may exist on the left. About one third of subjects have at least a partial mesentery of the right or left colon.

C. The sigmoid mesocolon remains unfixed to the posterior abdominal wall; the left ureter passes through its base.

Table: Synopsis of Anomalies of Cecum

Condition	Incidence	Symptoms
Undescended subhepatic cecum	Common; more frequent in males	Asymptomatic
Inverted cecum	Rare	Asymptomatic
Mobile cecum	Common; more frequent in males	Volvulus of cecum; recurrent right lower quadrant attacks; barium enema fails to fill ascending colon Volvulus of small intestine; recurrent lower or left lower quadrant attacks since childhood, hypertrophy of jejunum; variation in position of cecum
Anomalous fixation of cecum	Rare; sexes equally affected	Volvulus of small intestine; cecum constantly on left; barium meal may show duodenal dilatation and gastric retention; intermittent attacks
Retroperitoneal cecum	Common	Asymptomatic

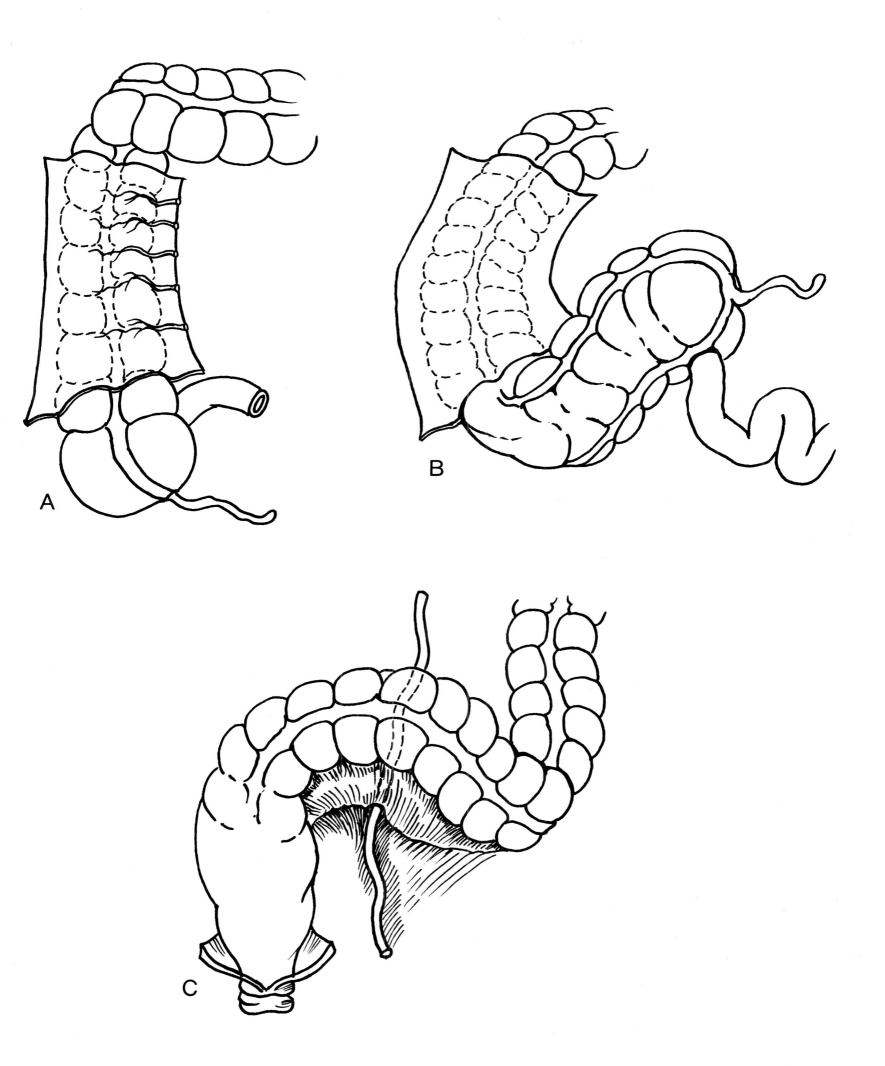

PLATE 9-3
Meckel's Diverticulum I

Meckel's diverticulum is a persistent portion of the embryonic yolk stalk (vitelline duct). It is present in about 2% of the population.

Most Meckel's diverticula (44%) arise from the ileum between 46 and 91 cm from the ileocecal valve (blue area). Not less than 5 feet of ileum should be examined in order not to miss a diverticulum.

Most diverticula are about 2 cm in diameter. Seventy-five percent will be from 1 to 5 cm long; the remainder will be longer. They always are antimesenteric and are supplied with blood from an extension of the superior mesenteric artery.

Remember:

1) Meckel's diverticulum occurs equally in males and females. Obstructing Meckel's diverticulum disease (usually intussusception) is more frequent in males.

2) Although 85% of intussusceptions in children are idiopathic, almost all intussusceptions caused by Meckel's diverticula occur in male children.

3) Ulceration of the diverticulum or adjacent ileum results from the presence of acid secreting parietal cells.

Meckel's Diverticulum Disease

Symptoms	Percent	Onset of Symptoms
1. Ulcerating	40	Infancy or childhood
2. Obstruction	32	Any age, but usually childhood
3. Inflammatory	17	Infancy or childhood
4. Umbilical	5	First few weeks of life
5. Neoplastic	6	Middle life

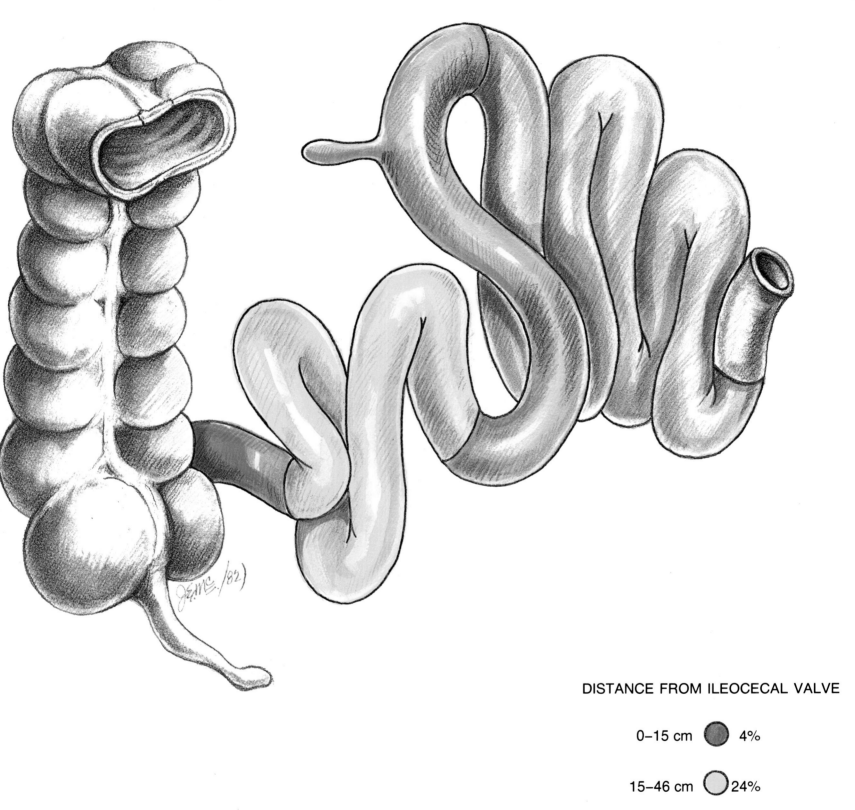

DISTANCE FROM ILEOCECAL VALVE

0–15 cm ⬤ 4%

15–46 cm ◯ 24%

46–91 cm ⬤ 44%

91–16.7 cm ⬤ 28%

PLATE 9-4
Meckel's Diverticulum II

A. Blind ending diverticulum, not attached to the anterior body wall.

B. Blind ending diverticulum, attached to the anterior body wall.

C. Omphaloileal fistula (patent Meckel's diverticulum).

D. The relation of the superior mesenteric artery to Meckel's diverticulum.

E. Vitelline cyst resulting from an unclosed midportion of the vitelline duct.

F–I. Stages of the prolapse of the ileum through an omphaloileal fistula. The mucosal surface presents at the umbilicus. This must not be confused with a diverticulum at the umbilicus (umbilical polyp); ligation could be catastrophic.

Remember:

A above is the most common form; Types A and B account for 82 to 96% of all Meckelian lesions.

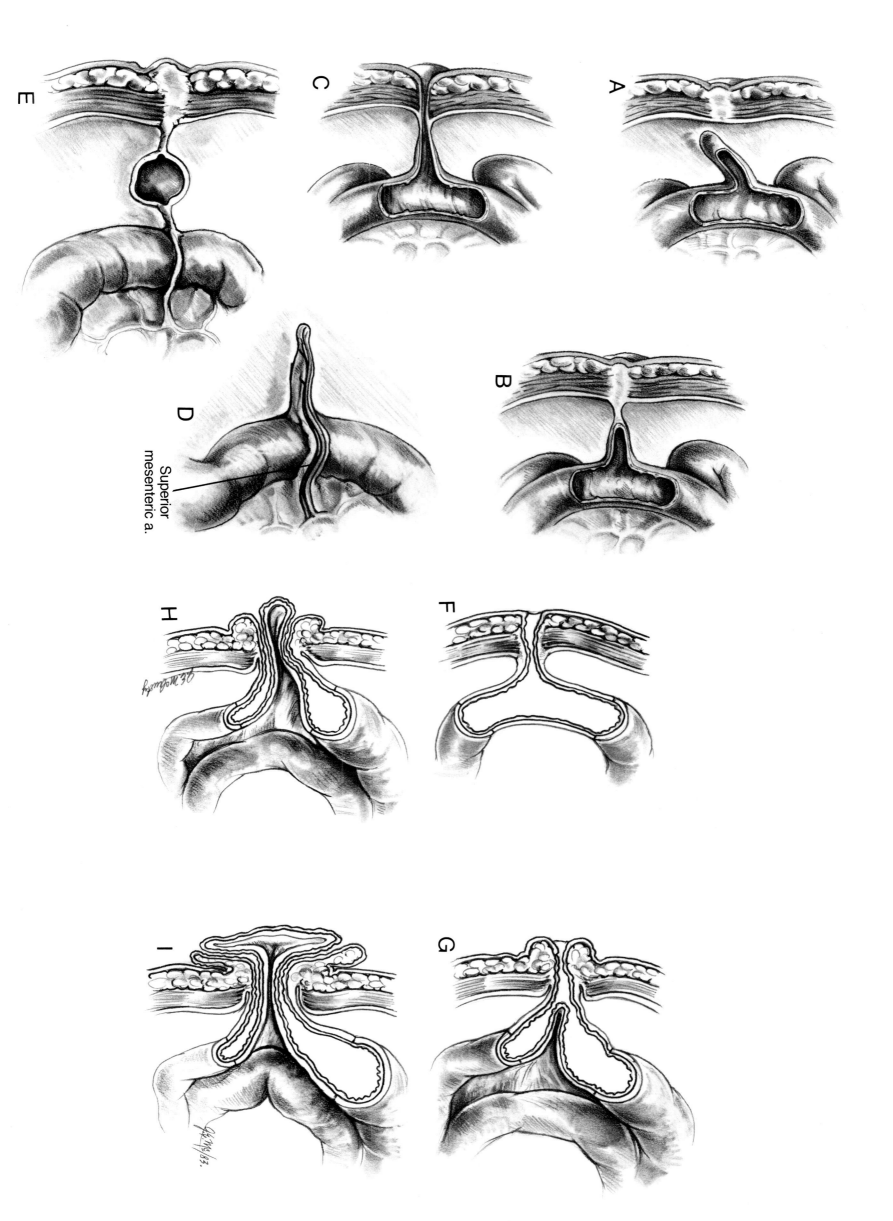

Superior
mesenteric a.

PLATE 9-5
Intestinal Obstructions

Three common causes of intestinal obstructions in infants and children are atresia or stenosis, congenital megacolon and intussusception. Atresias may occur in any portion of the small and large intestine; duodenum and ileum are more often affected than are jejunum and colon. In the duodenum, types A and B atresias predominate; in the ileum, types B and C are most frequent.

A. Membranous atresia from a mucosal diaphragm. The membrane may perforate and produce a stenosis with symptoms of chronic obstruction (type A).

B. Segmental atresia. A short segment of intestine is represented by a solid cord in the edge of the mesentery (type B).

C. Segmental atresia. A segment of intestine and mesentery is completely absent (type C).

D. Congenital megacolon (Hirschsprung's disease). The defect is the absence of myenteric ganglia, resulting in failure of peristalsis of the affected segment. The line of resection (broken line) must be through normally innervated but distended colon proximal to the narrowed, aganglionic segment. In 55% of patients the rectum and sigmoid colon only are affected. Very rarely, the entire colon is without ganglion cells.

E. Intussusception. The proximal intestinal segment (the intussusceptum) herniates into the intestinal segment just distal to it (the intussuscipiens) to form an intussusception. Meckel's diverticulum, polyps and stenoses may form the leading point of the intussusceptum, but 85% of cases in children are idiopathic, and about 85% of cases in adults are mechanical: polyps, cancer, endometriosis etc.

Inset: End-to-end anastomosis of resected intestine is the best. The small caliber of the distal segment may make end-to-side or side-to-side anastomoses necessary, but they increase the lines of potential leakage and the risk of the blind loop syndrome. A diagonal cut end of the smaller limb may make an end-to-end anastomosis feasible.

Remember:

1) As many of 25% of infants with segmental atresia may have one or more similar atresias distal to the first and obvious one.

2) Colonic aganglionosis must be confirmed by biopsy. Colonic distention may be caused by anal stenosis or atresia, afferent autonomic dysfunction (Riley's disease) or dysfunction associated with cretinism or mental retardation.

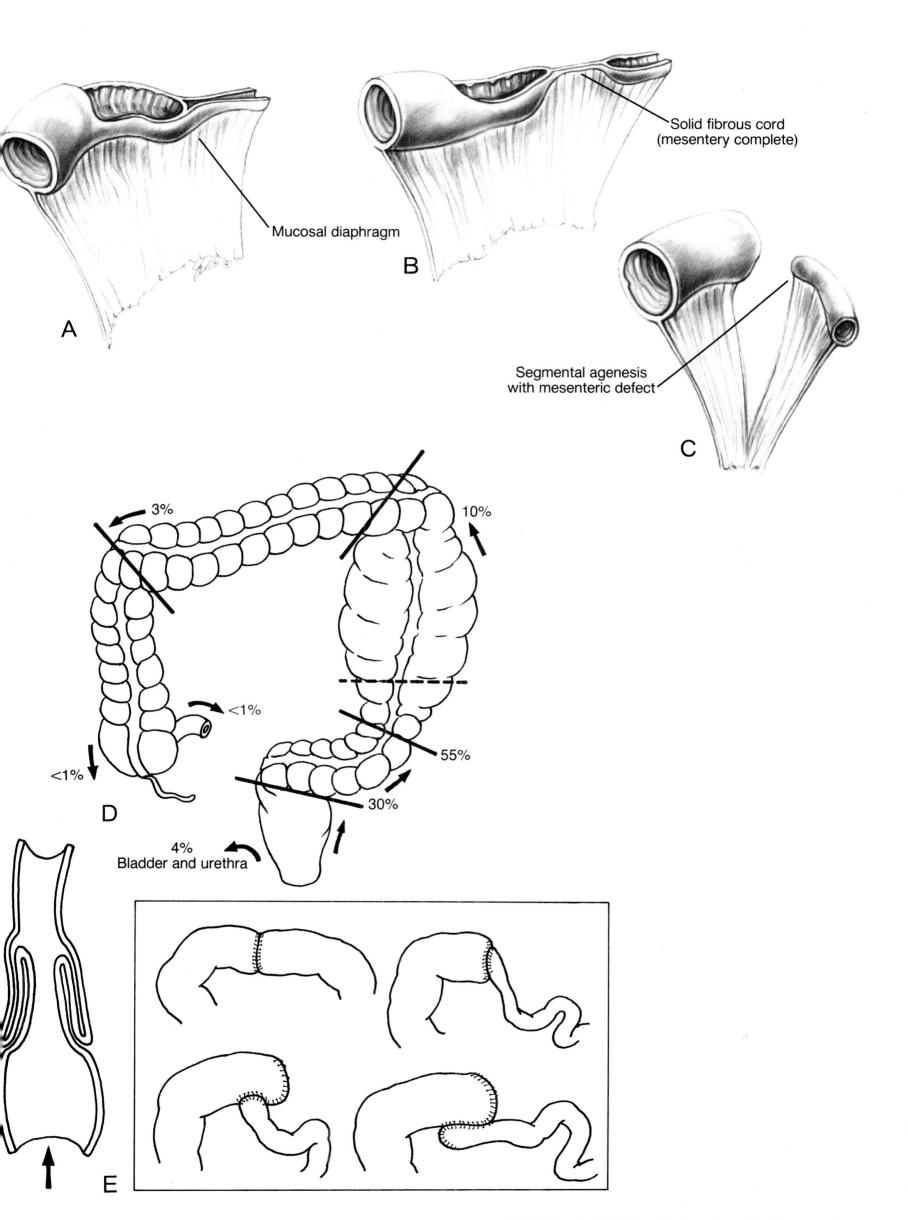

Mucosal diaphragm

A

B

Solid fibrous cord
(mesentery complete)

Segmental agenesis
with mesenteric defect

C

3%

10%

<1%

<1%

55%

30%

4%
Bladder and urethra

D

E

PLATE 9-6
Blood Supply to the Small Intestine

The vasa recta of the jejunum are long, whereas those of the ileum are shorter. They distribute vessels to both sides of the intestine (A), or to one side only (B, C). In the latter case, they pass to left or right alternately. They may supply the mesenteric side with a specific short vessel (C). There is no collateral circulation between the vasa recta or their branches at the surface of the intestine. After entering the intestinal wall the arteries form a small muscular plexus and a large submucosal plexus.

Remember:

1) The mesenteric side has a good blood supply; the antimesenteric side has a poorer blood supply.

2) The intestines elongate at least 100% after death. Measure the portion to be resected before resecting it. The length remaining is more important than the length resected. Record its length.

3) Resection of ileum is less well tolerated than resection of jejunum; it decreases vitamin B_{12}, D and potassium absorption and may increase the incidence of gall and kidney stones.

4) Try to spare the ileocecal valve if possible.

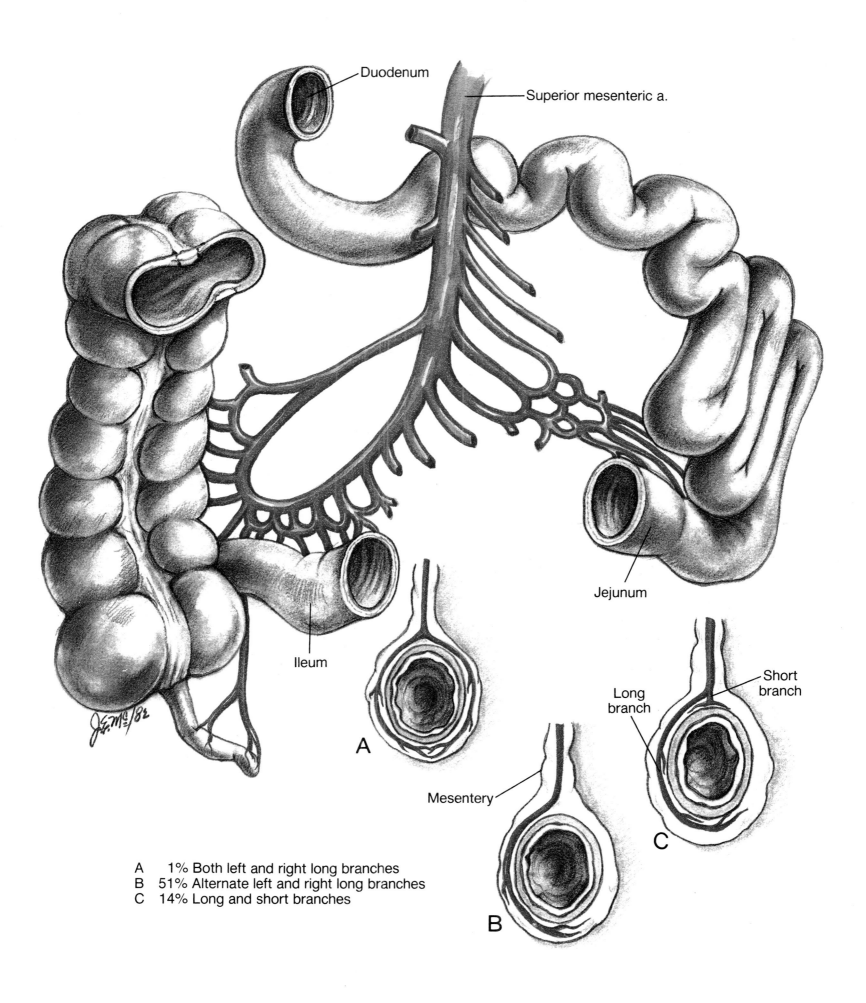

Duodenum

Superior mesenteric a.

Jejunum

Ileum

A

B

Mesentery

Long branch

Short branch

C

A 1% Both left and right long branches
B 51% Alternate left and right long branches
C 14% Long and short branches

PLATE 9-7
The Colon *in Situ*

A. The relations of the stomach, liver and pancreas to the transverse colon. The omentum shown is unusually short.

B. The peritoneal reflections of the transverse colon.

Remember:

1) Good surgery of the colon depends on three anatomical principles; a) Good mobilization; b) Protection of ureters, pancreas, duodenum, spleen and gonadal vessels; c) Good knowledge of the lymphatic drainage.

2) Before any colonic anastomosis, observe the colon for bleeding and arterial pulsation. If the viability is in doubt, resect even more. If there is any question of tension at the anastomosis, perform a proximal colostomy.

3) It is easier to mobilize the right colon than the left colon. On the left, phrenocolic ligament must be divided to free the splenic flexure. There is no such ligament on the right. Be gentle with the spleen.

4) The adult colon is separated from the kidney by abundant perinephric fat. In children there is no such fat.

5) Try not to resect any appendices epiploicae because their bases are close to the arteries of the colon wall. If they must be resected, ligate them without traction.

6) If the caliber of the distal colon is small, it may be increased by a small longitudinal incision at the antimesenteric border or by an oblique section of the distal limb.

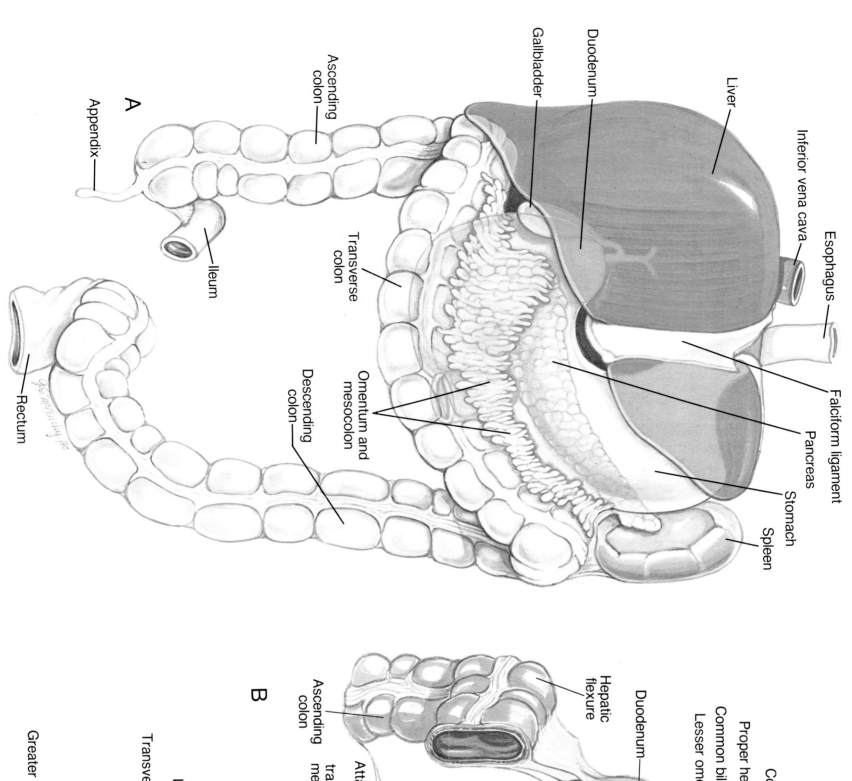

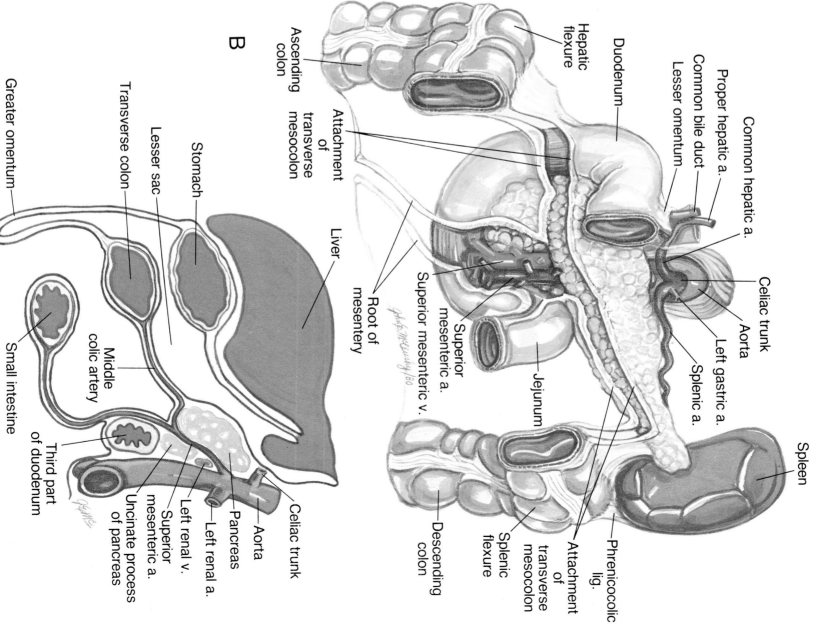

PLATE 9-8
Blood Supply to the Colon I

The arcades from the superior mesenteric artery on the right, and the inferior mesenteric artery on the left, form the marginal artery (of Drummond) from which arise the vasa recta.

Inset: The "long" vasa recta supply the epiploic appendices and the antimesenteric colon wall. "Short" branches of the vasa recta supply the mesenteric colon wall in most, but not all, vascular segments. Too much traction on epiploic appendages before ligation may injure the blood supply to the antimesenteric side of the colon.

Remember:

1) The blood supply of the antimesenteric border is poor. Try to preserve as many long branches of the vasa recta at the mesenteric border as possible. This can be done by an oblique incision.

2) Protect the blood supply of the remaining omentum so that when it is used to cap the anastomosis it is healthy, without infarcts or fat necrosis.

3) Sudeck's "critical point," above the origin of the last sigmoid artery, is no longer considered critical. The middle and inferior rectal arteries and the submucosal plexus are sufficient.

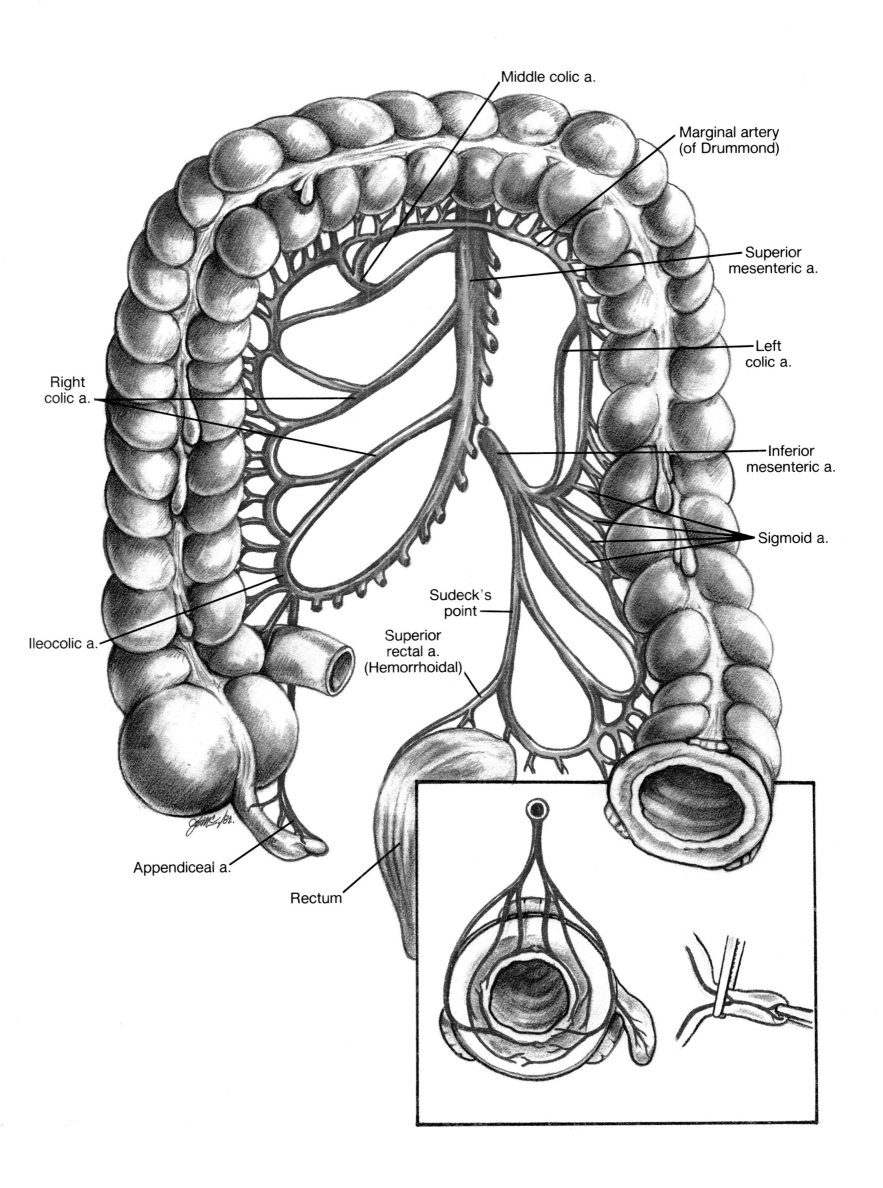

Middle colic a.

Marginal artery
(of Drummond)

Superior
mesenteric a.

Left
colic a.

Right
colic a.

Inferior
mesenteric a.

Sigmoid a.

Sudeck's
point

Ileocolic a.

Superior
rectal a.
(Hemorrhoidal)

Appendiceal a.

Rectum

PLATE 9-9
Blood Supply to the Colon II

A. The marginal artery is incomplete (at arrow).

B. The middle colic artery arises directly from the superior mesenteric artery. All of these arteries are variable.

Remember:

1) In cancer of the right colon, ligate the ileocolic and right colic arteries as high as possible.

2) In cancer of the transverse colon, ligate the middle colic artery as high as possible.

3) In cancer of the left colon, ligate the left colic artery at its origin.

4) In cancer of the sigmoid colon and rectum, ligate the inferior mesenteric artery at its origin. Keep in mind that the origin is covered by the third part of the duodenum. Do not injure the duodenum.

5) An adequate stoma with a good blood supply to both proximal and distal limbs is essential for any anastomosis.

6) Avoid torsion and tension at the anastomosis.

7) Avoid hematomas at the anastomotic site.

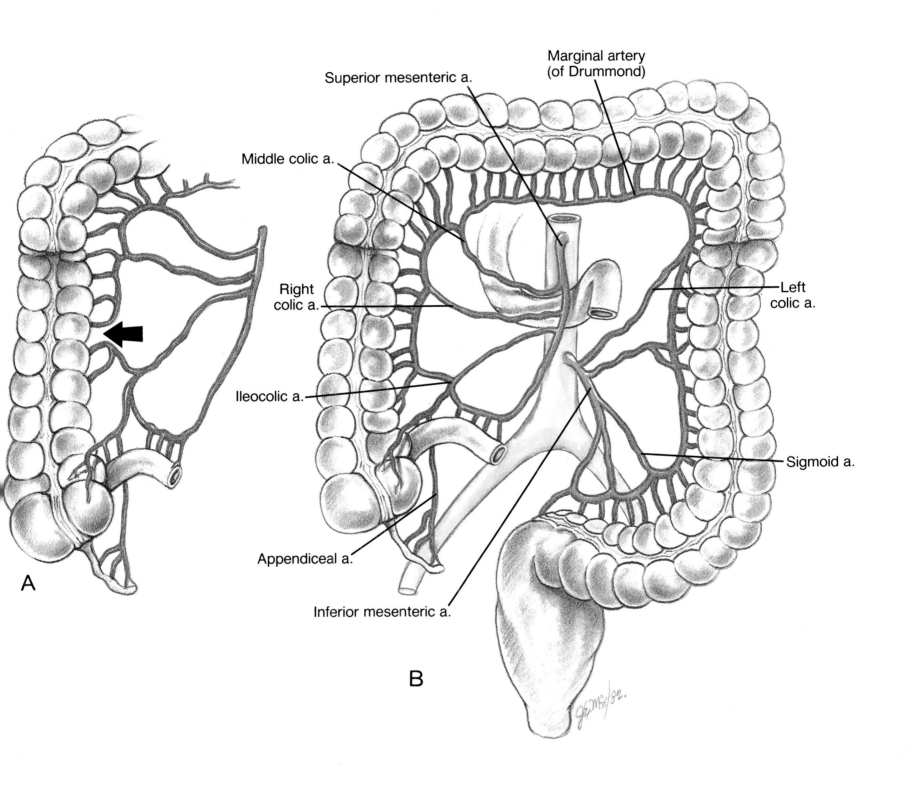

Superior mesenteric a.

Marginal artery
(of Drummond)

Middle colic a.

Right
colic a.

Left
colic a.

Ileocolic a.

Sigmoid a.

Appendiceal a.

Inferior mesenteric a.

A

B

PLATE 9-10
Lymph Nodes and Lymphatics of the Colon

A. Lymph nodes of the colon are (1) epicolic, beneath the colonic serosa, (2) paracolic, along the marginal artery, (3) intermediate, along the large arteries, and (4) principal, at the origins of the superior and inferior mesenteric arteries. There is an increase in the number of nodes from proximal to distal.

B. Diagram of the pathways of spread of primary carcinoma of the colon. Metastasis may be by veins, lymphatics or peritoneal seeding. The relative frequency is indicated by the breadth of the arrow.

Remember:

Occasionally, nodes from an inflamed appendix may drain to duodenal nodes producing upper abdominal discomfort.

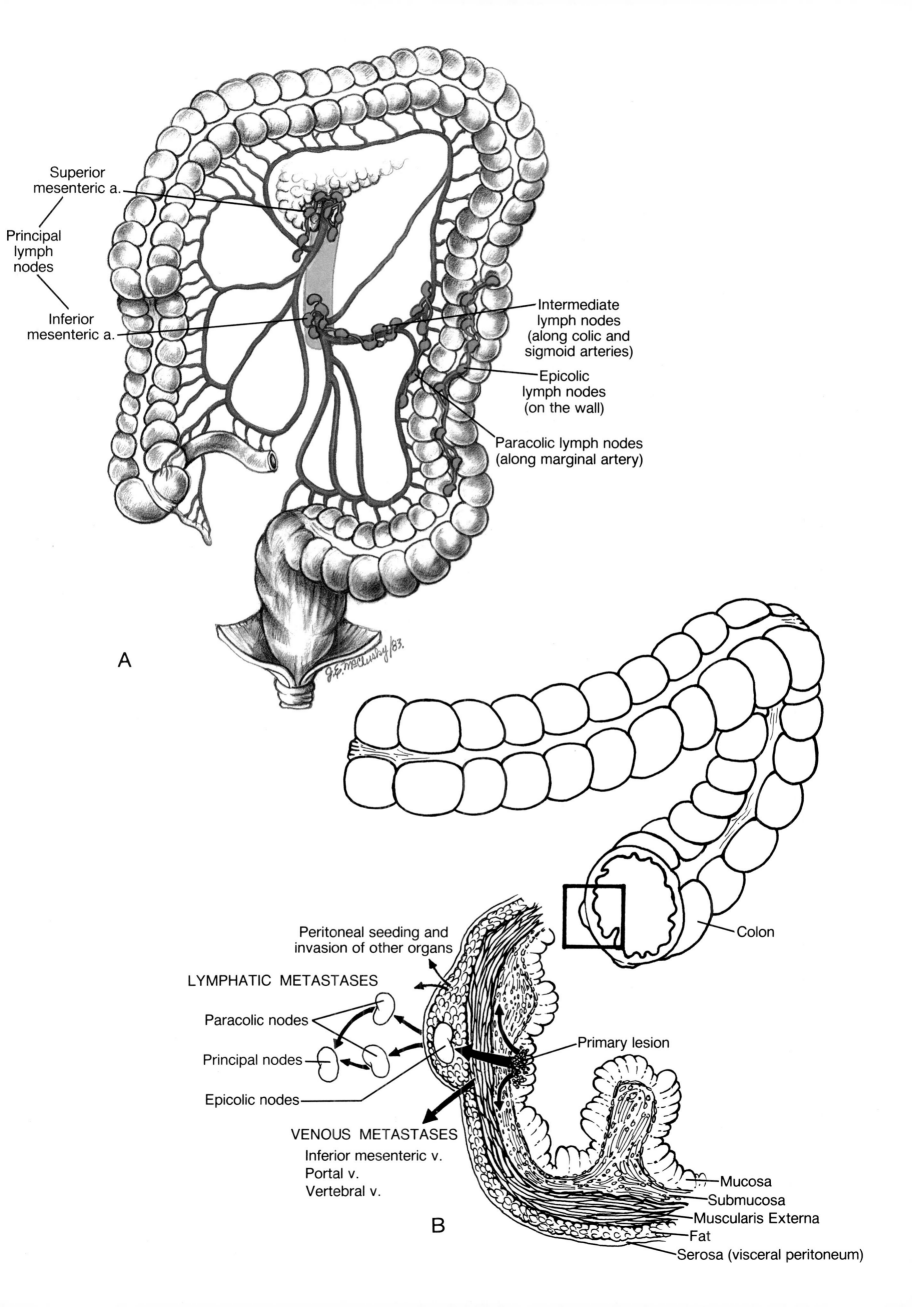

Superior
mesenteric a.

Principal
lymph
nodes

Inferior
mesenteric a.

Intermediate
lymph nodes
(along colic and
sigmoid arteries)

Epicolic
lymph nodes
(on the wall)

Paracolic lymph nodes
(along marginal artery)

J.E. McClusky/83.

A

Colon

Peritoneal seeding and
invasion of other organs

LYMPHATIC METASTASES

Paracolic nodes

Principal nodes

Epicolic nodes

Primary lesion

VENOUS METASTASES
Inferior mesenteric v.
Portal v.
Vertebral v.

Mucosa
Submucosa
Muscularis Externa
Fat
Serosa (visceral peritoneum)

B

PLATE 9-11
Three Types of Cecum and Appendix

A and B. "Infantile" types. The cecum and appendix are symmetrical.

C. "Adult" type. The appendix arises lateral to the tip of the cecum. The first cecal haustrum on the right (lateral) is larger than that on the left (medial).

Remember:

1) Absence of the appendix is very rare.

2) If more than four haustra are present, the last one may represent the appendix.

3) With an appendix on the left, the surgeon must distinguish situs inversus from malrotation of the intestine.

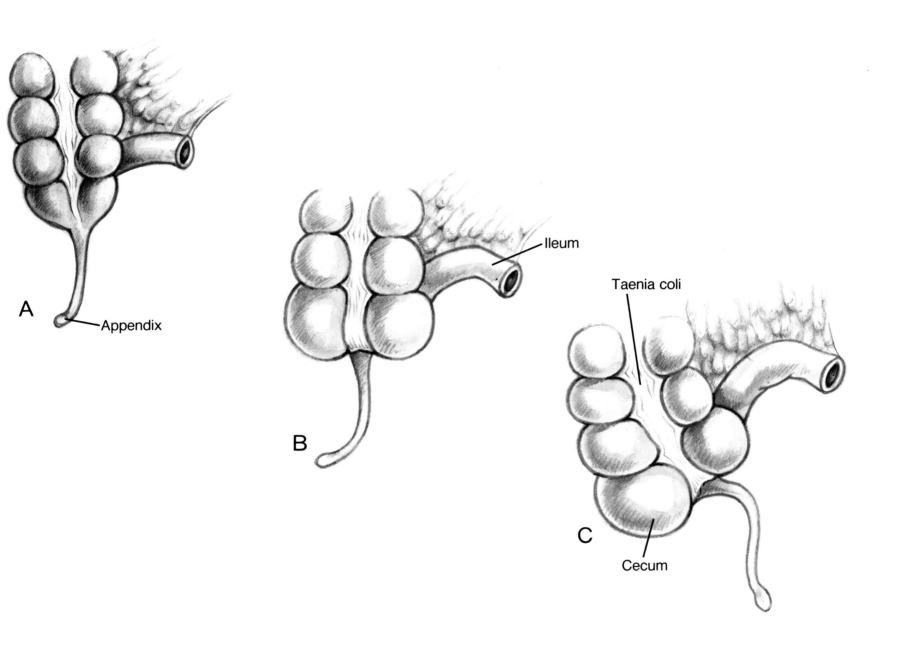

A

Appendix

B

Ileum

Taenia coli

C

Cecum

PLATE 9-12
Possible Positions of the Appendix

A. Directed upward, retrocecal and retrocolic

B. Directed downward into the pelvis.

C. Directed downward to the right beneath the cecum.

D. Directed downward to the left, anterior or posterior to the ileum;
   A and B are the most common locations.

E and *Inset*. The appendix in relation to the abdominal wall (McBurney's point). The "point" lies one third of the distance along a line from the iliac crest to the umbilicus.

Remember:

1) The appendix is a gypsy. If you can't find it, enlarge the incision and look for it. It may be (a) fixed with the cecum and covered with adhesions, (b) retrocecal, (c) fixed with the ileocecal mesentery, (d) scrotal or (e) intussuscepted.

2) To find the appendix, find the cecum. A taenia leads to the base of the appendix. A plain x-ray film will help. Malrotation (cecum on the left), undescended (subhepatic) cecum and mobile cecum are all possible.

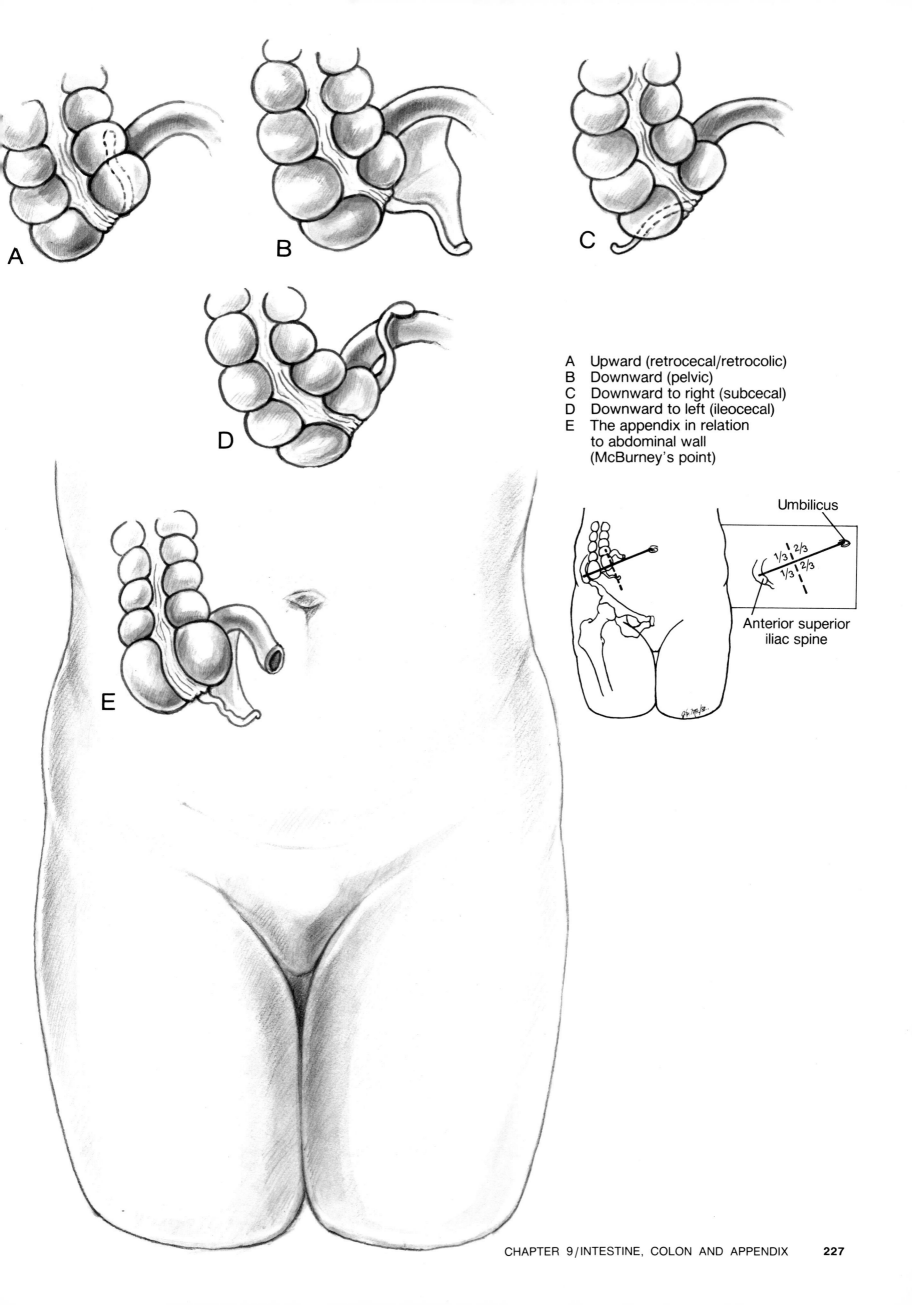

A   Upward (retrocecal/retrocolic)
B   Downward (pelvic)
C   Downward to right (subcecal)
D   Downward to left (ileocecal)
E   The appendix in relation
    to abdominal wall
    (McBurney's point)

Umbilicus

1/3 2/3
1/3 2/3

Anterior superior
iliac spine

PLATE 9-13
The Blood Supply to the Appendix

A. A single appendiceal artery arises from an ileal arcade of the superior mesenteric artery (marginal artery).

B. A single appendiceal artery arises high on the ileocolic artery.

C. Double appendiceal arteries. The two arteries may have different origins.

Remember:

1) With a short appendiceal mesentery, the appendiceal artery is short.

2) Be careful bringing the appendix up to avoid rupture of the mesentery and consequent bleeding. If possible, ligate *in situ*.

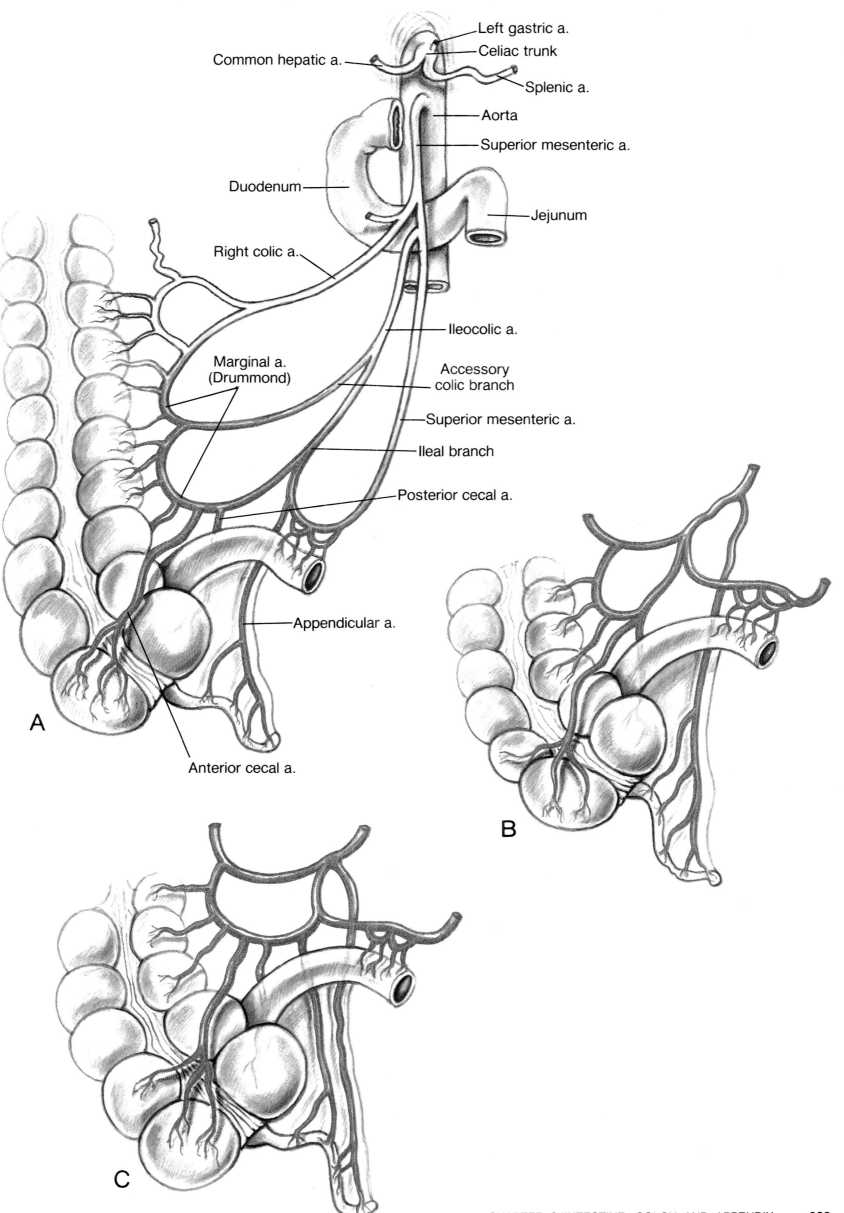

Left gastric a.

Celiac trunk

Common hepatic a.

Splenic a.

Aorta

Superior mesenteric a.

Duodenum

Jejunum

Right colic a.

Ileocolic a.

Accessory
colic branch

Marginal a.
(Drummond)

Superior mesenteric a.

Ileal branch

Posterior cecal a.

Appendicular a.

A

Anterior cecal a.

B

C

PLATE 9-14
Lymphatic Nodes and Lymphatic Drainage of the Appendix

A. General lymphatics of the appendix.

B. Diagram of the lymphatic drainage of the appendix.

Remember:

1) Primary drainage is to ileocolic lymph nodes.

2) Secondary drainage is to subpyloric lymph nodes anterior to the pancreas.

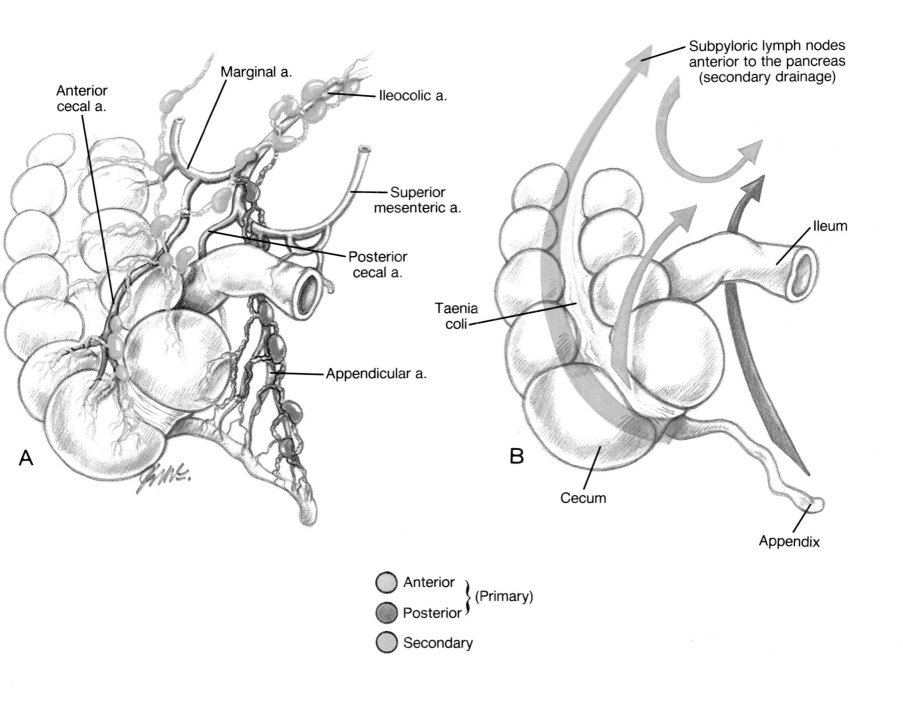

Anterior cecal a.

Marginal a.

Ileocolic a.

Superior mesenteric a.

Posterior cecal a.

Appendicular a.

A

Subpyloric lymph nodes anterior to the pancreas (secondary drainage)

Ileum

Taenia coli

B

Cecum

Appendix

○ Anterior } (Primary)
● Posterior
○ Secondary

PLATE 10-1
Formation of the Anus and Rectum

A. The embryonic cloaca at about the 5th week of gestation. The cloacal membrane (proctodeum) is intact, the tail and the tailgut are well developed.

B. Partitioning of the cloaca in the 6th week. A septum of mesoderm grows caudally, dividing the cloaca into a ventral urogenital sinus and a dorsal anal portion.

C. Partitioning is complete early in the 8th week. The cloacal membrane is divided into urogenital and anal membranes. The tailgut has disappeared; the ureters are present, and the bladder is indicated by a dilatation.

D. By the beginning of the 3rd month, the embryonic tail has been resorbed; the anal membrane has ruptured and the anus is in its definitive position. The bladder has not descended and the urachus is short.

Remember:

1) The rectum is derived from hindgut endoderm. The anus originates from ectoderm. The boundary is at the pectinate line in the adult (see also Plate 10-9).

2) The rectum and bladder have the same nerve supply (pelvic splanchnic nerve and hypogastric plexus).

3) The muscle fibers of the external sphincter form at the normal site of the anus if it is absent.

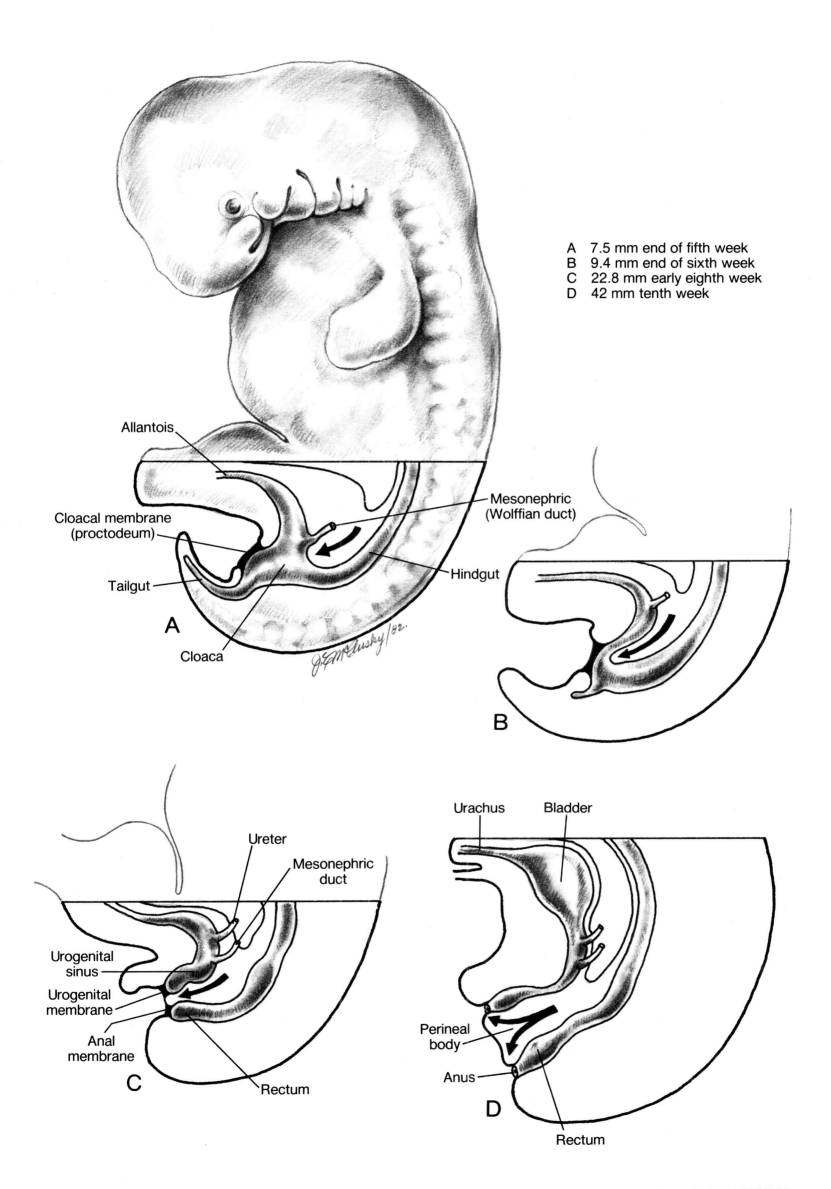

A   7.5 mm end of fifth week
B   9.4 mm end of sixth week
C   22.8 mm early eighth week
D   42 mm tenth week

Allantois

Mesonephric
(Wolffian duct)

Cloacal membrane
(proctodeum)

Hindgut

Tailgut

Cloaca

A

B

Ureter

Mesonephric
duct

Urogenital
sinus

Urogenital
membrane

Anal
membrane

Rectum

C

Urachus   Bladder

Perineal
body

Anus

Rectum

D

PLATE 10-2
Anomalies of the Anus and Rectum

A. Normal anatomy of anus and rectum in sagittal section.

B. Membranous atresia (low anal atresia, imperforate anus).

C. High rectal atresia without fistula.

D. Anal agenesis with fistula (low anal agenesis, anal ectopia).

E. Anorectal agenesis with fistula (high rectal atresia).

F. Anorectal agenesis without fistula in the female (high rectal atresia).

G. Anal stenosis at normal site.

H. Persistent cloaca. Common urethra, vagina and anal canal.

Portions of the external anal sphincter are almost always present even though the anus itself is absent.

Based on whether the rectum ends above or below the level of the puborectalis sling, the defects may be divided into: (1) anal or "low" defects (B, D, G); (2) anorectal or "high" defects (C, E, F); (3) cloacal defects (H).

Remember:

1) Most "imperforate" anus (78%) is anorectal agenesis (E) with fistula.

2) Fistulas are to vagina or uterus in females; to bladder in males.

3) About 80% of infants with anorectal defects (except anal stenosis) will have other severe defects. About 10% will have tracheoesophageal defects.

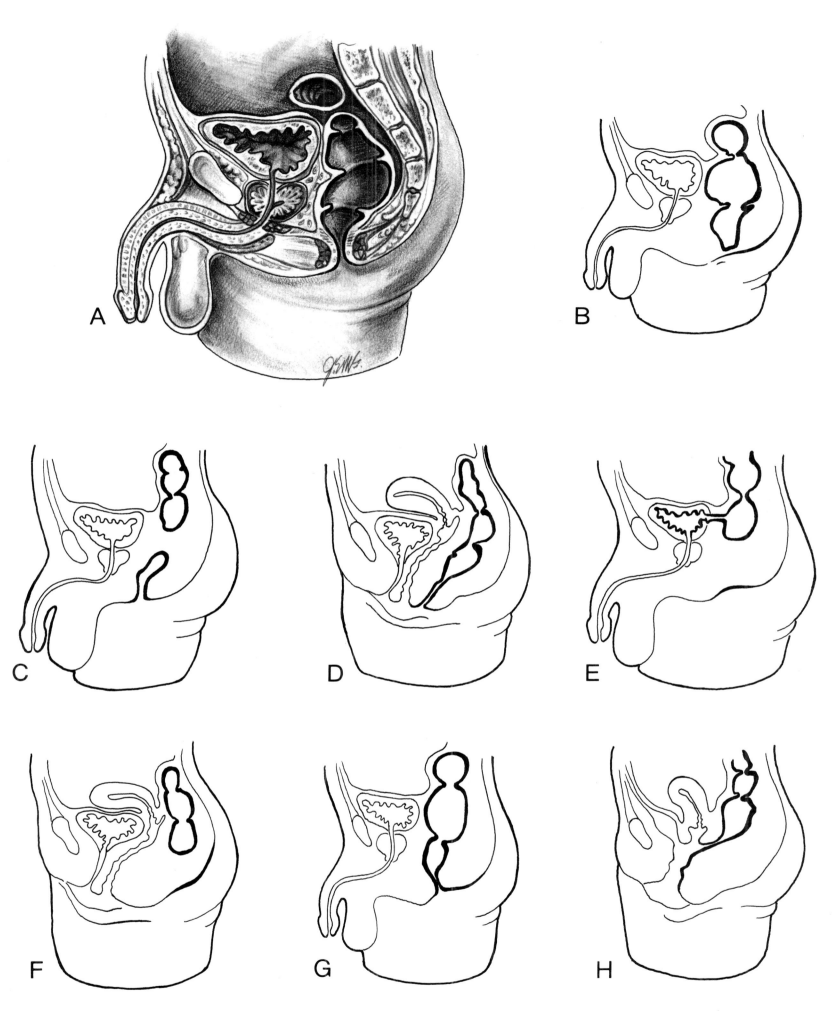

A. Normal anatomy in sagittal section
B. Membranous atresia (low anal atresia, imperforate anus)
C. High rectal atresia without fistula
D. Anal agenesis with fistula (low anal agenesis, anal ectopia)
E. Anorectal agenesis with fistula (high rectal atresia)
F. Anorectal agenesis without fistula in female (high rectal atresia)
G. Anal stenosis at normal site
H. Persistant cloaca, common urethra, vagina, and anal canal

PLATE 10-3
Coronal Section of Anus and Rectum

Both the inner circular and outer longitudinal smooth muscle coats of the colon become thickened as they reach the anal canal. They make up the involuntary internal anal sphincter.

The longitudinal layer, as described by Shafik, ends in a fibrous central tendon. Fibers from this tendon pierce the cutaneous portion of the external sphincter and attach to the skin to form the corrugator cutis ani.

The external sphincter is striated muscle of somatic rather than splanchnic origin. It is divided into deep, superficial and subcutaneous portions to form three slings around the rectum (see Plate 10-15).

Remember:

Anorectal support depends on: (a) anorectal sphincters; (b) anococcygeal body, (posterior); (c) perineal body, (anterior); (d) pelvic diaphragm.

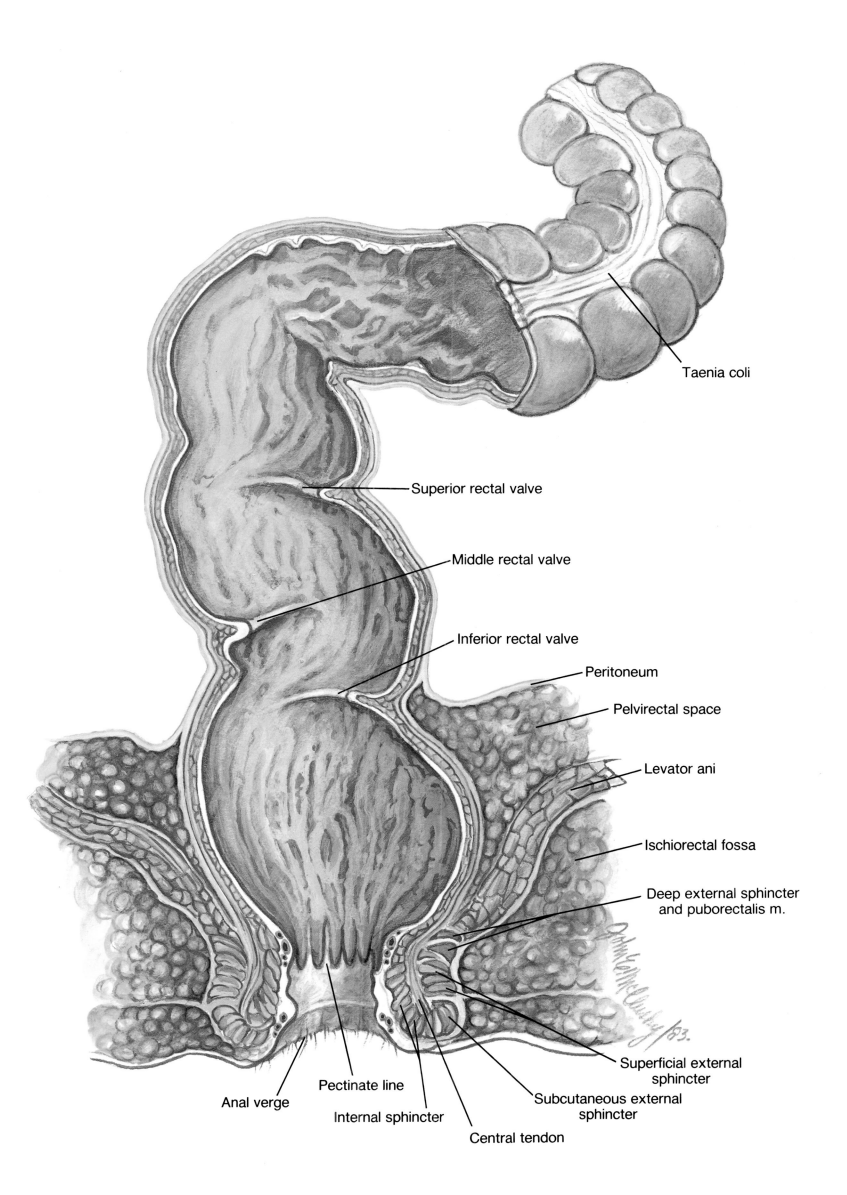

Taenia coli

Superior rectal valve

Middle rectal valve

Inferior rectal valve

Peritoneum

Pelvirectal space

Levator ani

Ischiorectal fossa

Deep external sphincter
and puborectalis m.

Superficial external
sphincter

Subcutaneous external
sphincter

Central tendon

Internal sphincter

Pectinate line

Anal verge

PLATE 10-4
The Surgical Anal Canal I

A. Coronal section through the anal canal showing the relations of the internal and external sphincters.

B. Coronal section through pelvis showing the spaces above and below the levator ani muscles.

Remember:

1) The striated external sphincter envelops the distal two thirds of the anal canal. In the middle one third, it overlaps the internal sphincter.

2) The smooth internal sphincter envelops the proximal two thirds of the anal canal.

3) The internal sphincter and the superficial portion of the external sphincter may be divided without loss of continence if the conjoined longitudinal muscle and the puborectalis muscle are intact.

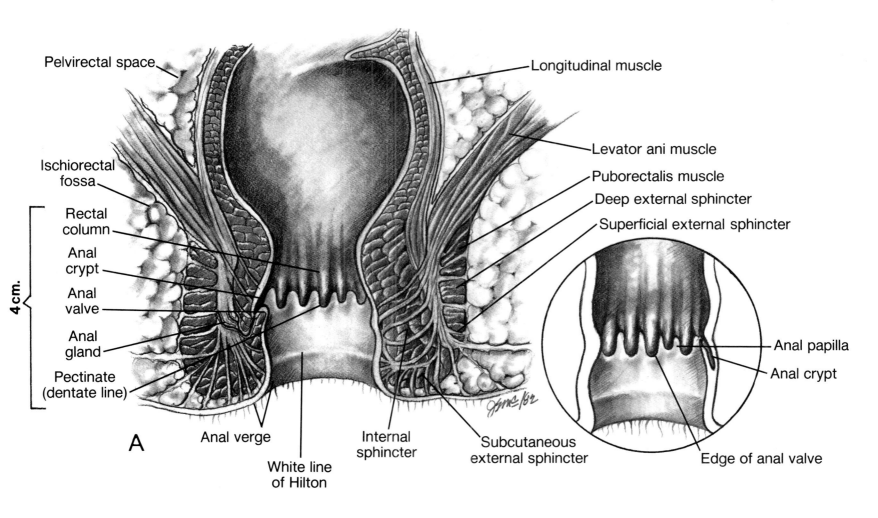

Pelvirectal space

Ischiorectal fossa

Rectal column

Anal crypt

Anal valve

Anal gland

Pectinate (dentate line)

4 cm.

Anal verge

White line of Hilton

Internal sphincter

Subcutaneous external sphincter

Longitudinal muscle

Levator ani muscle

Puborectalis muscle

Deep external sphincter

Superficial external sphincter

Anal papilla

Anal crypt

Edge of anal valve

A

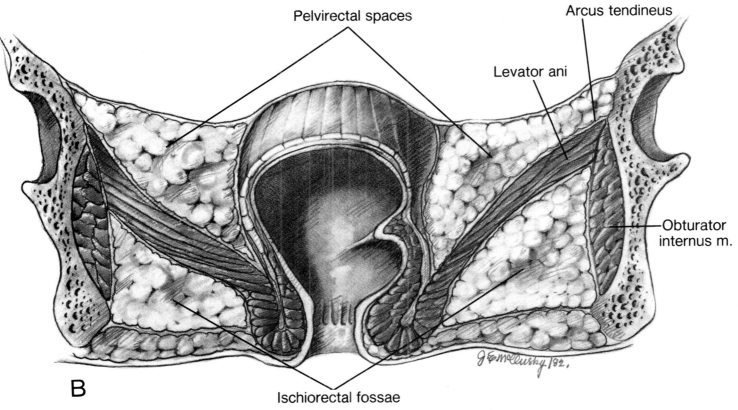

Pelvirectal spaces

Arcus tendineus

Levator ani

Obturator internus m.

Ischiorectal fossae

B

PLATE 10-5
The Surgical Anal Canal II

A. Coronal section through the anal canal with the sphincters relaxed.

   Inset: Engorged veins of the rectal plexus form hemorrhoids.

B. Conventional divisions of the rectum and anus.

   The lower rectum and the anal canal are not covered by peritoneum. The middle rectum is covered by peritoneum anteriorly only. Do not worry about a definite boundary between the sigmoid colon and the rectum.

Remember:

   1) In carcinoma of the lower rectum, about 8 cm above the anal verge, use an abdominoperineal resection or a sphincter saving procedure, performing an end-to-end anastomosis using the EEA stapling device.

   2) A curative resection of carcinoma of the rectosigmoid region must be 4 cm below the tumor to avoid any intramural extension.

   3) Avoid injury of the sphincteric mechanism.

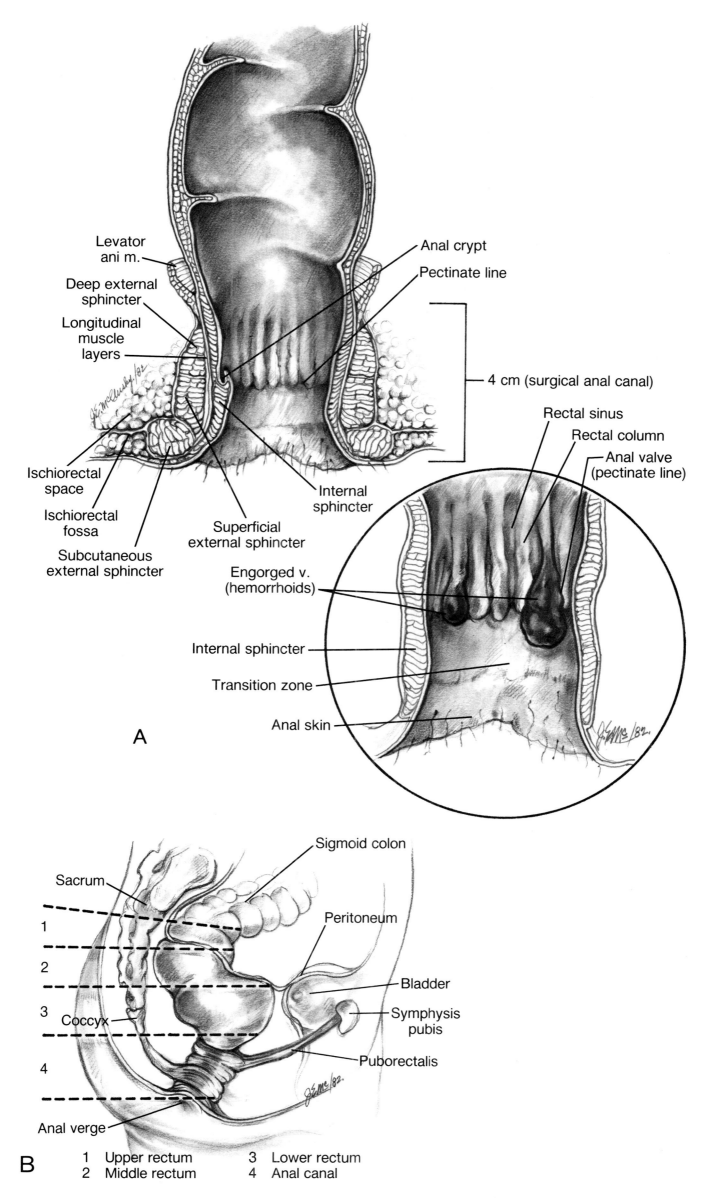

Levator
ani m.

Deep external
sphincter

Longitudinal
muscle
layers

Ischiorectal
space

Ischiorectal
fossa

Subcutaneous
external sphincter

Superficial
external sphincter

Internal
sphincter

Anal crypt

Pectinate line

4 cm (surgical anal canal)

Rectal sinus

Rectal column

Anal valve
(pectinate line)

Engorged v.
(hemorrhoids)

Internal sphincter

Transition zone

Anal skin

A

Sacrum

Sigmoid colon

Peritoneum

Bladder

Symphysis
pubis

Puborectalis

Coccyx

Anal verge

B

1	Upper rectum	3 Lower rectum
2	Middle rectum	4 Anal canal

PLATE 10-6
The Blood Supply to the Anus and Rectum

A. Anterior view of rectum and its arteries.

B. Posterior view of rectum and its arteries.

Remember:

1) There are eight sources of collateral circulation following bilateral internal iliac (hypogastric) artery ligation. Only the arteries in italics are illustrated.

a) Uterine and ovarian aa.

b) *Middle* and *superior rectal* aa.

c) *Obturator* and *inferior epigastric* aa.

d) *Inferior gluteal*, circumflex and perforating branches of the deep femoral a.

e) Iliolumbar and lumbar aa.

f) Lateral and *middle sacral* aa.

g) *Inferior external pudendal* aa.

h) Arteries of the bladder and the anterior body wall

2) The most common sites of ureteral injury during pelvic surgery are: (a) the pelvic wall lateral to the uterine vessels; (b) at the ureterovesical junction; (c) at the base of the infundibulopelvic ligament.

3) The middle rectal artery is often absent, especially in the female. In the male, this artery sends more blood to the prostate than to the rectum.

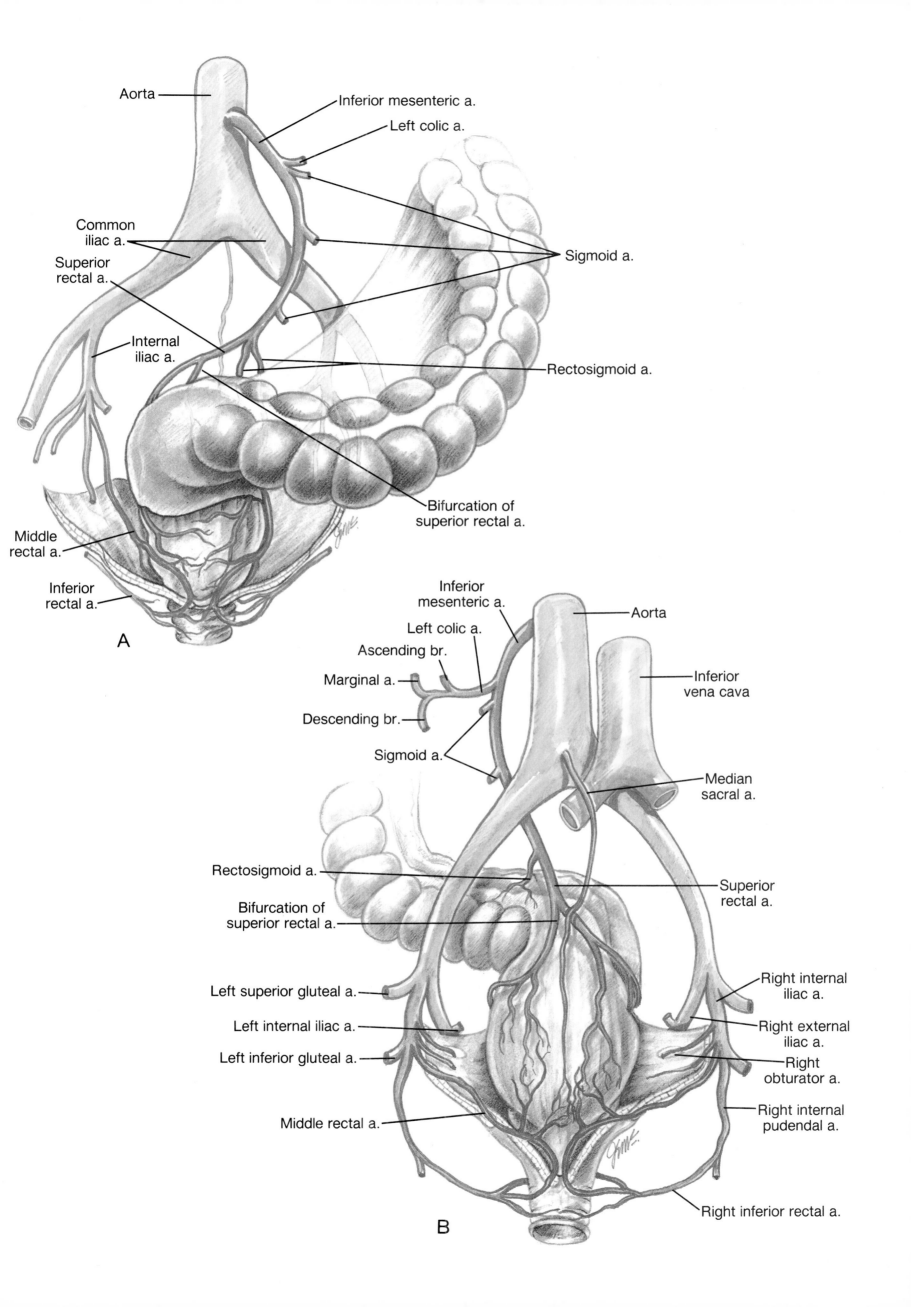

A

- Aorta
- Inferior mesenteric a.
- Left colic a.
- Common iliac a.
- Superior rectal a.
- Internal iliac a.
- Sigmoid a.
- Rectosigmoid a.
- Bifurcation of superior rectal a.
- Middle rectal a.
- Inferior rectal a.

B

- Inferior mesenteric a.
- Left colic a.
- Ascending br.
- Marginal a.
- Descending br.
- Sigmoid a.
- Aorta
- Inferior vena cava
- Median sacral a.
- Rectosigmoid a.
- Bifurcation of superior rectal a.
- Superior rectal a.
- Left superior gluteal a.
- Left internal iliac a.
- Left inferior gluteal a.
- Right internal iliac a.
- Right external iliac a.
- Right obturator a.
- Right internal pudendal a.
- Middle rectal a.
- Right inferior rectal a.

PLATE 10-7
Venous Drainage of the Anus and Rectum

The rectal venous plexus drains: (1) superiorly into the superior rectal vein, a tributary of the inferior mesenteric vein, and from there to the inferior mesenteric vein and to the portal system; (2) laterally into right and left middle rectal veins which enter the common iliac veins by way of the internal iliac veins to the inferior vena cava; (3) laterally to the internal pudendal veins and the iliac veins.

The pectinate line thus forms a watershed above which venous drainage is to the portal system, and below which drainage is to the systemic veins. The rectal plexus thus forms a natural portocaval shunt.

Remember:

1) The presacral (posterior) veins lie under the endopelvic fascia. Be careful not to tear them.

2) The internal vertebral plexus at the epidural fat of the spinal canal drains into the sacral veins and thence to the internal iliac vein.

3) Emboli, cancer metastases and infection may be carried by reflux into the internal vertebral plexus, to posterior intercostal veins, and by the azygos vein to the superior vena cava, bypassing the lungs to the brain.

4) Segmental resection of both hypogastric veins may be necessary with carcinoma of pelvic organs.

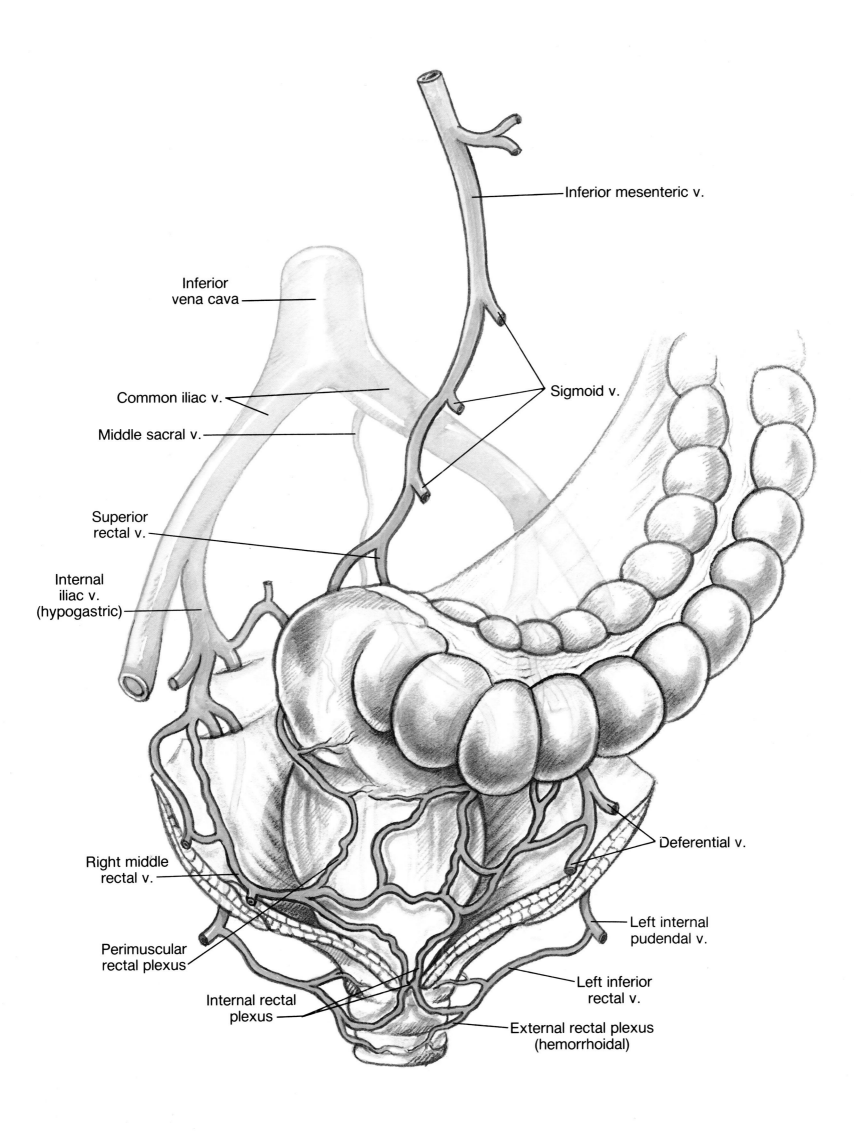

Inferior mesenteric v.

Inferior
vena cava

Sigmoid v.

Common iliac v.

Middle sacral v.

Superior
rectal v.

Internal
iliac v.
(hypogastric)

Deferential v.

Right middle
rectal v.

Left internal
pudendal v.

Perimuscular
rectal plexus

Left inferior
rectal v.

Internal rectal
plexus

External rectal plexus
(hemorrhoidal)

PLATE 10-8
Lymph Nodes and Lymphatic Drainage of the Anus and Rectum

Lymph nodes follow the superior rectal and middle rectal veins.

Inset: Below the pectinate line, lymphatic drainage is to inguinal nodes (see following Plate 10-9).

Remember:

1) Superior collecting channels are the most important. They drain that part of the rectum above the middle rectal valve to the pre- and para-aortic lymph nodes. They follow the superior rectal artery.

2) Middle collecting channels between the middle rectal valve and the pectinate line follow the middle rectal artery to the internal iliac nodes.

3) Inferior collecting channels follow the inferior rectal artery to the inguinal lymph nodes and the lateral wall of the pelvis.

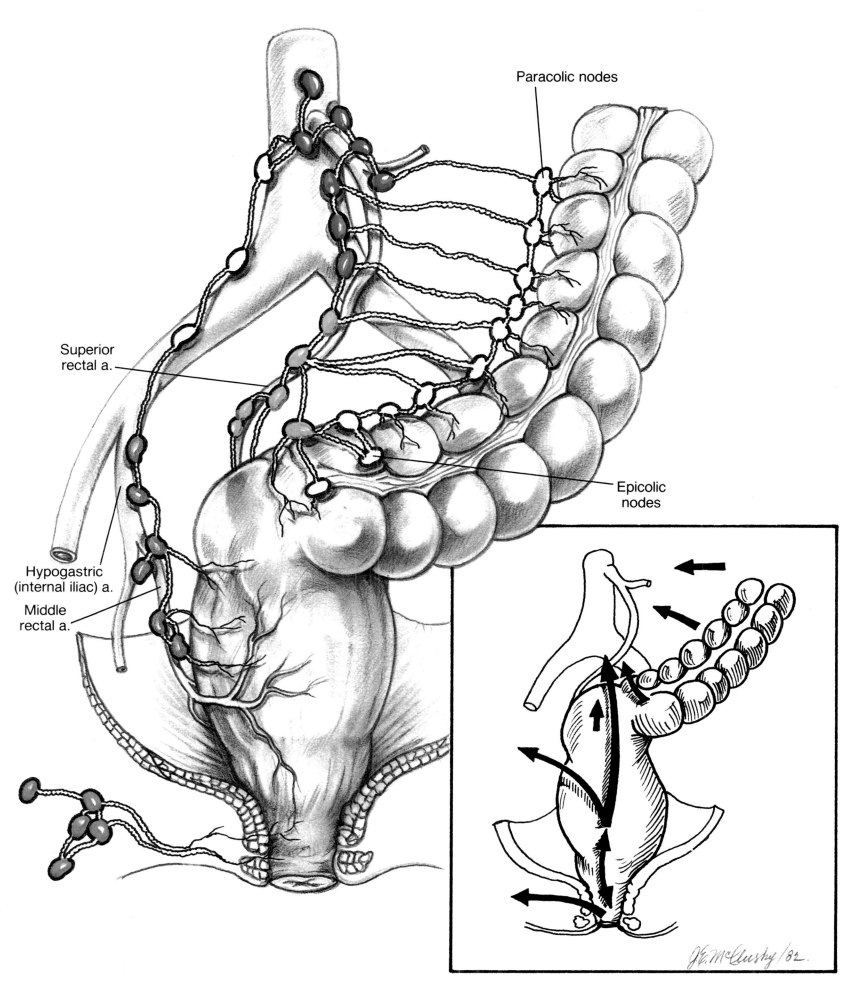

Left lumbar principal nodes

Intermediate nodes

Pararectal nodes

Inguinal nodes

Paracolic nodes

Superior rectal a.

Hypogastric (internal iliac) a.

Middle rectal a.

Epicolic nodes

PLATE 10-9
The Pectinate Line and Changes in the Surgical Anal Canal

	Above the Pectinate Line	**Below the Pectinate Line**
Embryonic Origin	Endoderm	Ectoderm
Anatomy		
Epithelial lining	Simple columnar	Stratified squamous
Arterial supply	Superior rectal artery	Inferior rectal artery
Venous drainage	Portal, by way of superior rectal vein	Systemic, by way of inferior rectal vein
External lymphatic drainage	To pelvic and lumbar nodes	To inguinal nodes
Nerve supply	Autonomic fibers (visceral)	Inferior rectal nerves (somatic)
Physiology	Sensation quickly diminishes	Excellent sensation
Pathology		
Cancer	Adenocarcinoma	Squamous cell carcinoma
Varices	Internal hemorrhoids	External hemorrhoids

IRA, inferior rectal artery; MRA, middle rectal artery; SRA, superior rectal artery; LRV, lower rectal valve; MRV, middle rectal valve; SRV, superior rectal valve.

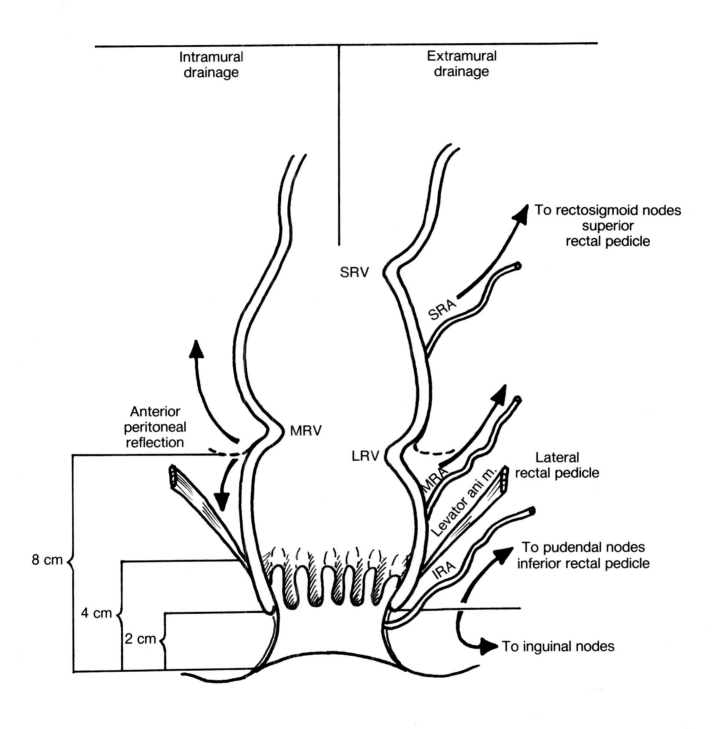

Intramural
drainage

Extramural
drainage

To rectosigmoid nodes
superior
rectal pedicle

SRV

SRA

Anterior
peritoneal
reflection

MRV

LRV

MRA

Levator ani m.

Lateral
rectal pedicle

IRA

To pudendal nodes
inferior rectal pedicle

8 cm

4 cm

2 cm

To inguinal nodes

PLATE 10-10
Paramedian Section of the Male Pelvis

The contents of the male pelvis. The levator ani muscle is shown in red. Compare with Plate 10-11.

Remember:

The pelvic wall from inside out consists of: (a) peritoneum; (b) internal iliac vessels; (c) parietal layer of pelvic fascia; (d) sacral plexus and branches; (e) muscles (obturator internal and piriformis); (f) bony wall.

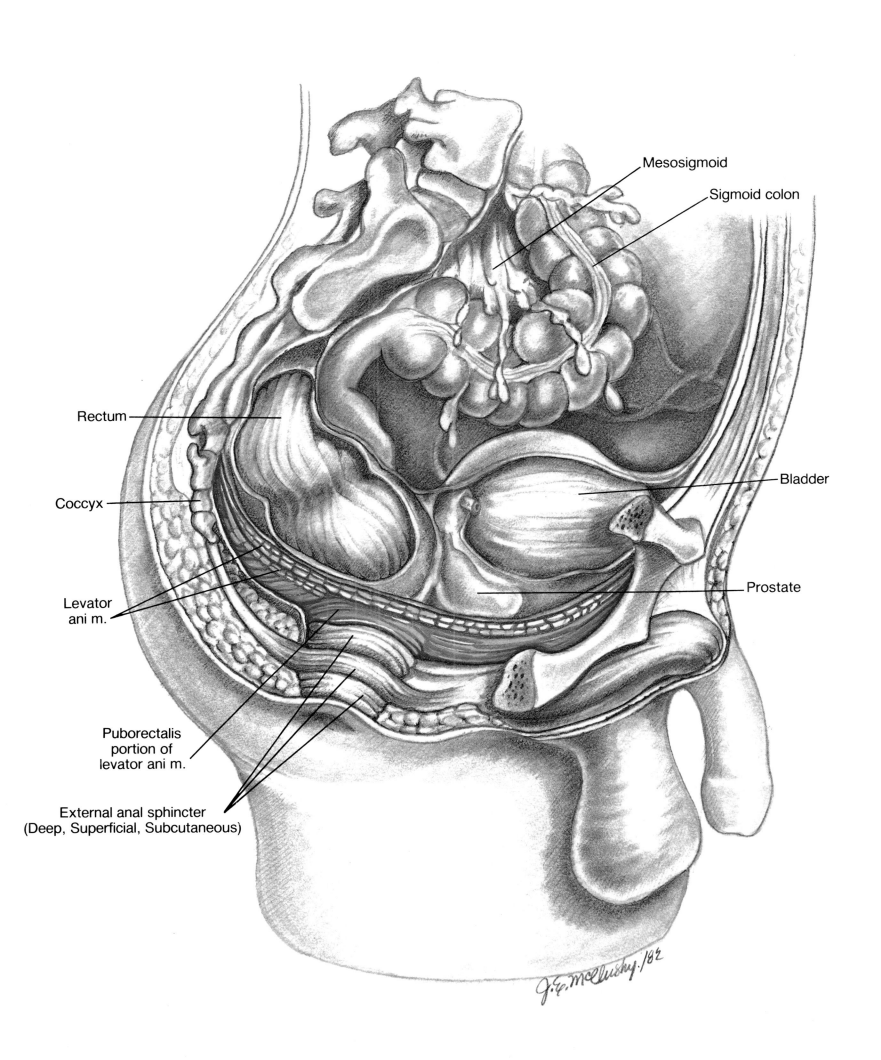

Mesosigmoid

Sigmoid colon

Rectum

Bladder

Coccyx

Levator
ani m.

Prostate

Puborectalis
portion of
levator ani m.

External anal sphincter
(Deep, Superficial, Subcutaneous)

PLATE 10-11
Paramedian Section of the Female Pelvis

The contents of the female pelvis.

Remember:

1) The pelvic floor slopes downward and forward to receive the lowest part of the fetus.

2) The passive stretching of the ileococcygeus will participate in the mechanisms of defecation and labor.

3) The pubococcygeus is responsible for the integrity of the pelvic floor.

4) The puborectalis forms a sling, which is responsible for the closing of the anorectal canal.

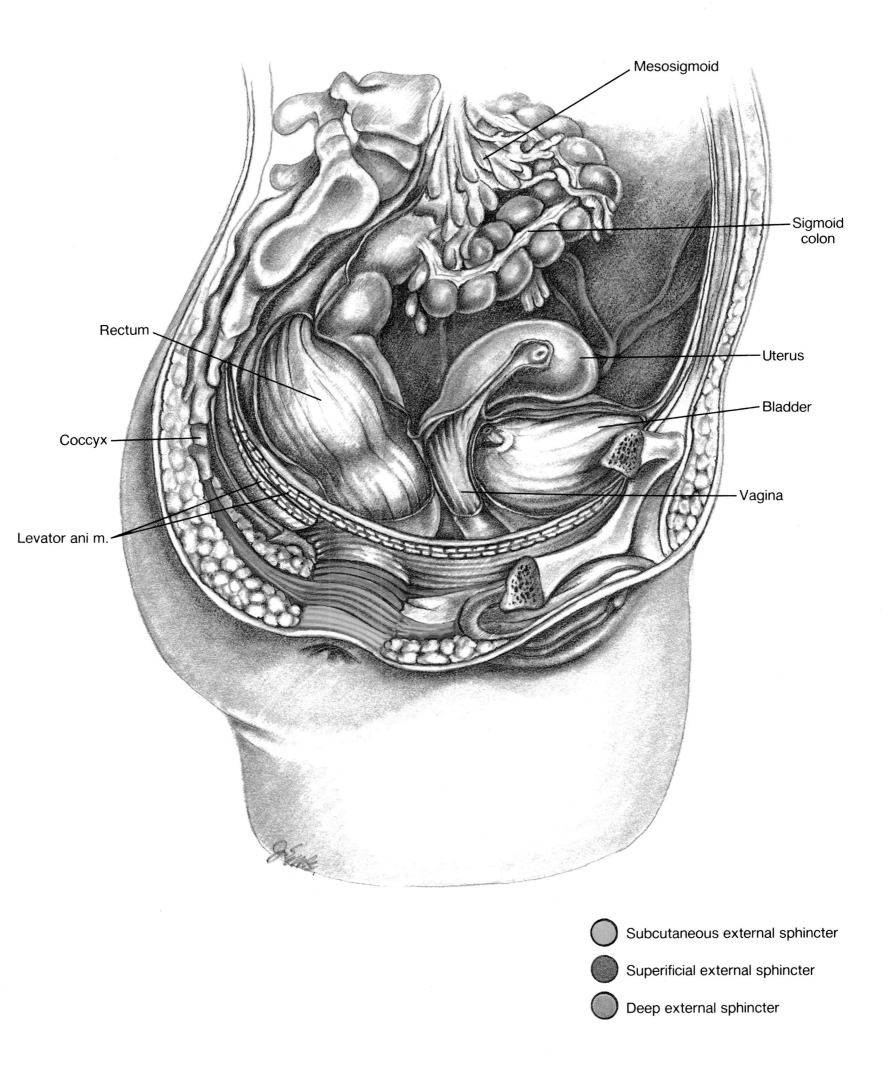

Mesosigmoid

Sigmoid
colon

Rectum

Uterus

Bladder

Coccyx

Vagina

Levator ani m.

Subcutaneous external sphincter

Superificial external sphincter

Deep external sphincter

PLATE 10-12
The Female Pelvic Diaphragm I

Remember:

1) The obturator nerve is the chief nerve supply in the pelvic wall.

2) The innervation of the visceral peritoneum is not known.

3) The pudendal nerve, the great splanchnic nerve, and the pudendal artery provide the innervation and blood supply to the rectum and urinary bladder.

4) The nerves to the pelvis are: (a) obturator nerve; (b) sacral sympathetic nerves; (c) sacral plexus; (d) pelvic plexus.

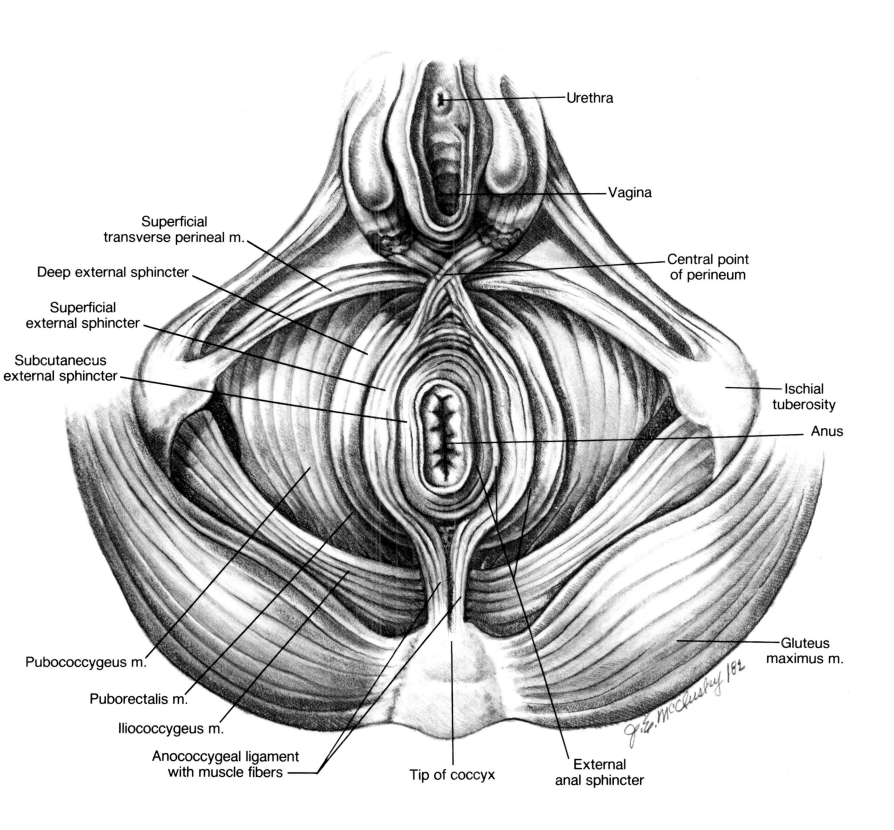

Urethra

Vagina

Central point
of perineum

Superficial
transverse perineal m.

Deep external sphincter

Superficial
external sphincter

Subcutanecus
external sphincter

Ischial
tuberosity

Anus

Pubococcygeus m.

Puborectalis m.

Iliococcygeus m.

Anococcygeal ligament
with muscle fibers

Tip of coccyx

External
anal sphincter

Gluteus
maximus m.

PLATE 10-13
The Female Pelvic Diaphragm II

A. The muscles of the pelvic diaphragm seen from above.

B. The muscles of the pelvic diaphragm seen from below.

Remember:

The sphincter vaginae or pubovaginalis muscle is part of the coccygeus muscle. It is a sling behind the vagina attaching to the perineal body. (In the male this sling is called levator prostatae).

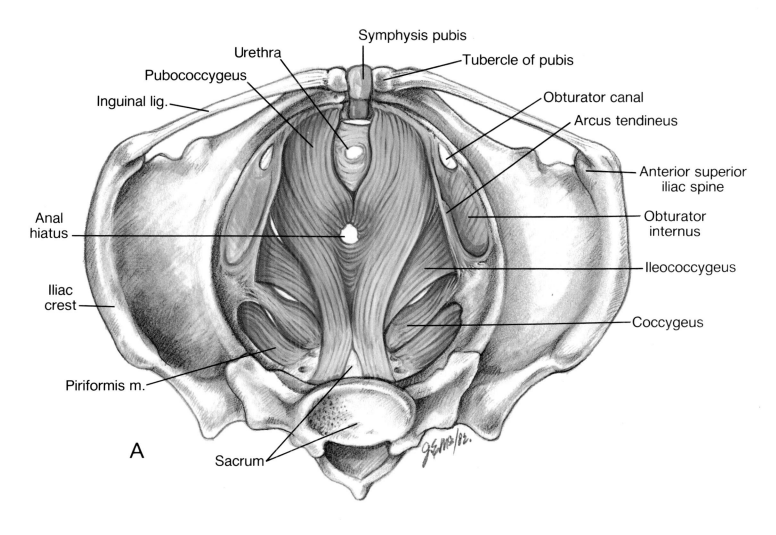

Symphysis pubis

Urethra

Pubococcygeus

Inguinal lig.

Tubercle of pubis

Obturator canal

Arcus tendineus

Anterior superior iliac spine

Obturator internus

Anal hiatus

Ileococcygeus

Iliac crest

Coccygeus

Piriformis m.

Sacrum

A

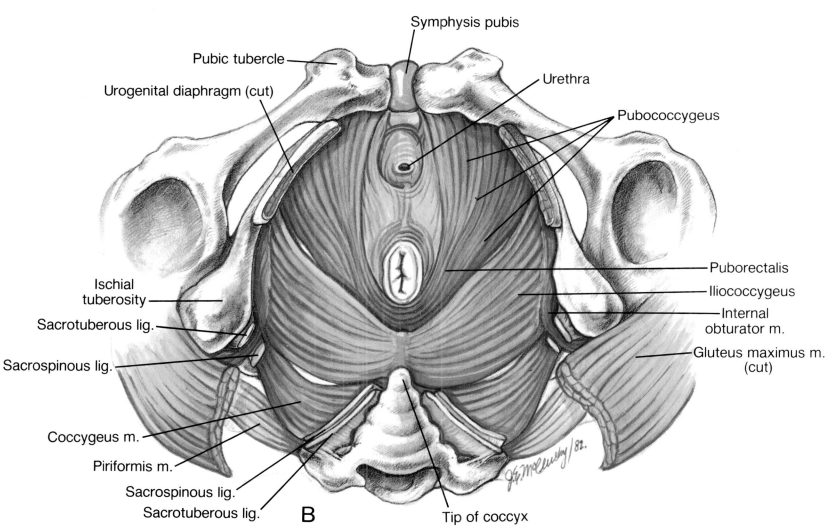

Symphysis pubis

Pubic tubercle

Urogenital diaphragm (cut)

Urethra

Pubococcygeus

Ischial tuberosity

Puborectalis

Sacrotuberous lig.

Iliococcygeus

Sacrospinous lig.

Internal obturator m.

Gluteus maximus m. (cut)

Coccygeus m.

Piriformis m.

Sacrospinous lig.

Sacrotuberous lig.

B

Tip of coccyx

PLATE 10-14
The Male Pelvic Diaphragm

A. The pelvic diaphragm and the components of the external anal sphincter seen from below.

B. Lateral view of the relationship of the components of the external sphincter and the anus and rectum.

The pelvic diaphragm, which never prolapses, prevents evisceration. Together with the anal sphincters, the anococcygeal body and the perineal body, it supports the anal canal.

Remember:

The pelvic diaphragm is the pelvic floor and is formed by the levator ani and coccygeus muscles.

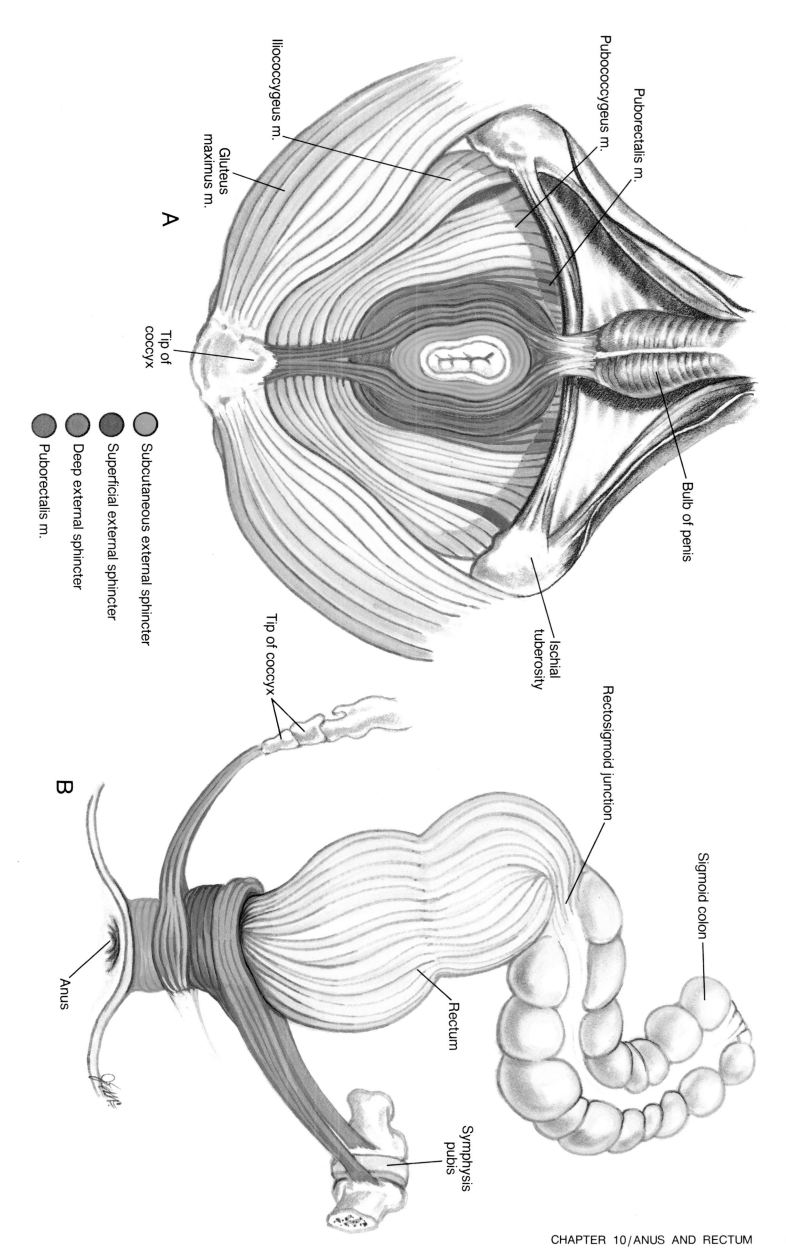

Iliococcygeus m.

Gluteus maximus m.

Pubococcygeus m.

Puborectalis m.

Tip of coccyx

Ischial tuberosity

Bulb of penis

A

Puborectalis m.

Deep external sphincter

Superficial external sphincter

Subcutaneous external sphincter

B

Tip of coccyx

Rectosigmoid junction

Sigmoid colon

Rectum

Anus

Symphysis pubis

PLATE 10-15
The External Anal Sphincter

A. Paramedial section of the male pelvis showing the components of the external anal sphincter.

B. The four components of the external anal sphincter and their attachments. The components are not as clearly demarcated as the illustration would suggest.

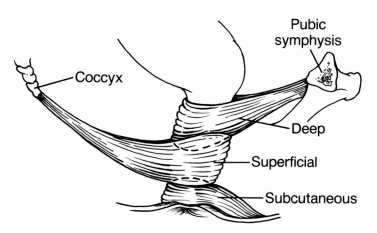

Diagram of the triple-loop system of Shafik (Invest. Urol. 12:412, 1975). The deep portion and puborectalis are considered to act as a unit:

	Composition	Nerve Supply
Upper loop	Puborectalis muscle and deep external sphincter.	Inferior rectal branch of the pudendal nerve
Middle loop	Superficial external sphincter.	Perineal branch of the fourth sacral nerve
Base loop	Subcutaneous external sphincter; those fibers insert on the perianal skin.	Inferior rectal nerve

Remember:

Any one of the three slings is capable of maintaining continence to solid stools, but not to fluid or gas.

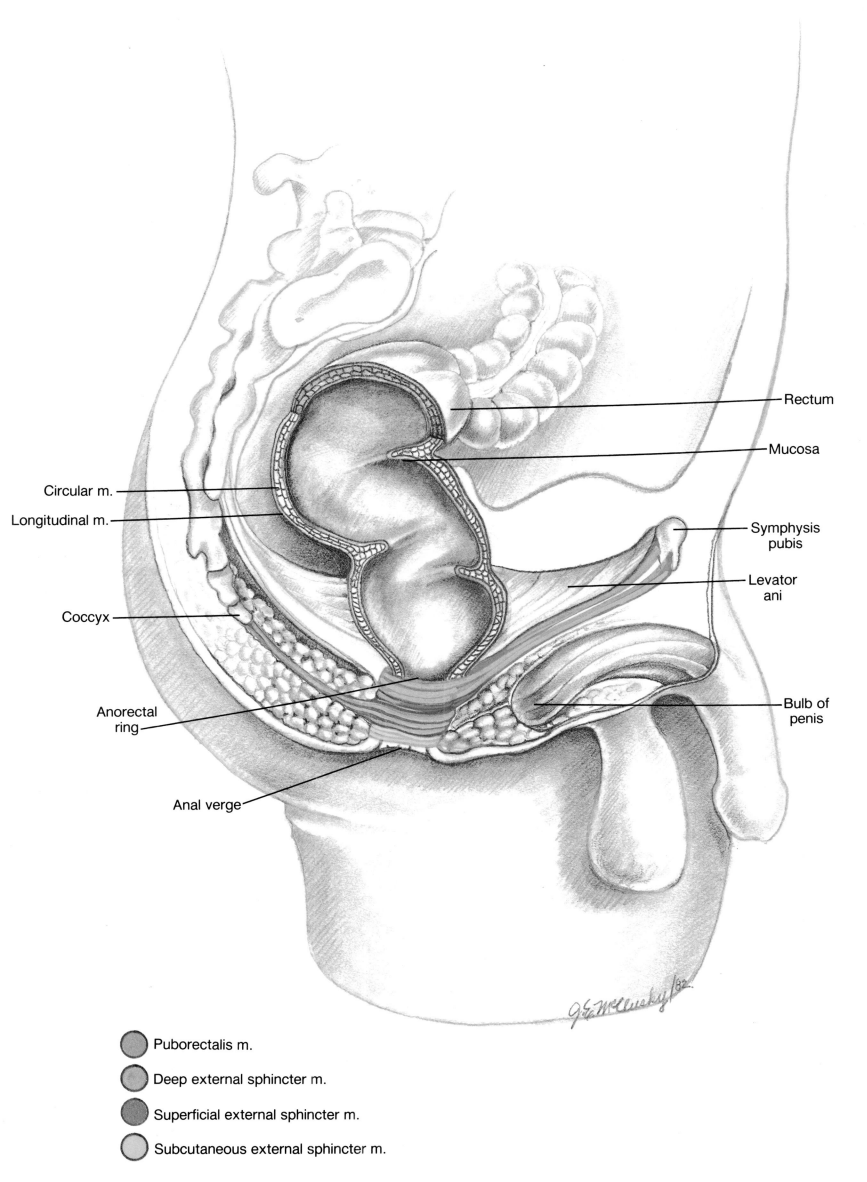

Rectum

Mucosa

Circular m.

Longitudinal m.

Symphysis pubis

Levator ani

Coccyx

Anorectal ring

Bulb of penis

Anal verge

Puborectalis m.

Deep external sphincter m.

Superficial external sphincter m.

Subcutaneous external sphincter m.

PLATE 10-16
Sympathetic Nerves to the Anus and Rectum

A. There are typically five lumbar ganglia on each side, but the number is variable; their specific segmental identification is often impossible. The longest and most constant ganglion is on the second lumbar vertebra. The sympathetic chain lies anterior to the lumbar vessels but occasionally it is posterior to them. Communication between right and left chains probably exists.

B. Neural pathways involved in continence. Rectal distension initiates relaxation of the internal sphincter and voluntary closure by the external sphincter.

C. Neural pathways involved in defecation. Voluntary relaxation of the external sphincter, relaxation of the internal sphincter, and contraction of the muscles of the rectal wall permit evacuation.

Remember:

1) Bladder dysfunction, failure of ejaculation and impotence may result from injury to sympathetic and parasympathetic nerves during separation of the posterior wall of the rectum from the sacrum. The scissors, and the palm of the dissecting hand, must stay close to the wall of the rectum to avoid the nerves during mobilization of anorectum.

2) In males undergoing bilateral sympathectomy, remove *only one* first lumbar ganglion to avoid failure of ejaculation, loss of libido and sterility. Both left and right second, third and fourth lumbar ganglia may be removed.

3) Be sure to protect the genitofemoral and the iliohypogastric nerves during lumbar sympathectomy.

4) The sympathetic trunk may bifurcate or trifurcate; branches may descend in the psoas-vertebral groove.

5) Continence is maintained by the pudendal and pelvic splanchnic nerves; evacuation by the pelvic splanchnic nerve alone.

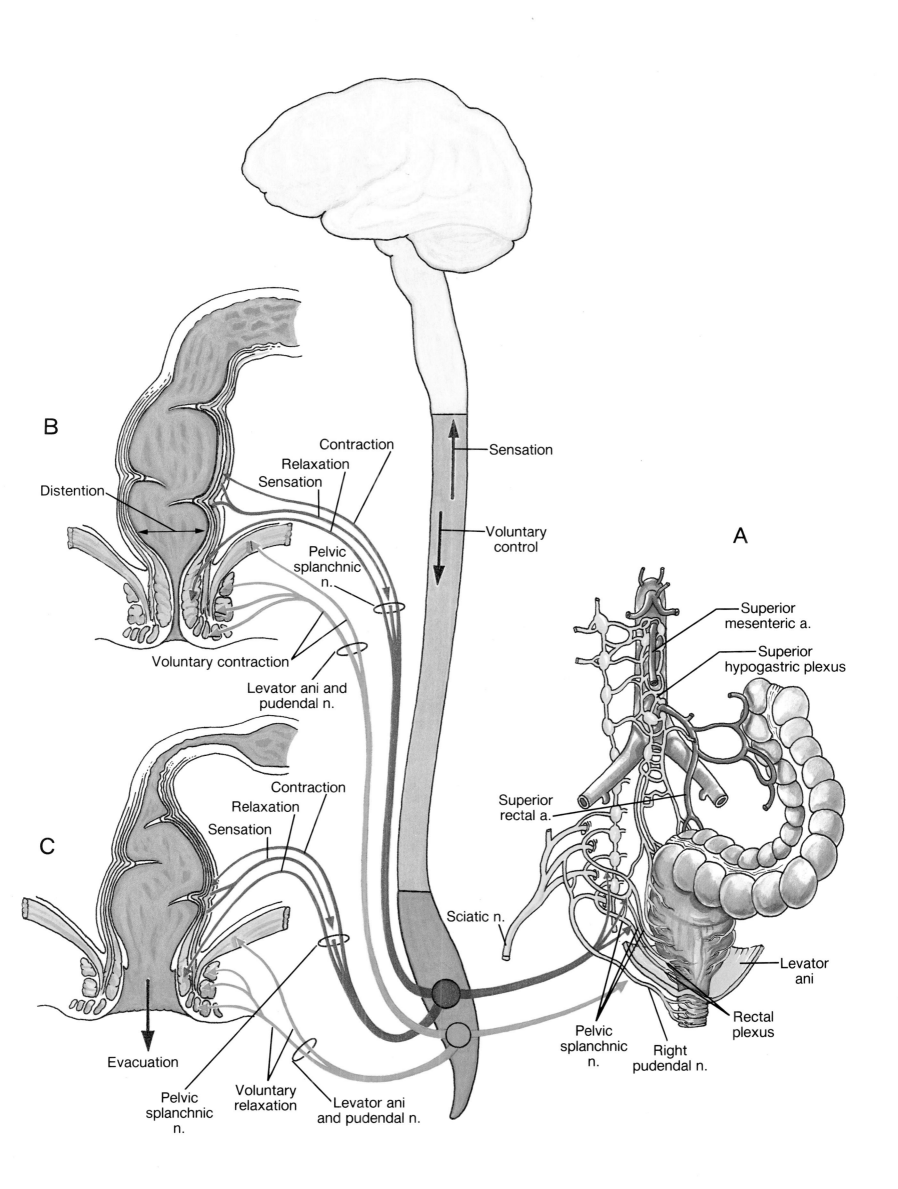

B

Distention

Contraction
Relaxation
Sensation

Pelvic
splanchnic
n.

Voluntary contraction

Levator ani and
pudendal n.

Sensation

Voluntary
control

A

Superior
mesenteric a.

Superior
hypogastric plexus

Superior
rectal a.

C

Contraction
Relaxation
Sensation

Sciatic n.

Evacuation

Pelvic
splanchnic
n.

Voluntary
relaxation

Levator ani
and pudendal n.

Pelvic
splanchnic
n.

Right
pudendal n.

Levator
ani

Rectal
plexus

PLATE 10-17
Examination of the Anal Canal and Rectum

A. The gloved and lubricated finger is inserted so that the distal interphalangeal joint is at the verge. The subcutaneous portion of the external sphincter is felt as a ring. The finger should feel the pectinate valves, 2 cm above the verge. External hemorrhoids, polyps and hypertrophic papillae are palpable if present.

B. The finger at the level of the middle interphalangeal joint brings the first joint to the ring formed by the deep portion of the external sphincter and its upper margin.

C. When the finger penetrates to the level of the metacarpophalangeal joint, the fingertip enters the rectum. The lowermost rectal fold may often be touched. Anterior to the rectum the examiner can palpate the bladder and the prostate gland in men and the cervix in women.

D. The sigmoidoscope, with its obturator in place, is directed toward the umbilicus. The tip is just past the anorectal ring.

E. With the obturator removed for direct observation, the middle rectal fold may be seen at about 8 cm from the verge. This is the level of the peritoneal reflection. The greatest risk of perforation by the instrument is between the middle and upper rectal folds just above the peritoneal reflection.

F. The superior rectal fold is from 8 to 12 cm from the verge. Beyond this, passage of the instrument is easy.

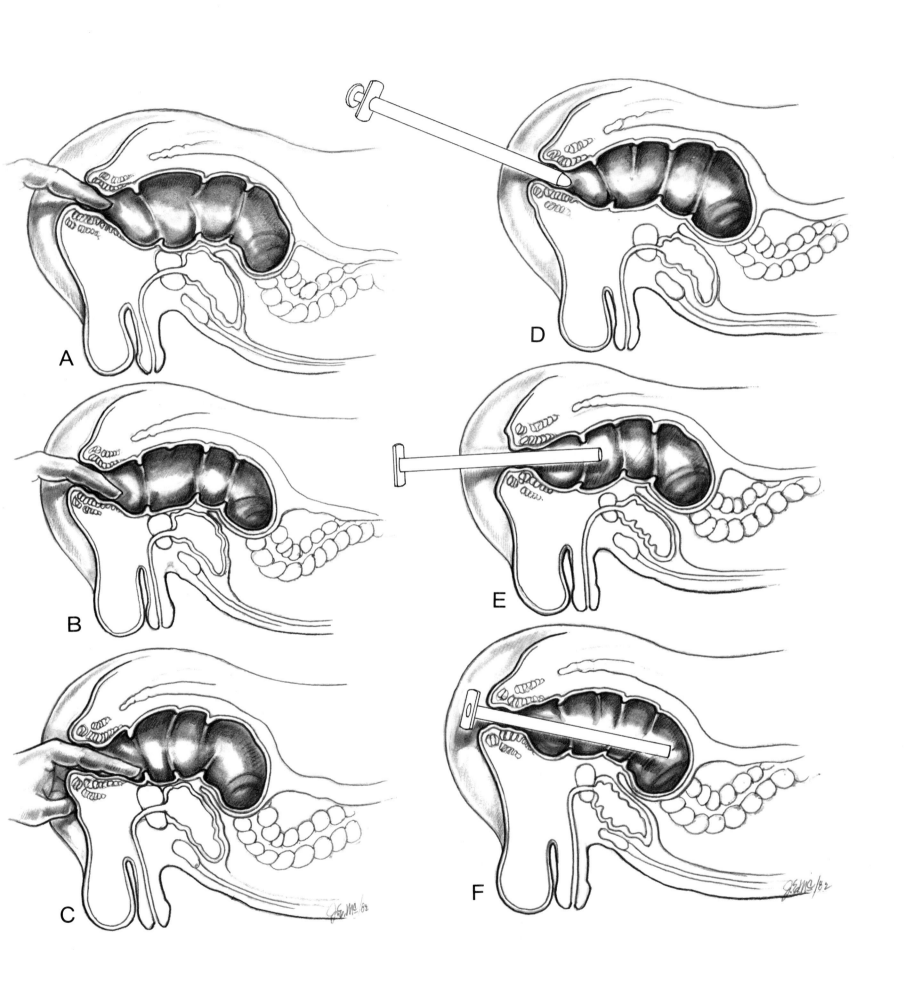

PLATE 11-1
The Development of the Adrenal (Suprarenal) Glands I

A. The adrenal glands arise from the coelomic epithelium early in the 4th week of gestation in the angle between the dorsal mesentery and the head of the mesonephros. Cords of epithelial cells grow into the mesoderm to form the future adrenal cortex. During the 5th week, migrating neural crest cells enter the adrenal primordium and differentiate into medullary chromaffin cells.

B to D. The adrenal glands remain close to their point of origin while the kidneys ascend from the pelvis during the 6th and 8th weeks until they meet the adrenal glands, which mold themselves to the contours of the upper poles of the kidneys at the 9th and 10th week. At birth the kidneys are externally lobulated.

Remember:

1) The adrenal glands develop *in situ*, not descending or ascending.

2) Occasionally the adrenal gland is beneath the renal or hepatic capsule (adrenorenal or adrenohepatic heterotopia). Adrenalectomy in such cases is very difficult.

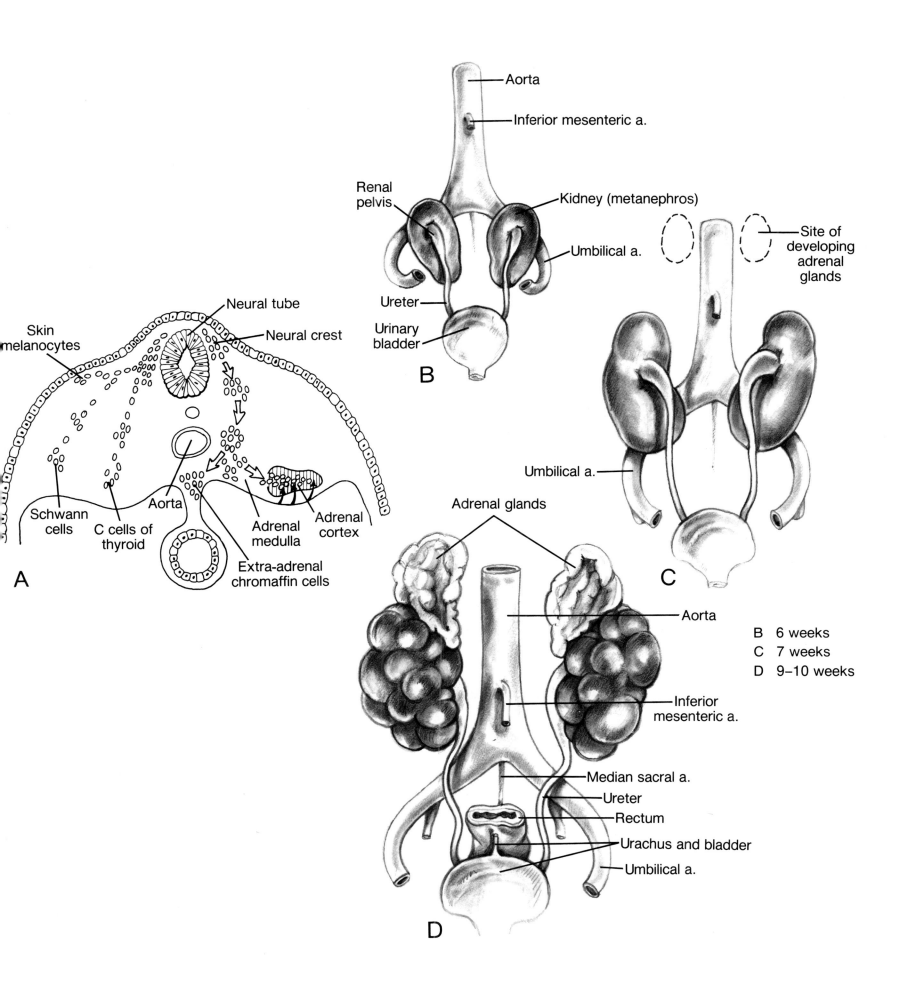

Skin melanocytes

Neural tube

Neural crest

Schwann cells

C cells of thyroid

Aorta

Adrenal medulla

Adrenal cortex

Extra-adrenal chromaffin cells

A

Aorta

Inferior mesenteric a.

Renal pelvis

Kidney (metanephros)

Umbilical a.

Ureter

Urinary bladder

B

Site of developing adrenal glands

Umbilical a.

C

Adrenal glands

Aorta

Inferior mesenteric a.

Median sacral a.

Ureter

Rectum

Urachus and bladder

Umbilical a.

D

B 6 weeks
C 7 weeks
D 9–10 weeks

PLATE 11-2
The Development of the Adrenal (Suprarenal) Glands II

A. Right adrenal gland and right kidney with diagrammatic sections through the adrenal gland to show changes in the relative volume of the layers: (1) at the 5th fetal month, (2) at birth, and (3) in the adult. The large fetal cortex disappears with an absolute decrease in adrenal mass up to puberty. Adult proportions are not reached until after puberty.

B. Sites of heterotopic adrenal glands and cortical tissue.

Inset: Sites of heterotopic medullary tissue (paraganglia). These are formed by neural crest cells that did not reach the cortical primordium.

Remember:

1) Accessory adrenal tissue, cortical, medullary or both, may be found throughout the abdomen. These are true accessory glands. The most common location is on the aorta, celiac artery or superior mesenteric artery.

2) Cortical tissue alone can be found under the renal capsule, the broad ligament and the spermatic cord.

3) The largest extra-adrenal chromatin structure is the organ of Zuckerkandl close to the aortic bifurcation.

Table: Anomalies of the Adrenal Glands

Defect	Origin	Frequency	Remarks
Adrenal agenesis	4th week	Uncommon	Associated with ipsilateral absence of kidney
Adrenal fusion	6th week	Rare	Associated with fused kidneys
Adrenal hypoplasia	?	Rare	Associated with anencephaly (usually lethal)
Adrenal heterotopia	8th week	Uncommon	Within capsule of liver or kidney; asymptomatic
Accessory adrenal tissue	4–5th week	Common	Usually cortical tissue only, asymptomatic

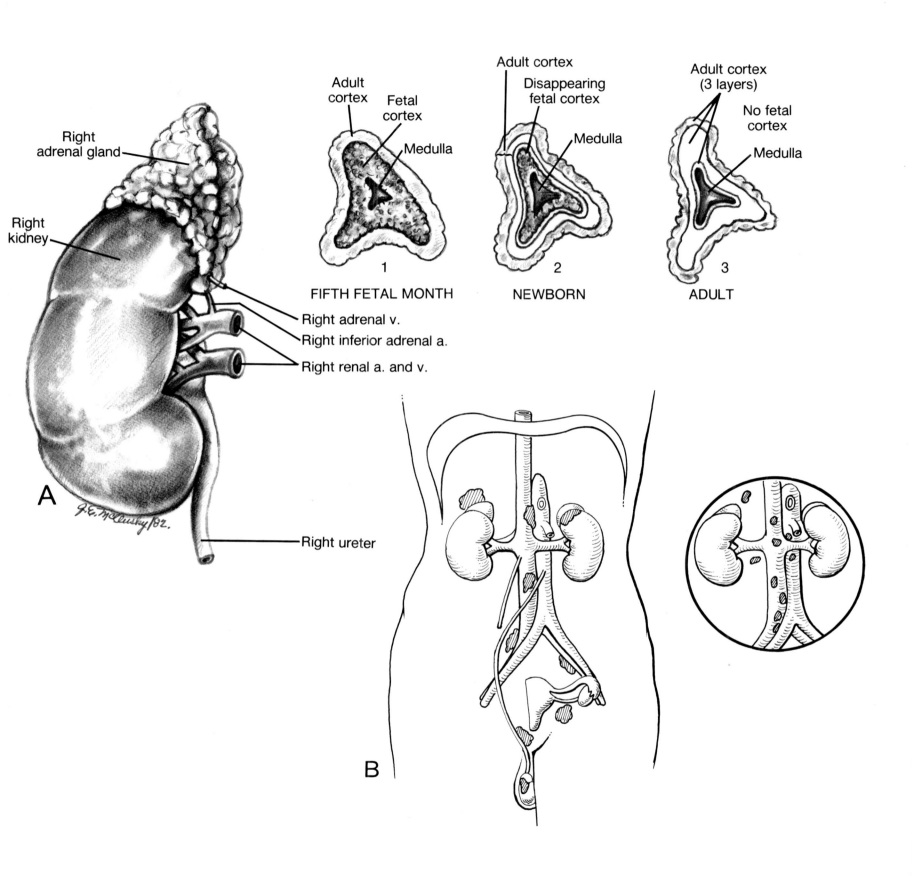

Right
adrenal gland

Right
kidney

Right adrenal v.
Right inferior adrenal a.
Right renal a. and v.

A

Right ureter

Adult
cortex   Fetal
cortex
            Medulla

1

FIFTH FETAL MONTH

Adult cortex
Disappearing
fetal cortex
            Medulla

2

NEWBORN

Adult cortex
(3 layers)
            No fetal
            cortex
            Medulla

3

ADULT

B

PLATE 11-3
The Left and Right Adrenal (Suprarenal) Glands *in Situ*

In this figure, the stomach has been removed and the liver retracted upward.

Remember:

1) Careful dissection is necessary during left adrenalectomy to avoid injuries to the inferior mesenteric vein, middle and left colic arteries, superior renal polar arteries, renal artery and vein, spleen, pancreas, renal capsule and left colon.

2) During right adrenalectomy avoid injury to the hepatic veins, inferior vena cava, superior renal artery, gastroduodenal artery, liver and duodenum.

3) The right adrenal vein is very short and must be dissected and ligated very carefully.

4) Avoid excessive retraction when performing right or left adrenalectomy through an anterior or posterior approach.

5) Variations in the number and positions of veins may occur, but are rare. Be careful.

6) The right adrenal gland is usually higher than the left (reverse of the relation of the kidneys).

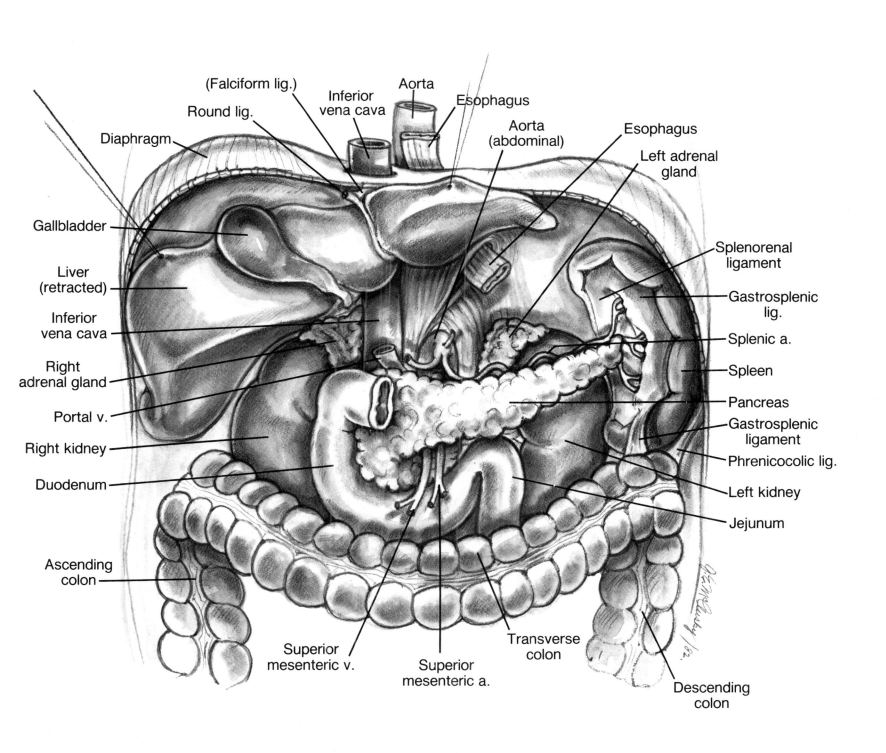

(Falciform lig.)

Round lig.

Diaphragm

Inferior vena cava

Aorta

Esophagus

Aorta (abdominal)

Esophagus

Left adrenal gland

Gallbladder

Liver (retracted)

Inferior vena cava

Right adrenal gland

Portal v.

Right kidney

Duodenum

Ascending colon

Splenorenal ligament

Gastrosplenic lig.

Splenic a.

Spleen

Pancreas

Gastrosplenic ligament

Phrenicocolic lig.

Left kidney

Jejunum

Superior mesenteric v.

Superior mesenteric a.

Transverse colon

Descending colon

PLATE 11-4
Vessels and Nerves of the Adrenal (Suprarenal) Glands

A. The adrenal arteries and veins. Note that the arteries divide before entering the gland. There are more branches than are shown in the drawing.

B. The nerves of the adrenal glands.

Remember:

1) The short right adrenal vein empties into the inferior vena cava. Be gentle during dissection. The left adrenal vein is longer and empties into the left renal vein. Both may drain abnormally.

2) Accessory veins are rare. They may enter the inferior phrenic or the right renal vein. The right accessory vein in this figure is larger than usual to emphasize the possibility of such an aberrant vessel.

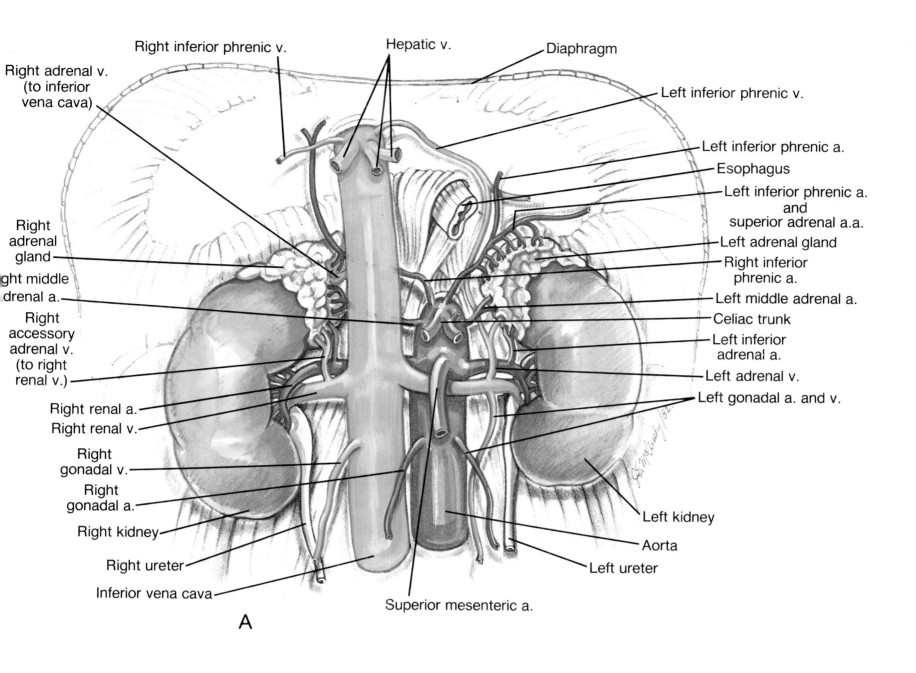

Right inferior phrenic v.

Hepatic v.

Diaphragm

Right adrenal v.
(to inferior
vena cava)

Left inferior phrenic v.

Left inferior phrenic a.

Esophagus

Left inferior phrenic a.
and
superior adrenal a.a.

Right
adrenal
gland

Left adrenal gland

Right inferior
phrenic a.

ght middle
drenal a.

Left middle adrenal a.

Celiac trunk

Right
accessory
adrenal v.
(to right
renal v.)

Left inferior
adrenal a.

Left adrenal v.

Left gonadal a. and v.

Right renal a.

Right renal v.

Right
gonadal v.

Right
gonadal a.

Right kidney

Left kidney

Right ureter

Aorta

Left ureter

Inferior vena cava

Superior mesenteric a.

A

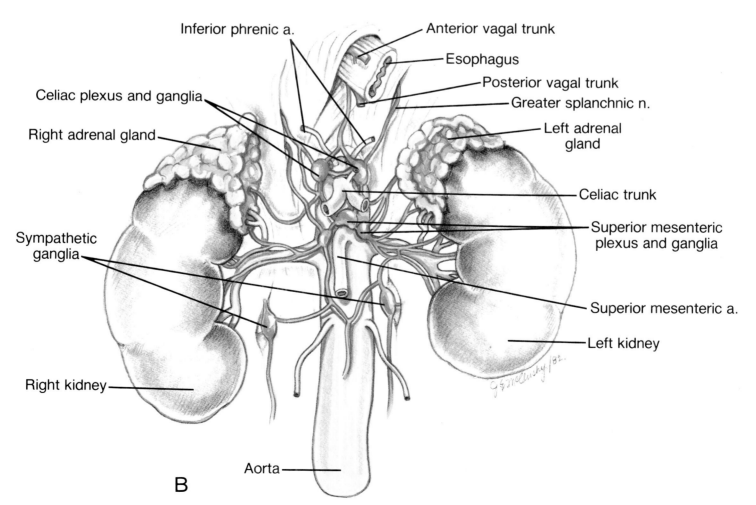

Inferior phrenic a.

Anterior vagal trunk

Esophagus

Celiac plexus and ganglia

Posterior vagal trunk

Greater splanchnic n.

Right adrenal gland

Left adrenal
gland

Celiac trunk

Superior mesenteric
plexus and ganglia

Sympathetic
ganglia

Superior mesenteric a.

Left kidney

Right kidney

Aorta

B

PLATE 11-5
The Lymphatic Drainage of the Adrenal (Suprarenal) Glands

Both adrenal glands drain to periaortic (red) and renal hilar lymph nodes (green) (shown for the left adrenal gland only). The right adrenal gland drains also the liver (orange). The left adrenal gland drains also to mediastinal lymph nodes (blue).

Remember:

This lymphatic connection between abdomen and thorax may explain metastases from cancer of the liver to the adrenal gland.

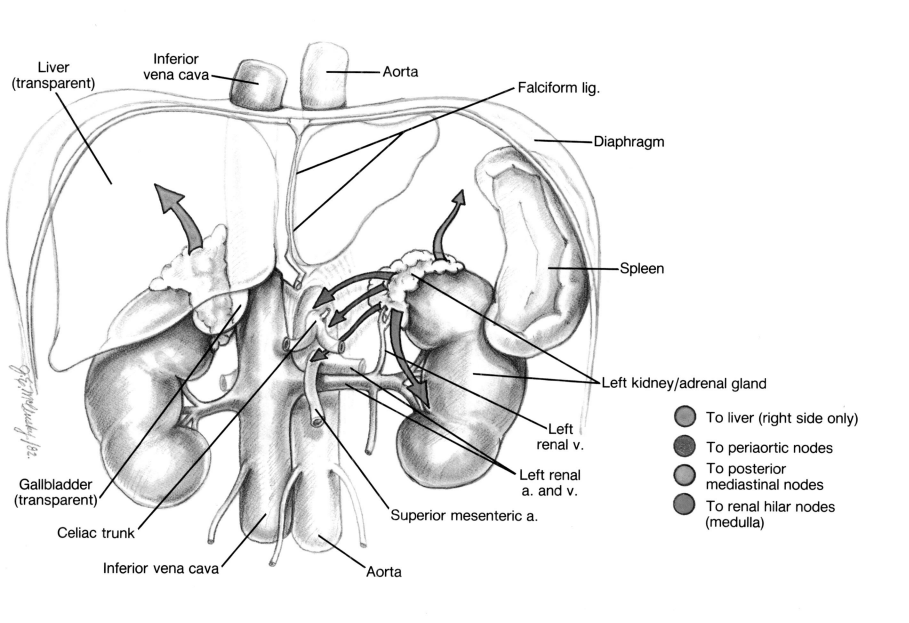

Liver
(transparent)

Inferior
vena cava

Aorta

Falciform lig.

Diaphragm

Spleen

Left kidney/adrenal gland

Left
renal v.

Left renal
a. and v.

Superior mesenteric a.

Gallbladder
(transparent)

Celiac trunk

Inferior vena cava

Aorta

To liver (right side only)

To periaortic nodes

To posterior
mediastinal nodes

To renal hilar nodes
(medulla)

PLATE 11-6
Adrenalectomy

A. Removal of the left adrenal gland. The gland is being dissected from the kidney and retracted upward and to the right.

B. Removal of the right adrenal gland. Following a Kocher maneuver, the right adrenal gland and the upper pole of the kidney are exposed. Notice the superior position of the right adrenal vein. The numerous adrenal arteries must be ligated and divided. The inferior vena cava may be gently retracted to expose the arteries more fully.

Remember:

1) The renal fascia (of Gerota) completely envelops each adrenal gland, separating the adrenal from the kidney. In extremely rare cases this separation does not exist, and the gland is heavily fixed to the kidney.

2) When the arterial blood supply is reached, dissection must be slow and careful. As many as 50 or 60 small arteries may enter the capsule.

3) Major divisions of the left renal vein may be ligated *close* to the hilus with impunity. Intrarenal collaterals will save the left kidney.

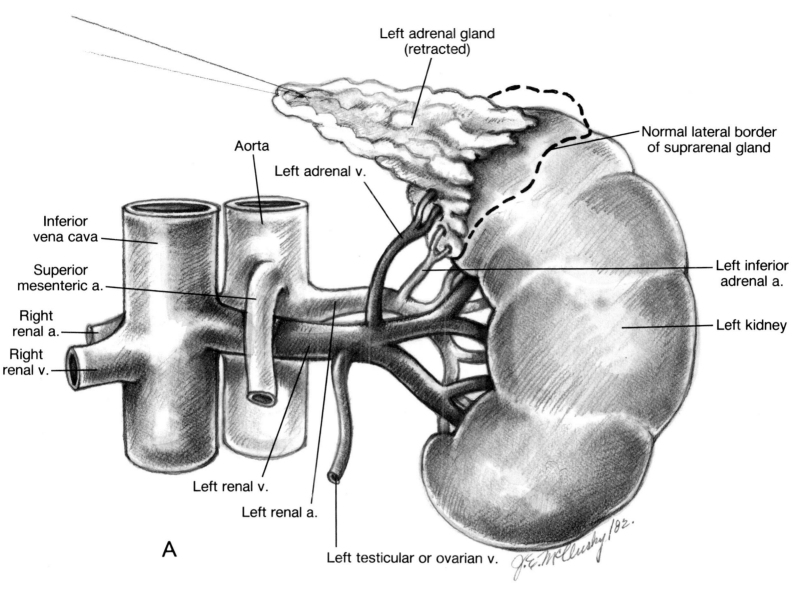

Left adrenal gland
(retracted)

Aorta

Left adrenal v.

Normal lateral border
of suprarenal gland

Inferior
vena cava

Superior
mesenteric a.

Right
renal a.

Right
renal v.

Left inferior
adrenal a.

Left kidney

Left renal v.

Left renal a.

Left testicular or ovarian v.

A

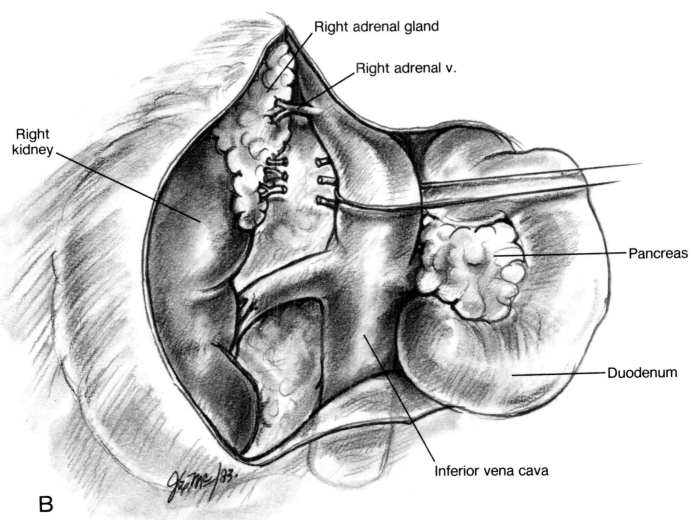

Right adrenal gland

Right adrenal v.

Right
kidney

Pancreas

Duodenum

Inferior vena cava

B

PLATE 12-1
The Urogenital Tract of the Male

A. Diagrammatic anterior view of the male urogenital system showing the blood supply to the testis.

B. Lateral view of right testis. The parietal layer of the tunica vaginalis has been opened to reveal the spermatic cord, testis and epididymis. The appendix testis (hydatid of Morgagni) is a vestige of the Müllerian duct which forms the uterine tube in the female. The appendix epididymis represents part of the Wolffian duct not incorporated in the adult epididymis.

C. Cross section of testes and scrotum showing the scrotal layers.

D. Anterior view of left testis. The parietal layer of the tunica vaginalis and the spermatic cord has been opened.

There are anastomoses between the testicular and deferential arteries, and, in two thirds of subjects, anastomosis with the cremasteric artery also. This collateral circulation will permit ligation of the testicular artery without necrosis in all but 2% of cases. Testicular atrophy may be expected in 80% of patients.

Remember:

1) Do not sacrifice spermatic vessels to increase the available length of spermatic cord.

2) The ductus deferens is always long enough for a good testicular mobilization and scrotal placement. If the testicle or ductus is not found, look again. Congenital testicular absence is very rare.

3) Collateral blood supply of the normal testis is *not* available to the newly transplanted testis.

4) Following herniorrhaphy, the lymph drainage of the testis passes to the preaortic lymph nodes as well as to the inguinal nodes. Keep this in mind when diagnosing a malignant testicular tumor.

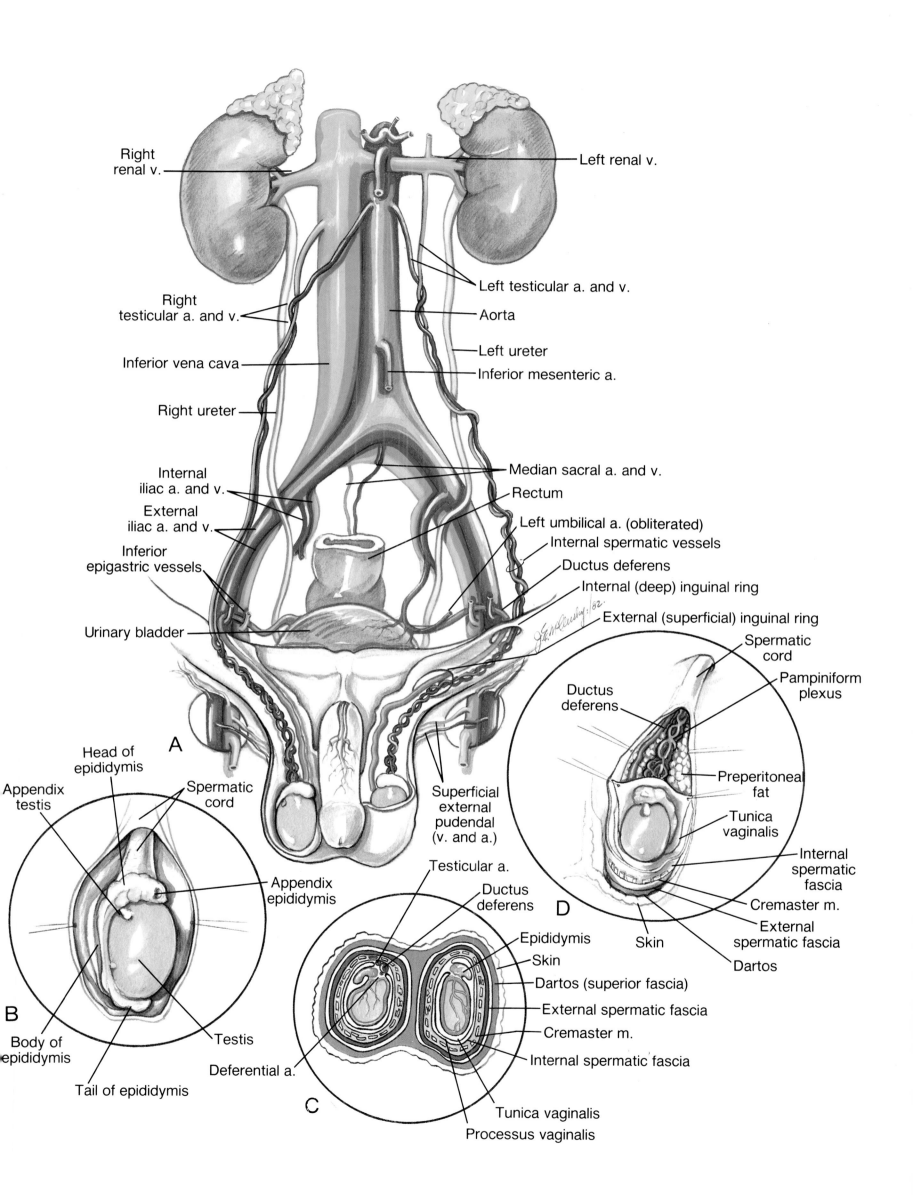

Right
renal v.

Left renal v.

Right
testicular a. and v.

Left testicular a. and v.

Aorta

Left ureter

Inferior mesenteric a.

Inferior vena cava

Right ureter

Median sacral a. and v.

Rectum

Internal
iliac a. and v.

Left umbilical a. (obliterated)

External
iliac a. and v.

Internal spermatic vessels

Inferior
epigastric vessels

Ductus deferens

Internal (deep) inguinal ring

External (superficial) inguinal ring

Urinary bladder

Spermatic
cord

Pampiniform
plexus

Ductus
deferens

Preperitoneal
fat

Tunica
vaginalis

Internal
spermatic
fascia

Cremaster m.

External
spermatic fascia

Superficial
external
pudendal
(v. and a.)

Skin

Dartos

D

Head of
epididymis

Appendix
testis

Spermatic
cord

Appendix
epididymis

Testicular a.

Ductus
deferens

Epididymis

Skin

Dartos (superior fascia)

External spermatic fascia

Cremaster m.

Internal spermatic fascia

Tunica vaginalis

Processus vaginalis

B

Body of
epididymis

Testis

Deferential a.

Tail of epididymis

C

PLATE 12-2
Closure of the Processus Vaginalis

A. Normal closure following descent of the testis and epididymis.

B. Superior (funicular) portion of the processus remains unclosed. This is an invitation to indirect inguinal hernia of the "acquired" type.

C. Entire processus remains unclosed. This is an invitation to indirect inguinal hernia of the "congenital" type (even if it appears late in life).

Remember:

1) Normal descent of the testis does not ensure normal closure of the processus vaginalis.

2) With the cranial part partially open, a hydrocele may develop.

3) If the midportion of the processus vaginalis is unclosed, a cyst may develop.

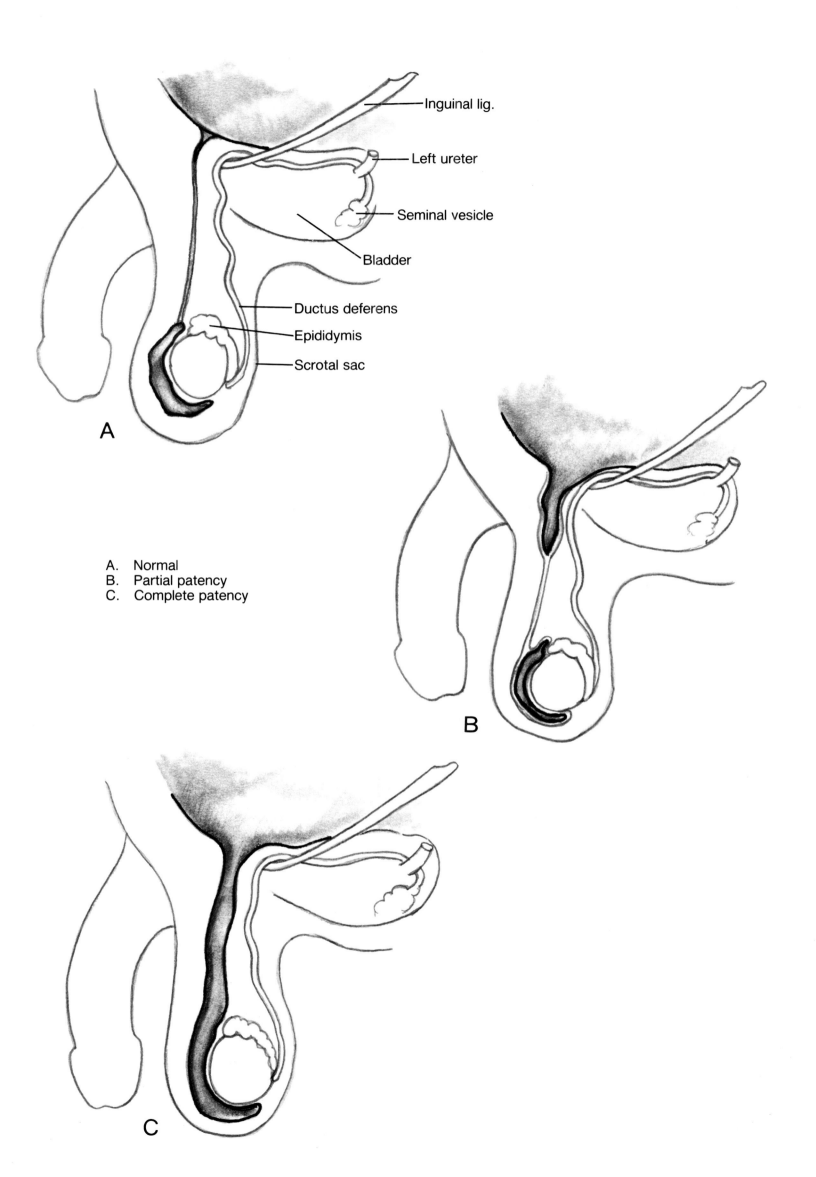

Inguinal lig.

Left ureter

Seminal vesicle

Bladder

Ductus deferens

Epididymis

Scrotal sac

A

A. Normal
B. Partial patency
C. Complete patency

B

C

PLATE 12-3
Descent of the Testes

A. The testes are entering the internal inguinal ring. The scrotal ligaments (gubernacula) connect the lower poles with the bottom of the scrotal sacs.

B. The right testis is in the inguinal canal. On the left, the processus vaginalis is opened to show its relation to the testis.

C. Both testes have descended, the gubernacula have almost vanished. The left processus is still open into the abdominal cavity. Normal closure (see Plate 12-2A) will follow.

Remember:

1) The lymphatics of the testes, epididymis, ductus deferens and tunica vaginalis drain to the periaortic nodes with frequent crossover to the opposite side.

2) The blood supply of the testicle:
  (a) Main
    (i) testicular artery ⎫
    (ii) deferential artery ⎭ anastomoses are always present
  (b) Secondary
    (i) cremasteric
    (ii) posterior scrotal
    (iii) external pudendal

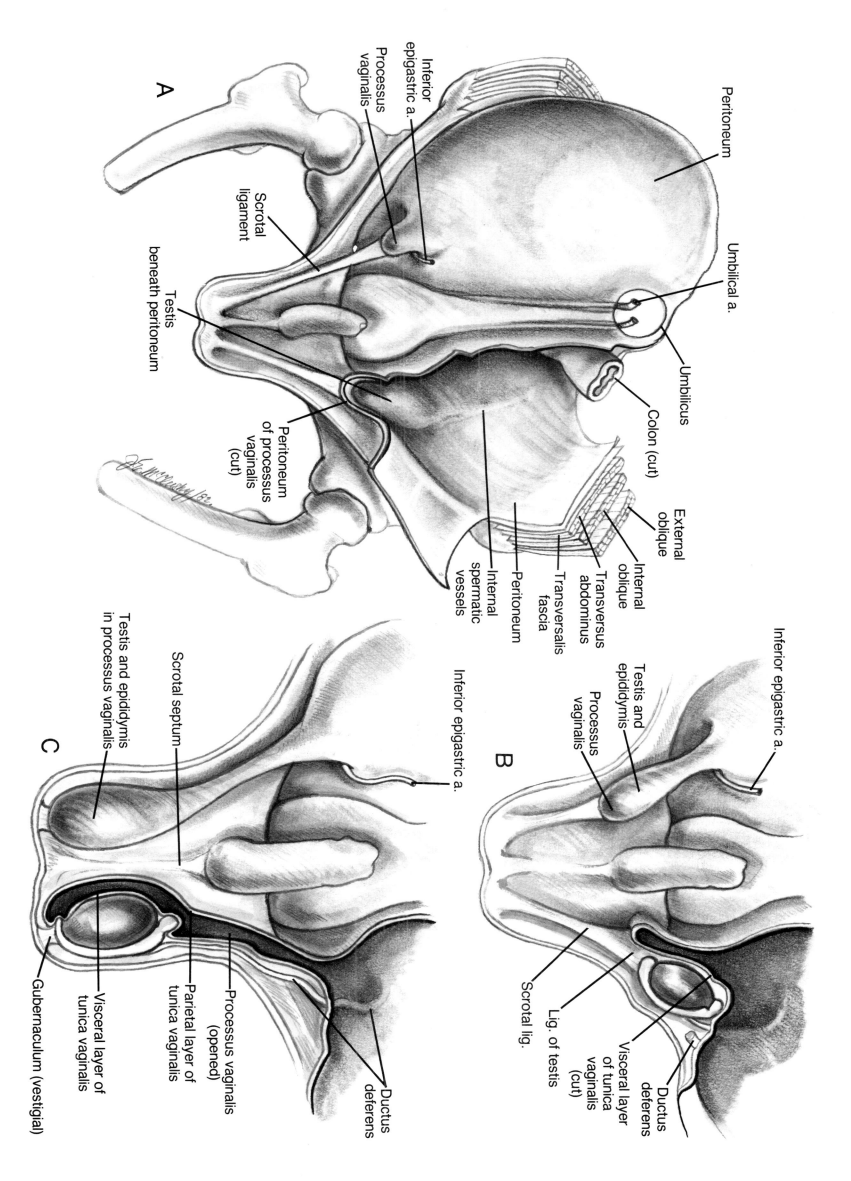

A

Peritoneum

Umbilical a.

Umbilicus

Colon (cut)

Inferior
epigastric a.

Processus
vaginalis

Scrotal
ligament

Testis
beneath peritoneum

Peritoneum
of processus
vaginalis
(cut)

External
oblique

Internal
oblique

Transversus
abdominus

Transversalis
fascia

Peritoneum

Internal
spermatic
vessels

B

Inferior epigastric a.

Testis and
epididymis

Processus
vaginalis

Inferior epigastric a.

Scrotal lig.

Lig. of testis

Visceral
layer
of tunica
vaginalis
(cut)

Ductus
deferens

C

Testis and epididymis
in processus vaginalis

Scrotal septum

Gubernaculum (vestigial)

Visceral layer of
tunica vaginalis

Parietal layer of
tunica vaginalis

Processus
vaginalis
(opened)

Ductus
deferens

PLATE 12-4
Undescended and Maldescended Testes

A. Maldescended (ectopic) testes. Retained testes not in the normal path of descent. Perineal ectopia is not shown. Most undescended and ectopic testes are not functional.

B. Undescended testes. Percentage of testes arrested along the normal path of descent. The great majority are retained in the inguinal canal.

Remember:

1) Scarpa's fascia is well developed and may be mistaken for the aponeurosis of the external oblique muscle. Therefore, the diagnosis of absent testis is wrong because the surgeon did not open the inguinal canal.

2) A CT scan preferably, or if not available a gonadal venogram, will be useful for localization of the testis.

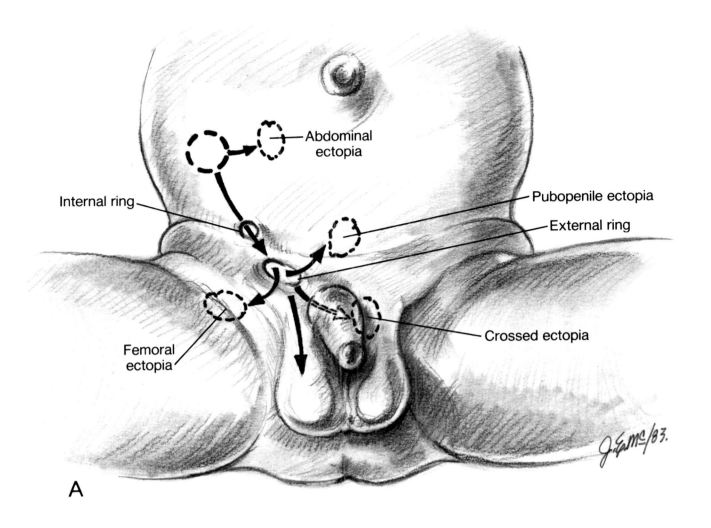

A

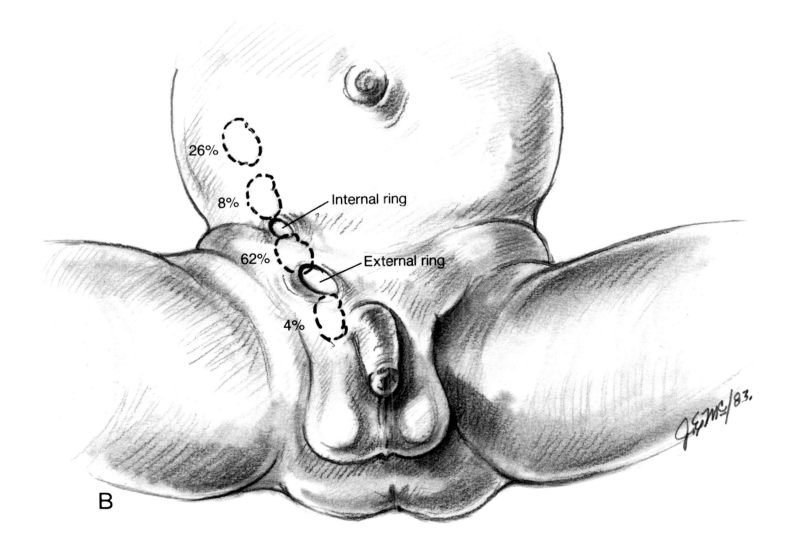

B

PLATE 12-5
Epididymectomy

A. Branches of the testicular artery.

B. Dissection of the epididymis. An epididymal branch of the testicular artery is revealed. The testicular artery bifurcates at the upper one third of the testicle into a medial (testicular) branch and a lateral (epididymal) branch. The latter gives off a superior (epididymal) and an inferior (testicular) branch. The branch to the testis must be preserved; the branch to the epididymis may be ligated. Dissection should start at the lower pole of the testis and stop 2.5 cm above the lower pole to avoid this testicular branch. The length of the epididymis is 4 cm.

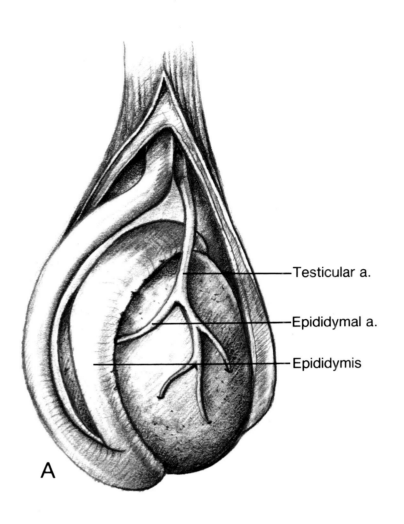

Testicular a.

Epididymal a.

Epididymis

A

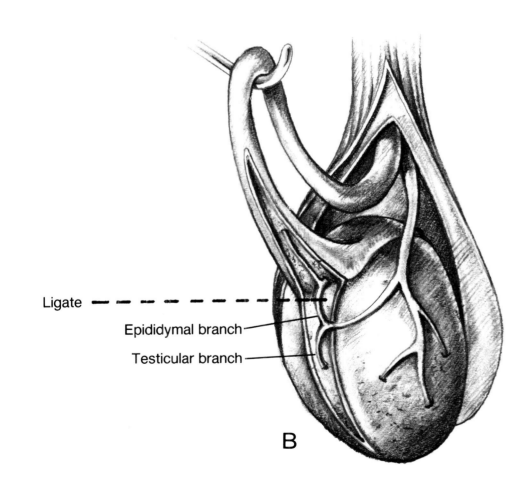

Ligate

Epididymal branch

Testicular branch

B

PLATE 13-1
The Inferior Vena Cava and Its Tributaries

The inferior vena cava begins with the junction of the right and left common iliac veins at the level of the fifth lumbar vertebra, and ends in the right atrium of the heart.

The vena cava in its upward course receives blood from three sources: (1) Lumbar veins from the body wall (see Plate 13-3); (2) Veins of the three paired glands: (gonads, kidneys and adrenals); (3) Hepatic veins and inferior phrenic veins.

Remember:

There are no valves in the inferior vena cava or the common iliac veins that form it. One valve in the external iliac vein is present in 80% of subjects.

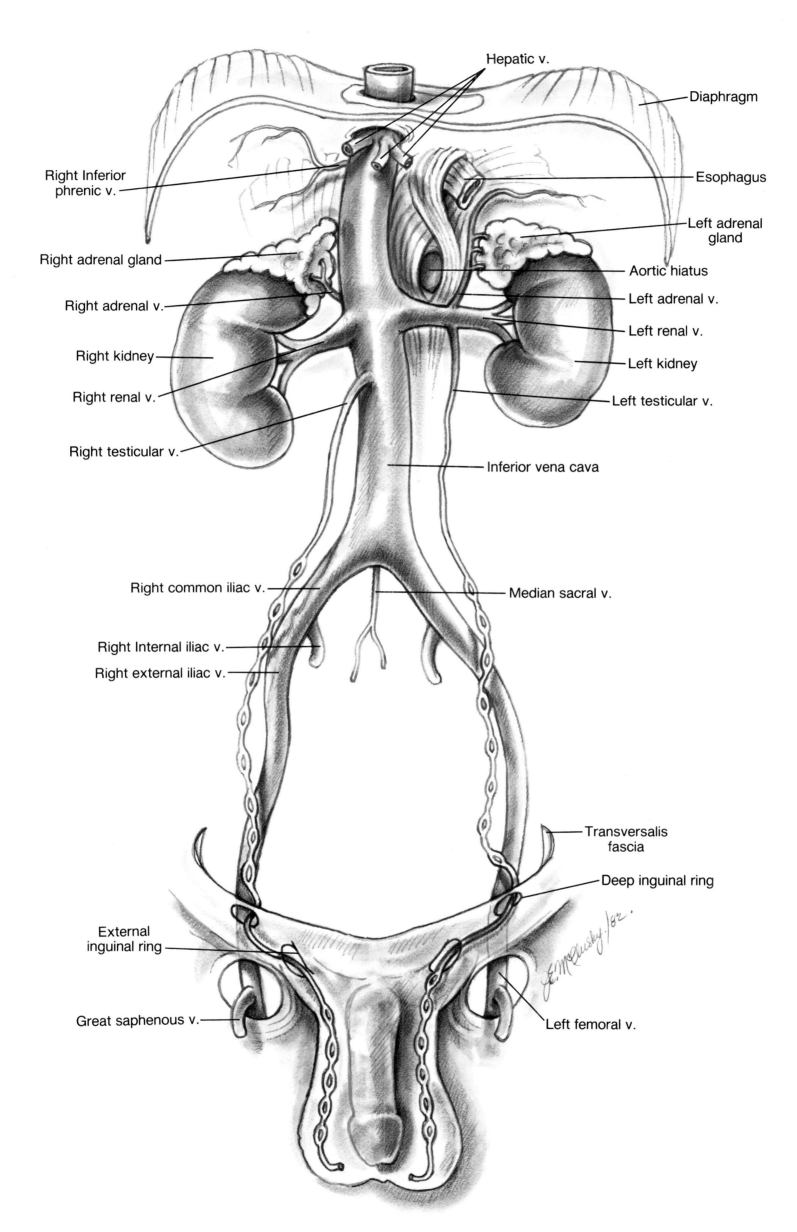

Hepatic v.

Diaphragm

Right Inferior phrenic v.

Esophagus

Left adrenal gland

Right adrenal gland

Aortic hiatus

Right adrenal v.

Left adrenal v.

Left renal v.

Right kidney

Left kidney

Right renal v.

Left testicular v.

Right testicular v.

Inferior vena cava

Right common iliac v.

Median sacral v.

Right Internal iliac v.

Right external iliac v.

Transversalis fascia

Deep inguinal ring

External inguinal ring

Great saphenous v.

Left femoral v.

PLATE 13-2
The Inferior Vena Cava at the Diaphragm

A. Diagram of the relations of the inferior vena cava to the esophagus and aorta at the diaphragm. The right inferior phrenic vein enters the inferior vena cava; the left phrenic vein may enter the vena cava, the adrenal vein or both (see Plate 3-8A).

B. An anomalous double inferior vein is found in 2 to 3% of individuals. In the case illustrated, the right vessel is the larger and receives all of the lumbar veins.

  A single, left-sided vena cava is less common, but not unknown. These anomalies are always associated with septation defects of the heart. Left-sided and double inferior cava are usually the result of a persistent left embryonic subcardinal vein, or the persistence of both embryonic supracardinal veins.

C. Relations of the inferior vena cava to the aorta, celiac trunk, superior mesenteric artery and the renal vein.

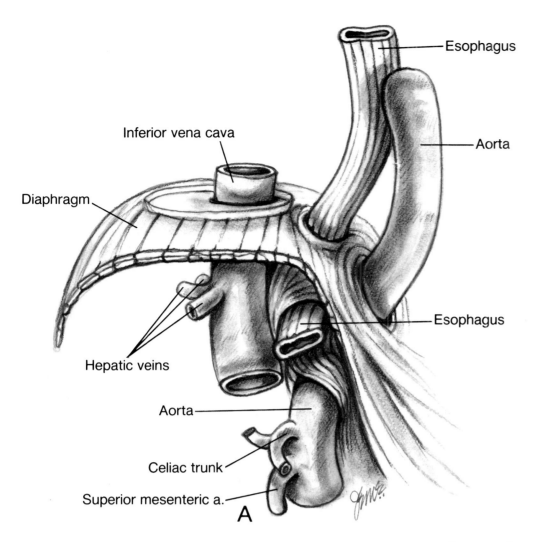

Esophagus

Inferior vena cava

Aorta

Diaphragm

Esophagus

Hepatic veins

Aorta

Celiac trunk

Superior mesenteric a.

A

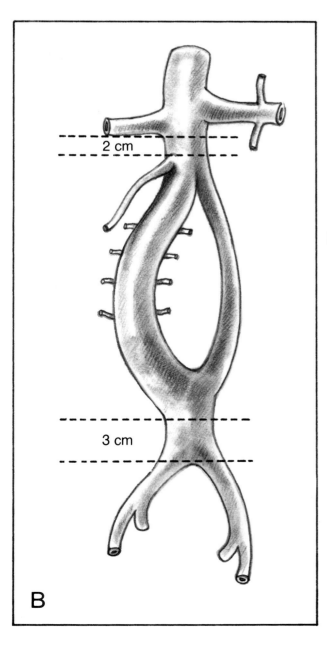

2 cm

3 cm

B

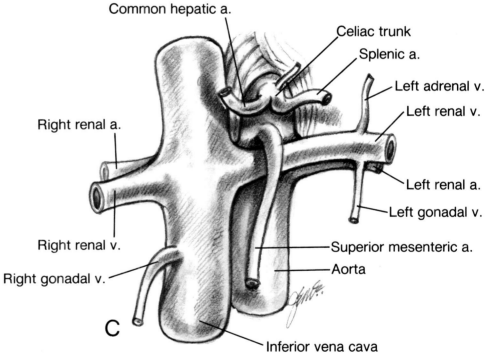

Common hepatic a.

Celiac trunk

Splenic a.

Left adrenal v.

Left renal v.

Right renal a.

Left renal a.

Left gonadal v.

Right renal v.

Superior mesenteric a.

Right gonadal v.

Aorta

C

Inferior vena cava

PLATE 13-3
Diagram of the Inferior Vena Cava with Measurements

A. Anterior view of the inferior vena cava. It may be ligated about 3 cm above the bifurcation or 1 cm below the right renal vein. In the latter procedure, the ligature must lie between the right renal vein and the gonadal vein. Collateral circulation after ligation is by way of the lumbar veins, the vertebral veins and the azygos vein. The left gonadal vein must be ligated.

The inferior vena cava may be divided into a infrarenal segment (purple) and an iliofemoral segment (dark blue). The measurements of distances between landmarks are averages.

B and C. The lumbar veins enter the vena cava posteriorly, never laterally or anteriorly. They may be paired (50%), or unpaired (50%). If paired, they may join to form a common trunk before entering the posterior side of the vena cava (25%).

D. The inferior vena cava showing the sites of entrance of 591 lumbar veins observed in 132 cadavers. Note that the right gonadal vein itself is a segmental lumbar vein.

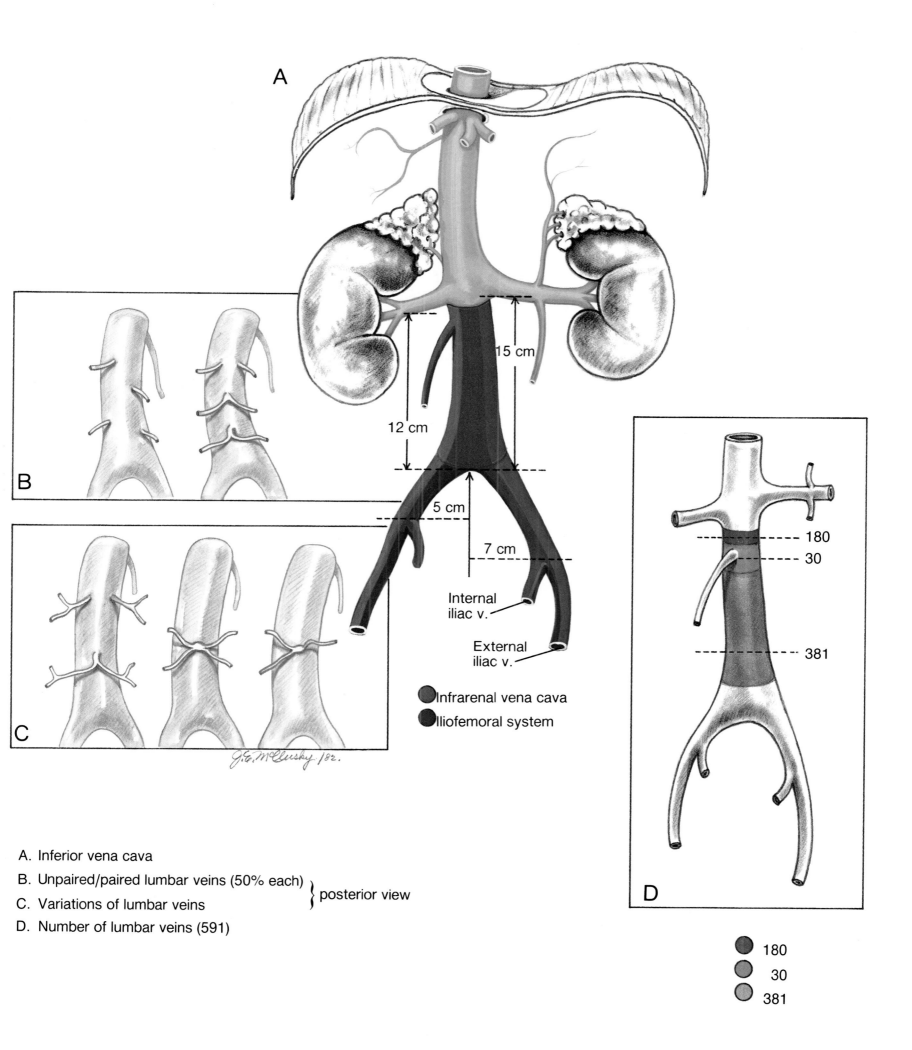

A

B

15 cm

12 cm

5 cm

7 cm

Internal
iliac v.

External
iliac v.

C

● Infrarenal vena cava
● Iliofemoral system

D

180
30

381

J.E. McClusky '82.

A. Inferior vena cava

B. Unpaired/paired lumbar veins (50% each) ⎫
                                             ⎬ posterior view
C. Variations of lumbar veins   ⎭

D. Number of lumbar veins (591)

● 180
● 30
● 381

PLATE 13-4
Superficial Veins of the Thigh and Leg

A. Anterior aspect of the thigh. The superficial tributaries of the femoral vein. Superficial veins of the lower limb are numerous and variable. They lie in the superficial fascia beneath the skin. It is not practical to name more than a few of the larger, more constant vessels.

B. The superficial veins of the thigh and leg communicate with the deep veins by valved venous shunts (perforating veins) that pass through the deep fascia. The largest of these shunts are the superior ends of the greater and lesser saphenous veins.

In addition to the saphenous shunts, there are several smaller shunts in the thigh and leg. The most constant of these are the "direct" perforating veins: (1) in the lower portion of the thigh, a vein connects the greater saphenous or a tributary with the femoral vein in the adductor canal, (2) in the leg, just below the knee, a vein connects the greater saphenous with the posterior tibial vein, (3) on the lateral side of the leg at the junction of the middle and lower thirds, a vein connects the lesser saphenous vein with the peroneal vein, and (4) in the lower portion of the leg, three medial perforating veins connect the greater saphenous or the posterior arch vein with the posterior tibial vein.

Numerous small, inconstant "indirect" perforating veins pass through the deep fascia to the cavenous plexus in the muscles of the thigh and leg. From these muscles, blood drains into the deep veins.

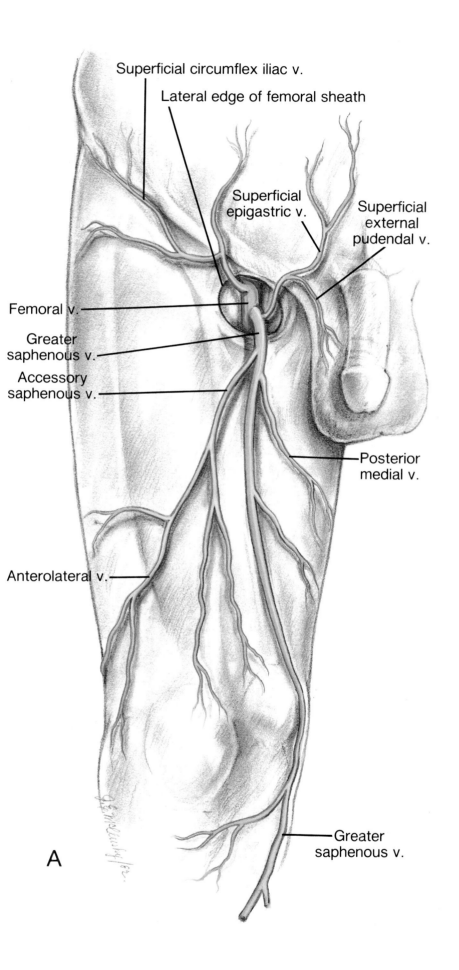

Superficial circumflex iliac v.

Lateral edge of femoral sheath

Superficial epigastric v.

Superficial external pudendal v.

Femoral v.

Greater saphenous v.

Accessory saphenous v.

Posterior medial v.

Anterolateral v.

Greater saphenous v.

A

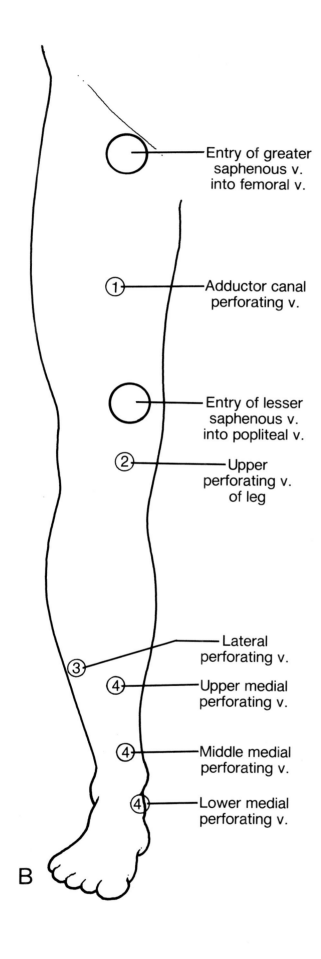

Entry of greater saphenous v. into femoral v.

① Adductor canal perforating v.

Entry of lesser saphenous v. into popliteal v.

② Upper perforating v. of leg

Lateral perforating v.

③

④ Upper medial perforating v.

④ Middle medial perforating v.

④ Lower medial perforating v.

B

PLATE 13-5
Superficial Veins and Nerves of the Leg

A. Anterior aspect of the leg.

B. Medial aspect of the leg.

C. Posterolateral aspect of the leg.

D. Direct perforating veins arise from tributaries of the superficial veins and pass through the fascia to enter the deep veins. Valves are present in the perforating, deep and superficial veins.

E. Indirect perforating veins arise from the superficial venous plexus, pass through the fascia and enter the venous plexus of the underlying muscles. This plexus drains to the deep veins.

Remember:

1) Protect the nerves associated with the veins: the saphenous nerve accompanies the greater saphenous vein, the sural nerve accompanies the lesser saphenous vein, the posterior cutaneous nerve accompanies the lesser saphenous vein in the popliteal area.

2) Be sure to ligate all perforating veins and obvious tributary veins. Sparing the lesser saphenous vein may permit recurrence of varicosities.

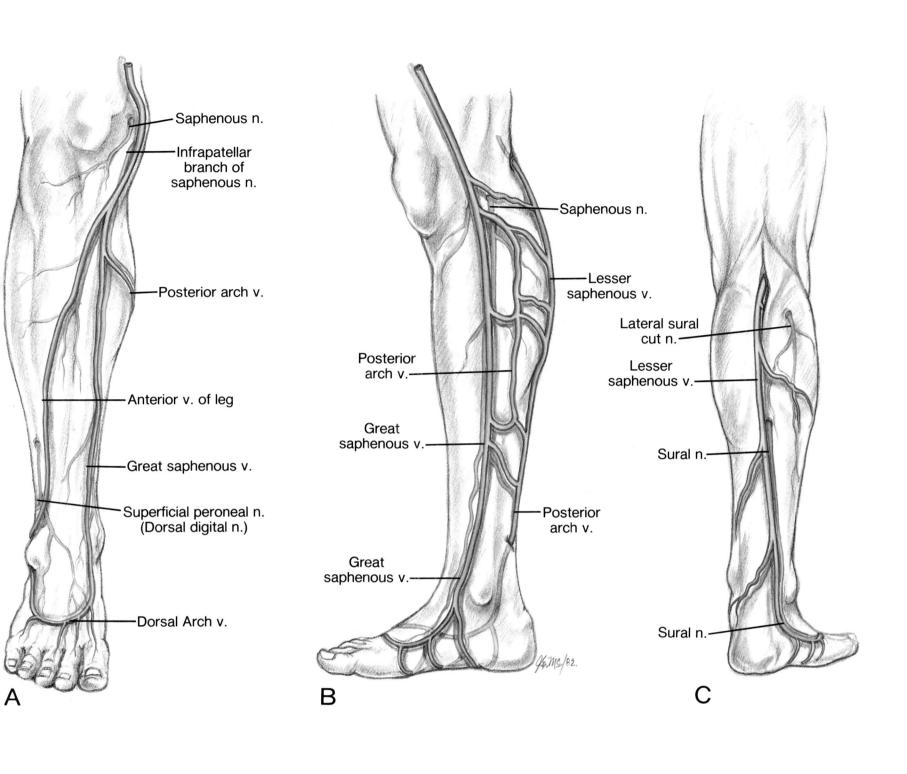

A

Saphenous n.

Infrapatellar branch of saphenous n.

Posterior arch v.

Anterior v. of leg

Great saphenous v.

Superficial peroneal n. (Dorsal digital n.)

Dorsal Arch v.

B

Saphenous n.

Lesser saphenous v.

Posterior arch v.

Great saphenous v.

Posterior arch v.

Great saphenous v.

C

Lateral sural cut n.

Lesser saphenous v.

Sural n.

Sural n.

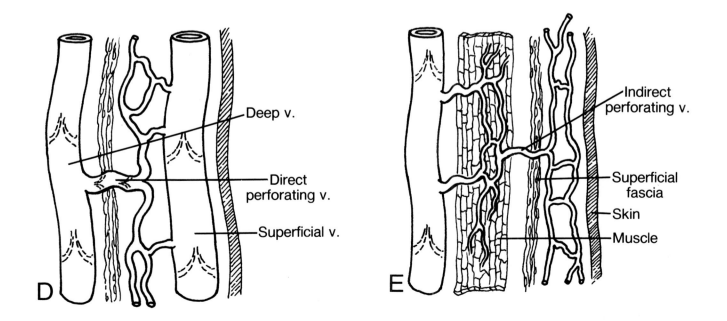

D

Deep v.

Direct perforating v.

Superficial v.

E

Indirect perforating v.

Superficial fascia

Skin

Muscle

PLATE 14-1
The Inguinal Region I

A. The skin has been removed to show the superficial external pudendal, superficial circum-flex and superficial epigastric arteries and their origin from the femoral artery.

B. The skin, superficial fascia (Camper's and Scarpa's) and aponeurosis of the external oblique muscle have been removed to reveal the internal oblique muscle.

Remember:

1) Some of these vessels may be too large for electrocoagulation. They should be ligated to avoid postoperative inguinal or scrotal hematoma during herniorrhaphy.

2) In the inguinal region, the internal oblique is muscular and the transversus abdominis is aponeurotic.

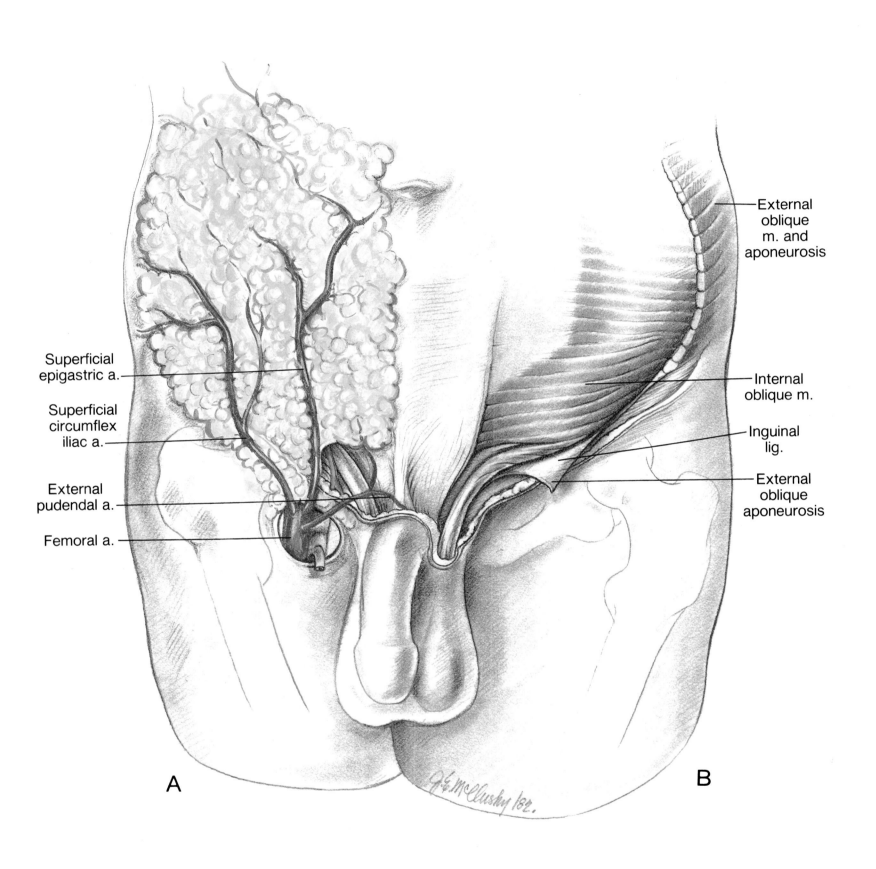

Superficial
epigastric a.

Superficial
circumflex
iliac a.

External
pudendal a.

Femoral a.

A

External
oblique
m. and
aponeurosis

Internal
oblique m.

Inguinal
lig.

External
oblique
aponeurosis

B

PLATE 14-2
The Inguinal Region II

A. Relations of the external inguinal ring and spermatic cord are shown.

B. The external oblique aponeurosis is cut to show the inferior border of the internal oblique muscle, and the ilioinguinal nerve. The inguinal ligament is reflected laterally and the external oblique aponeurosis is reflected medially.

Remember:

The inguinal canal is 4 to 5 cm long, located just above the inguinal ligament. The canal has four walls and two openings:

Anterior wall	Aponeurosis of external oblique muscle; lateral one third of internal oblique muscle.
Posterior wall (floor)	Lateral portion of fused aponeurosis of the transversus abdominis muscle and the transversalis fascia. Medial portion of transversalis fascia and the conjoined tendon area (see Plate 14-3).
Superior wall (roof)	Lower edge (arched fibers) of the internal oblique muscle and the transversus abdominis muscle and aponeurosis.
Inferior wall	Inguinal and lacunar ligaments.
Internal inguinal ring	Opening through the transversalis fascia.
External inguinal ring	Opening in the aponeurosis of the external oblique muscle.

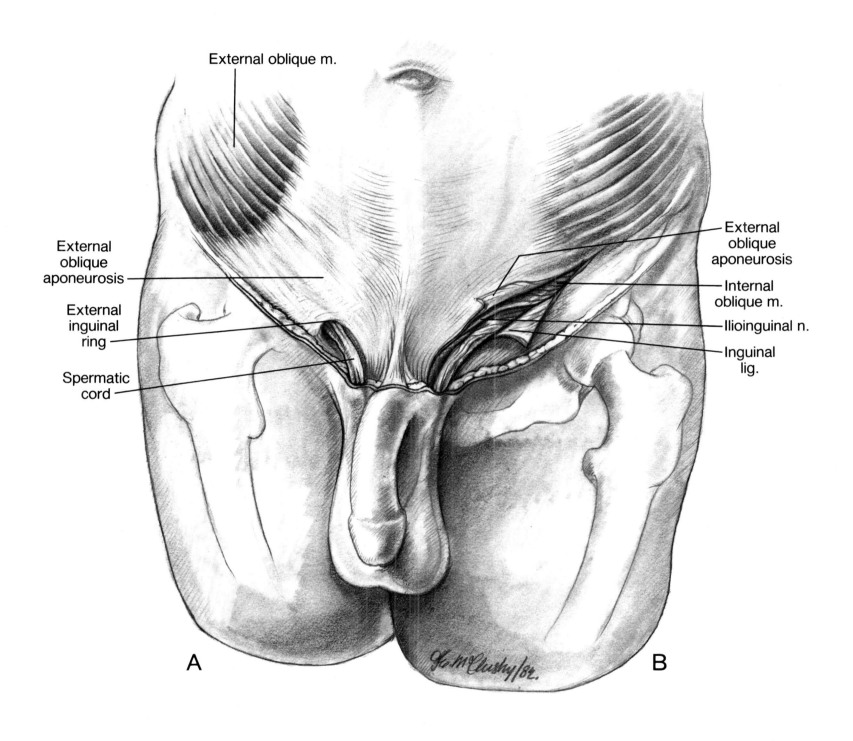

External oblique m.

External oblique aponeurosis

External inguinal ring

Spermatic cord

External oblique aponeurosis

Internal oblique m.

Ilioinguinal n.

Inguinal lig.

A

B

PLATE 14-3
The Inguinal Region III

A. The "conjoined area" of the inguinal region.

Inset: The conjoined area contains the transversus abdominis aponeurosis, inferior fibers of internal oblique muscle or aponeurosis, the lateral border of the rectus sheath, the reflected inguinal ligament, and the ligament of Henle.

The concept of the "conjoined area" must replace that of the "conjoined tendon" of older surgeons and anatomists. The "tendon" is defined as the fusion of lower fibers of the internal oblique aponeurosis with similar fibers from the aponeurosis of the transversus abdominis as they insert on the pubic tubercle and superior ramus of the pubis. This configuration, easily described but rarely encountered, is present in fewer than 5% of individuals. For practical purposes the conjoined tendon does not exist.

B. Hesselbach's triangle (purple), the site of direct inguinal hernia. The medial border of the triangle is related to the lateral border of the rectus abdominis, the site of supravesical hernia.

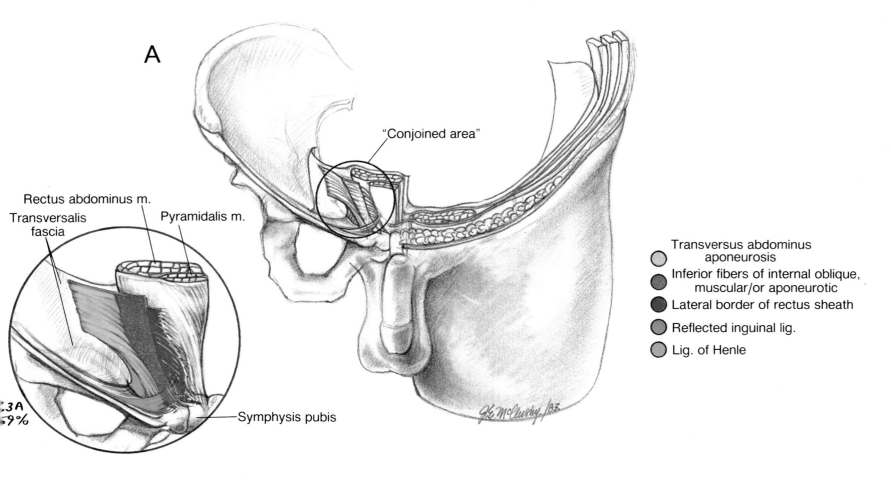

A

"Conjoined area"

Rectus abdominus m.
Transversalis fascia
Pyramidalis m.

3A
9%

Symphysis pubis

Transversus abdominus aponeurosis
Inferior fibers of internal oblique, muscular/or aponeurotic
Lateral border of rectus sheath
Reflected inguinal lig.
Lig. of Henle

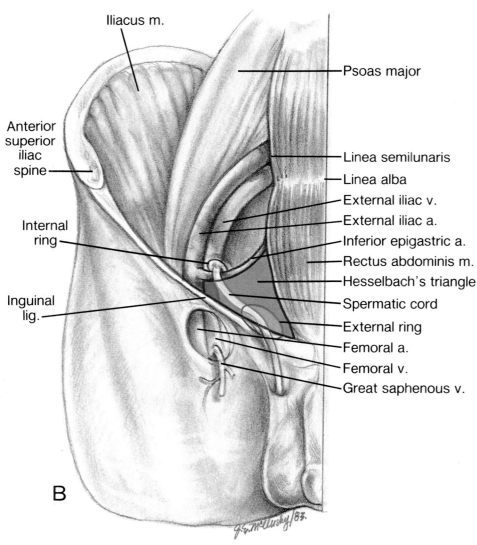

Iliacus m.

Psoas major

Anterior superior iliac spine

Linea semilunaris
Linea alba
External iliac v.
External iliac a.
Inferior epigastric a.
Rectus abdominis m.
Hesselbach's triangle
Spermatic cord
External ring
Femoral a.
Femoral v.
Great saphenous v.

Internal ring

Inguinal lig.

B

PLATE 14-4
The Inguinal Region IV

The left half of the figure shows the typical arrangement of structures seen when the external oblique muscle and aponeurosis are removed. The internal oblique and transversus abdominis muscles are visible.

The right half of the drawing is an atypical arrangement of the same structures.

Inset: The inguinal canal and its contents.

Remember:

The inguinal canal in the male contains the spermatic cord and its coverings:

Three Fasciae	External spermatic (from external oblique muscle)
	Cremasteric (from internal oblique and transversus abdominis muscles)
	Internal spermatic (from transversalis fascia)
Three Arteries	Testicular artery
	Cremasteric artery
	Deferential artery
Three Veins	Pampiniform plexus and testicular vein
	Cremasteric vein
	Deferential vein
Three Nerves (See Plate 14-7,8)	Genitofemoral nerve
	Ilioinguinal nerve
	Sympathetic and parasympathetic nerves (testicular plexus)
Lymphatics	

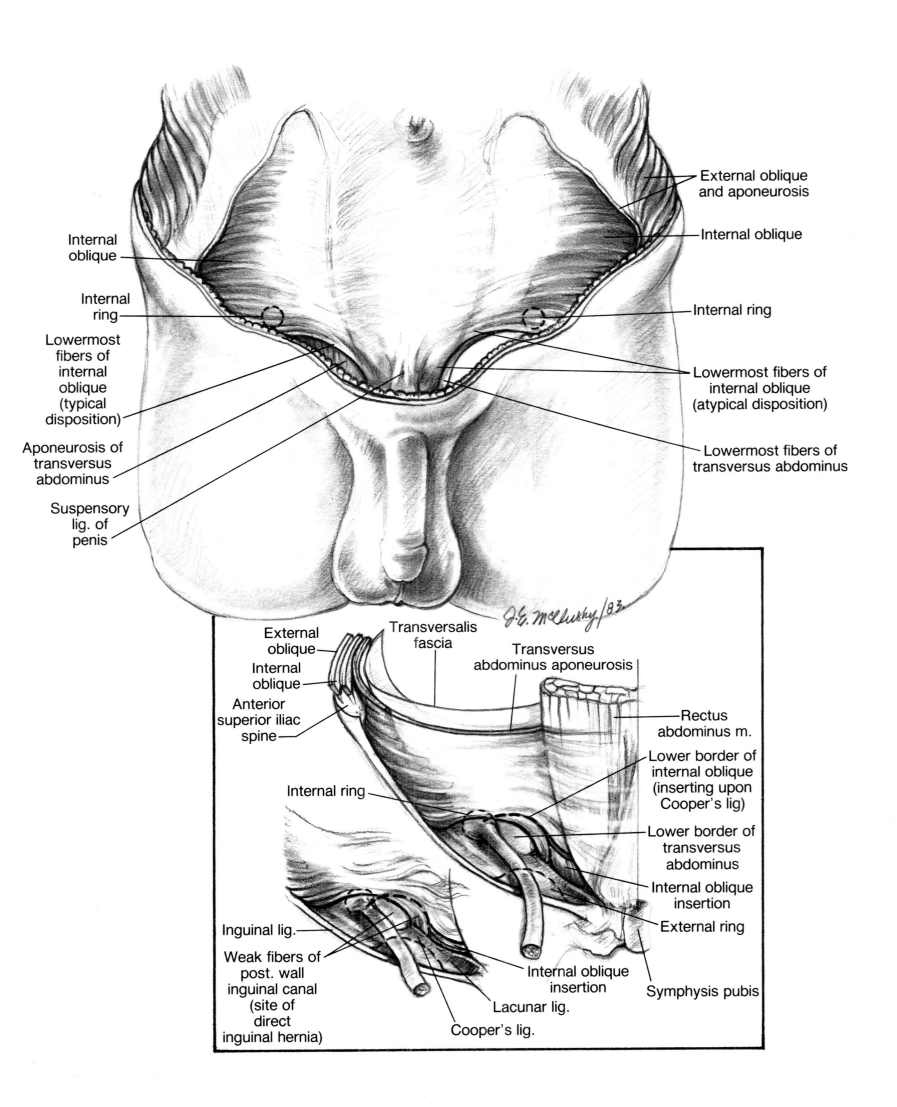

Internal
oblique

Internal
ring

Lowermost
fibers of
internal
oblique
(typical
disposition)

Aponeurosis of
transversus
abdominus

Suspensory
lig. of
penis

External oblique
and aponeurosis

Internal oblique

Internal ring

Lowermost fibers of
internal oblique
(atypical disposition)

Lowermost fibers of
transversus abdominus

J.E. McClusky/83.

External
oblique

Internal
oblique

Anterior
superior iliac
spine

Transversalis
fascia

Transversus
abdominus aponeurosis

Rectus
abdominus m.

Lower border of
internal oblique
(inserting upon
Cooper's lig)

Internal ring

Lower border of
transversus
abdominus

Internal oblique
insertion

External ring

Inguinal lig.

Weak fibers of
post. wall
inguinal canal
(site of
direct
inguinal hernia)

Internal oblique
insertion

Lacunar lig.

Cooper's lig.

Symphysis pubis

PLATE 14-5
The Inguinal Region V

A. The normal anatomy of the posterior wall of the inguinal canal.

B. Direct inguinal hernia. Note the iliopubic tract.

Inset: The femoral sheath and its contents.

Remember:

1) The posterior wall (floor) of the inguinal canal is formed by fusion of the transversalis fascia and the aponeurosis of the transversus abdominis muscle.

2) The most important layer of the abdominal wall is the transversus abdominis muscle and aponeurosis.

3) The spermatic cord is covered by the external spermatic fascia only distal to the external inguinal ring.

4) The inguinal ligament is the lower edge of the external oblique aponeurosis. There are no muscles that insert or originate from the inguinal ligament; the internal oblique and transversus abdominis muscles are but fellow travelers. The internal oblique muscle is related to the lateral half of the inguinal ligament. The transversus abdominis muscle is related to the lateral one third of the ligament; both muscles arise from the iliopsoas fascia.

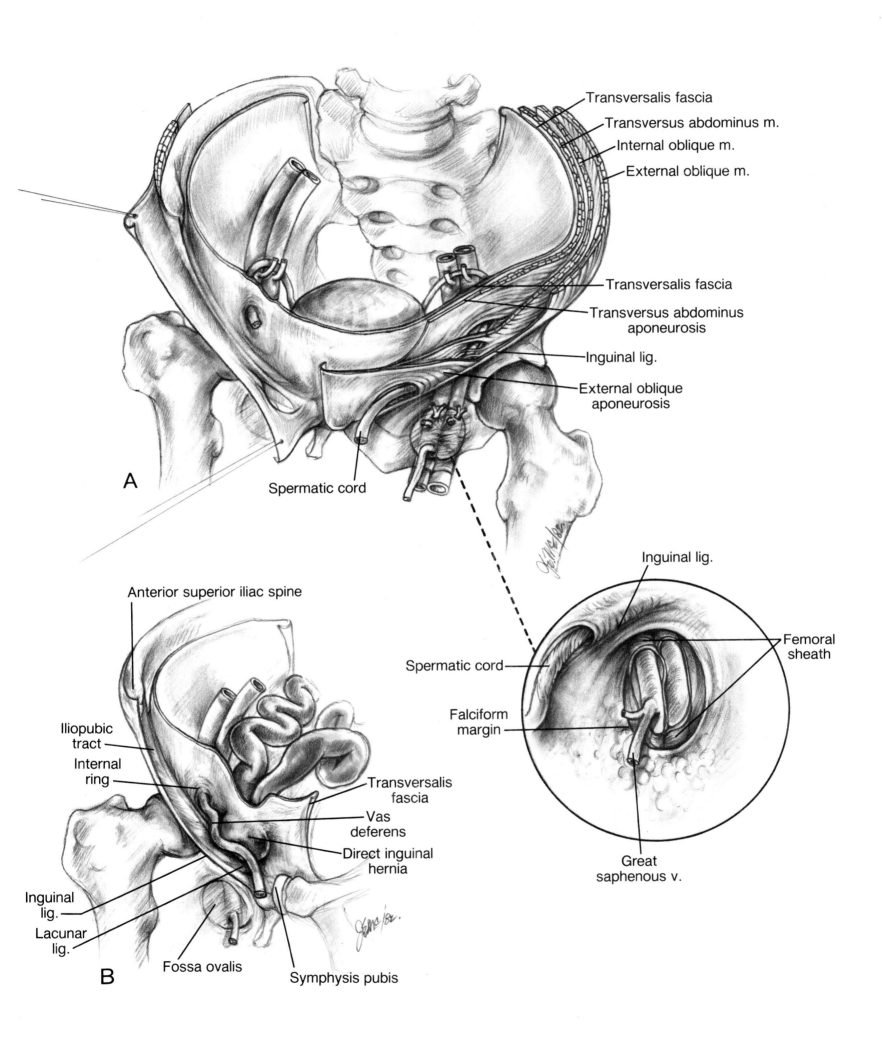

Transversalis fascia

Transversus abdominus m.

Internal oblique m.

External oblique m.

Transversalis fascia

Transversus abdominus aponeurosis

Inguinal lig.

External oblique aponeurosis

Spermatic cord

A

Inguinal lig.

Spermatic cord

Femoral sheath

Falciform margin

Great saphenous v.

Anterior superior iliac spine

Iliopubic tract

Internal ring

Transversalis fascia

Vas deferens

Direct inguinal hernia

Inguinal lig.

Lacunar lig.

Fossa ovalis

Symphysis pubis

B

PLATE 14-6
The Inguinal Region VI

A. Femoral hernia. The fossa ovalis is the site of femoral hernias. The femoral canal, just under the medial end of the inguinal ligament, is 1.5 to 2.5 cm long and lies in the pectineal fascia. It opens into the peritoneal cavity as the femoral ring. The boundaries of the ring are: (1) Anterior: inguinal ligament, iliopubic tract, or both; (2) Posterior: pectineal ligament (of Cooper); (3) Medial: lacunar ligament; (4) Lateral: femoral vein.

Remember:

The femoral sheath is an extension of the transversalis fascia which encloses the femoral artery, vein and the femoral canal.

B. Indirect inguinal hernias. Incarceration may occur at either the internal or external ring. The external ring is a triangular opening of the aponeurosis of the external oblique muscle; the base is part of the pubic crest and the margins are formed by the two crura. The superior crus is the aponeurosis itself and the inferior crus is formed by the inguinal ligament.

Inset: An aberrant obturator artery may produce serious bleeding if the lacunar ligament is incised during herniorrhaphy.

C. Cross section of the spermatic cord containing an indirect hernial sac located between the pampiniform venous plexus (anterior) and the ductus deferens (posterior).

Remember:

If the indirect hernial sac reaches the scrotum, leave the distal part of the sac open in place to avoid hydrocele.

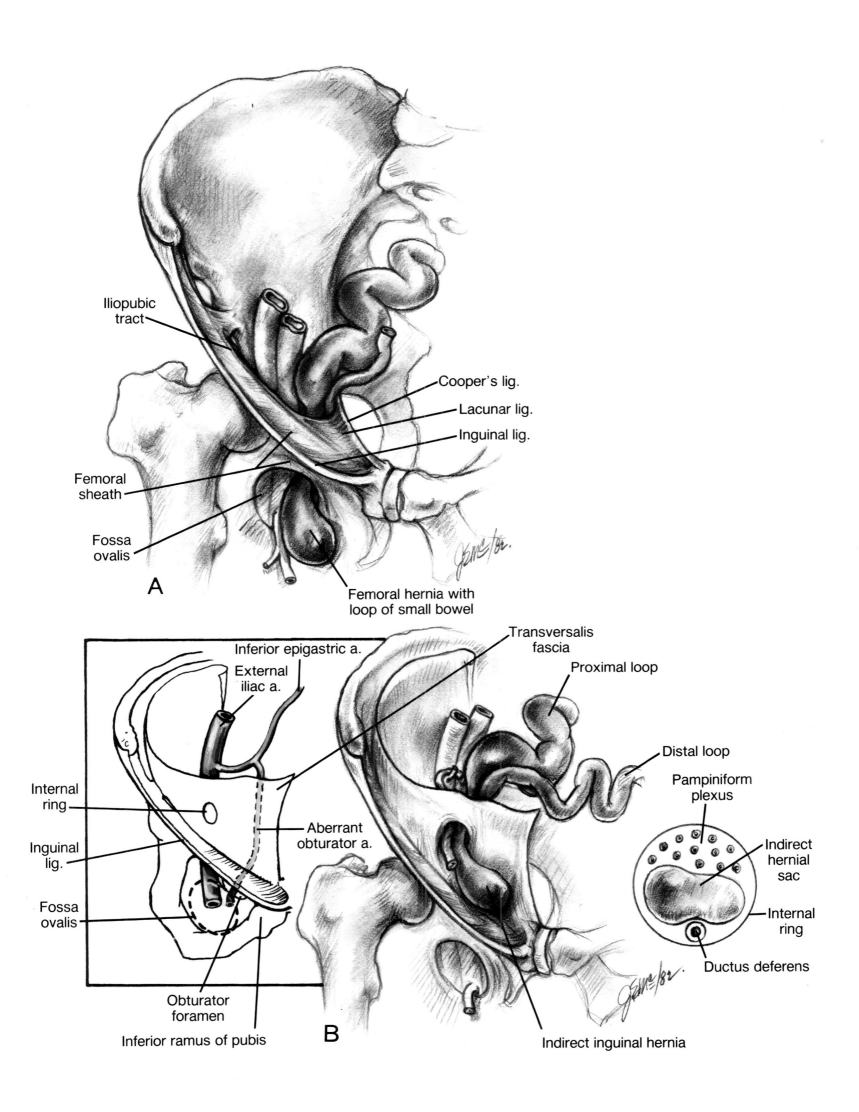

A

Iliopubic tract

Cooper's lig.

Lacunar lig.

Inguinal lig.

Femoral sheath

Fossa ovalis

Femoral hernia with loop of small bowel

B

Inferior epigastric a.

External iliac a.

Transversalis fascia

Proximal loop

Internal ring

Distal loop

Pampiniform plexus

Inguinal lig.

Aberrant obturator a.

Indirect hernial sac

Fossa ovalis

Internal ring

Obturator foramen

Ductus deferens

Inferior ramus of pubis

Indirect inguinal hernia

PLATE 14-7
Nerves of the Inguinal Region I
Nerves with which the surgeon should be familiar.

Nerve	Origin	Location	Structures Innervated
Genitofemoral	L_1–L_2	Genital branch in inguinal canal Femoral branch close to femoral artery under inguinal ligament	Cremaster muscle, skin of scrotum or labia Skin of upper part of thigh
Lateral femoral cutaneous	L_2–L_3	Anterior surface of iliacus muscle and under inguinal ligament (see also Plate 14–8)	Anterior branch to skin of lateral anterior thigh Posterior branch to skin of lateral posterior thigh
Ilioinguinal	L_1	Under fascia of external oblique muscle closely related to spermatic cord	Skin of upper medial thigh, root of penis, scrotum or labia majora
Iliohypogastric (not shown)	T_{12}–L_1	Under fascia of external oblique muscle	Skin of upper lateral thigh and over symphysis pubis

Remember:

Injury to these nerves by section or entrapment with sutures may produce pain or sensory loss in the areas of skin innervated.

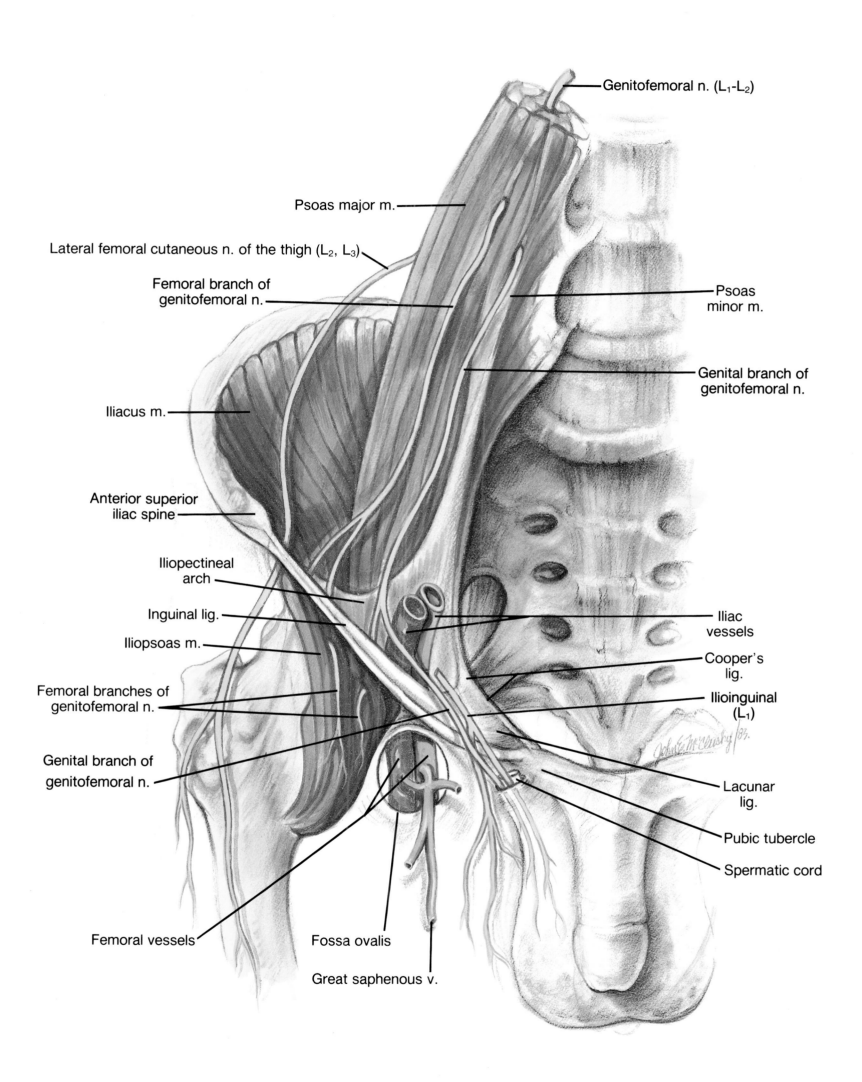

Genitofemoral n. (L$_1$-L$_2$)

Psoas major m.

Lateral femoral cutaneous n. of the thigh (L$_2$, L$_3$)

Femoral branch of genitofemoral n.

Psoas minor m.

Iliacus m.

Genital branch of genitofemoral n.

Anterior superior iliac spine

Iliopectineal arch

Inguinal lig.

Iliac vessels

Iliopsoas m.

Cooper's lig.

Femoral branches of genitofemoral n.

Ilioinguinal (L$_1$)

Genital branch of genitofemoral n.

Lacunar lig.

Pubic tubercle

Spermatic cord

Femoral vessels

Fossa ovalis

Great saphenous v.

PLATE 14-8
Nerves of the Inguinal Region II

Relations of the lateral femoral cutaneous nerve. Entrapment of this nerve may result in neuralgia, burning, tingling or numbness of the anterolateral aspect of the thigh.

Remember:

The lateral femoral cutaneous nerve arises from the second and third lumbar vertebrae nerves or as a branch of the femoral nerve. It travels downward across the iliac artery, penetrating the most lateral part of the inguinal ligament.

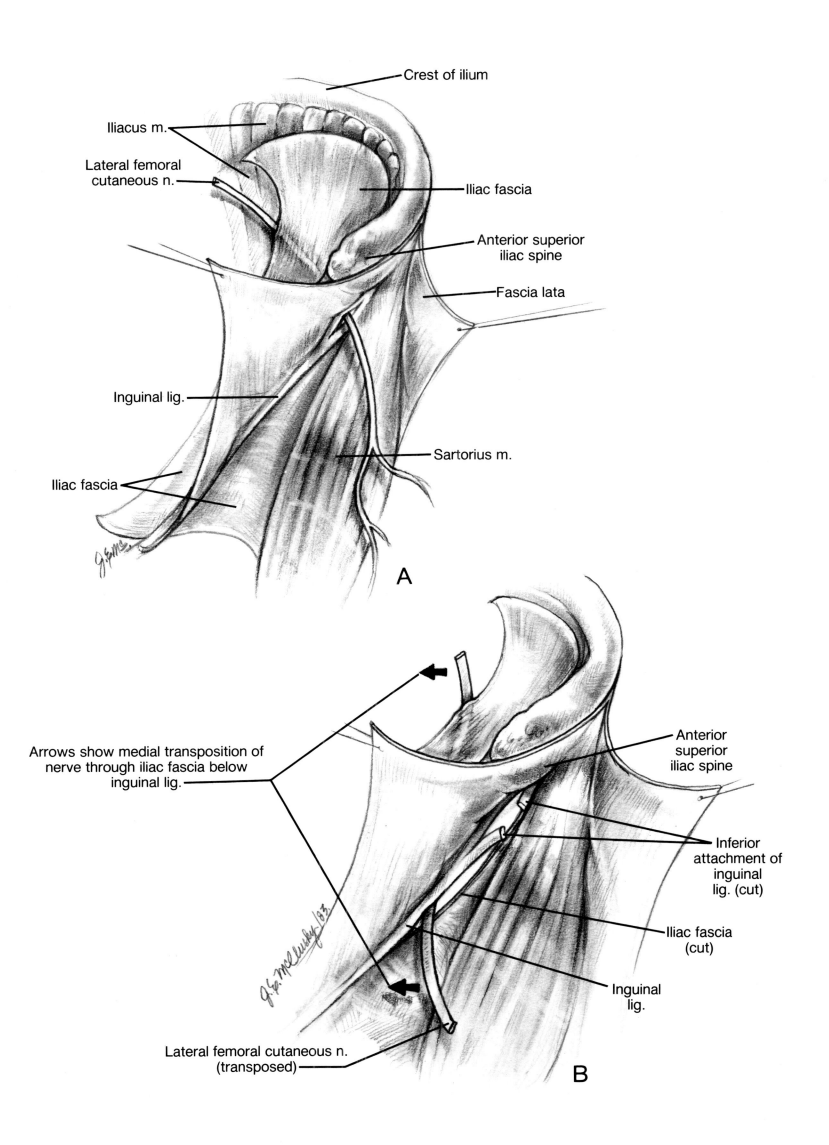

Crest of ilium

Iliacus m.

Lateral femoral
cutaneous n.

Iliac fascia

Anterior superior
iliac spine

Fascia lata

Inguinal lig.

Sartorius m.

Iliac fascia

A

Arrows show medial transposition of
nerve through iliac fascia below
inguinal lig.

Anterior
superior
iliac spine

Inferior
attachment of
inguinal
lig. (cut)

Iliac fascia
(cut)

Inguinal
lig.

Lateral femoral cutaneous n.
(transposed)

B

PLATE 14-9
Interparietal Hernia

This is a variety of indirect inguinal hernia. The sac enters the internal ring and may pass between any two layers of the abdominal wall. The sac may be single or multilocular, often with an indirect hernial component which emerges through the inguinal ring. The incision is that for an indirect inguinal hernia.

A. Properitoneal interparietal hernia. The sac lies between the peritoneum and transversus abdominis muscle.

B. Interstitial interparietal hernia. The sac lies between muscle layers of the abdominal wall. Arrowheads indicate other intermuscular planes through which herniation may take place.

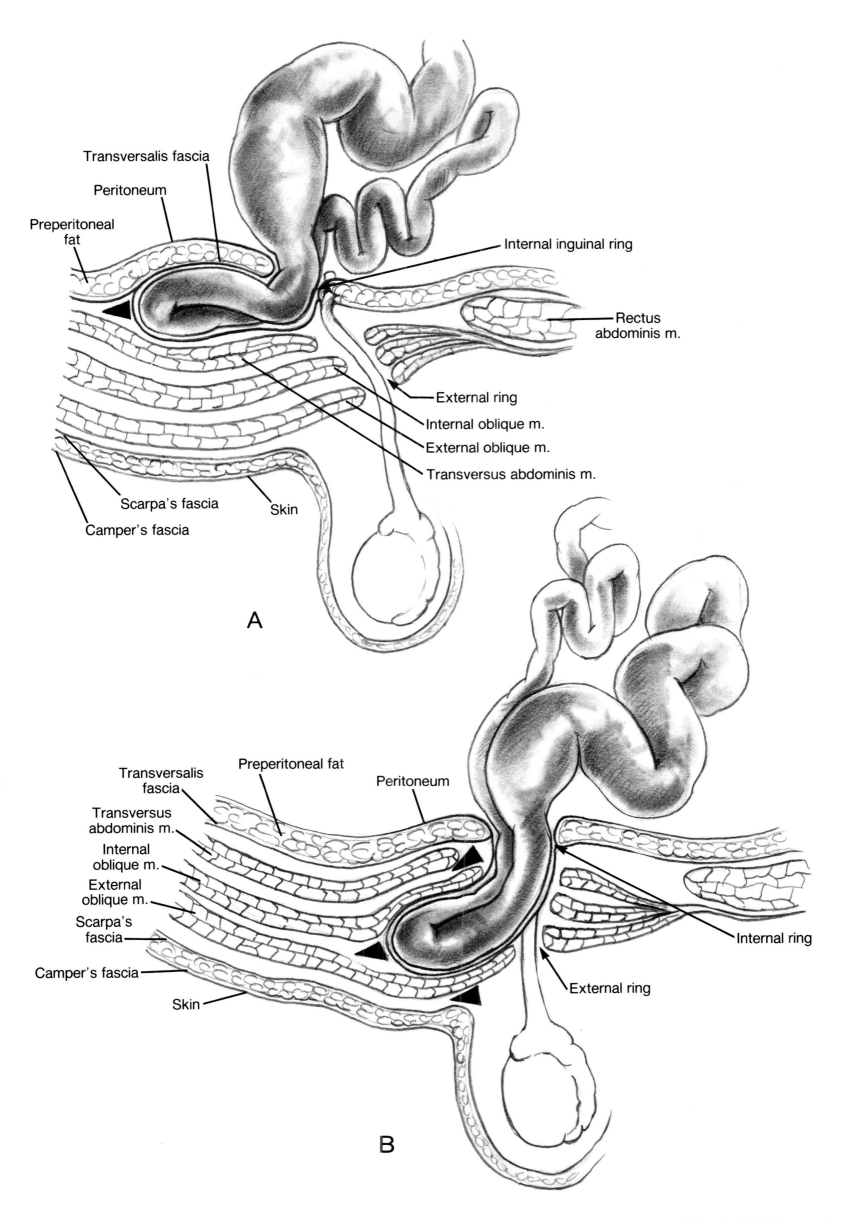

Transversalis fascia

Peritoneum

Preperitoneal fat

Internal inguinal ring

Rectus abdominis m.

External ring

Internal oblique m.

External oblique m.

Transversus abdominis m.

Scarpa's fascia

Skin

Camper's fascia

A

Transversalis fascia

Preperitoneal fat

Peritoneum

Transversus abdominis m.

Internal oblique m.

External oblique m.

Scarpa's fascia

Camper's fascia

Internal ring

External ring

Skin

B

PLATE 14-10
Supravesical Hernia I

The anterior abdominal wall is viewed from the posterior surface. An external supravesical hernia may pass in front of the bladder (prevesical), beside the bladder (paravesical) or behind the bladder (retrovesical). These hernias result from loss of integrity of the transversus abdominis muscle and the transversalis fascia. Most of these hernias pass downward as direct inguinal or femoral hernias and are termed *external* supravesical hernias.

About half of direct inguinal hernias originate in the supravesical fossa between the middle umbilical ligament and the medial umbilical fold.

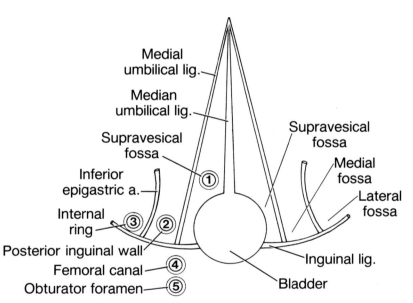

Diagram of the sites of groin hernias in relation to the anterior abdominal wall and the bladder.

1. indirect inguinal hernia
2. direct inguinal hernia
3. supravesical hernia
4. femoral hernia
5. obturator hernia

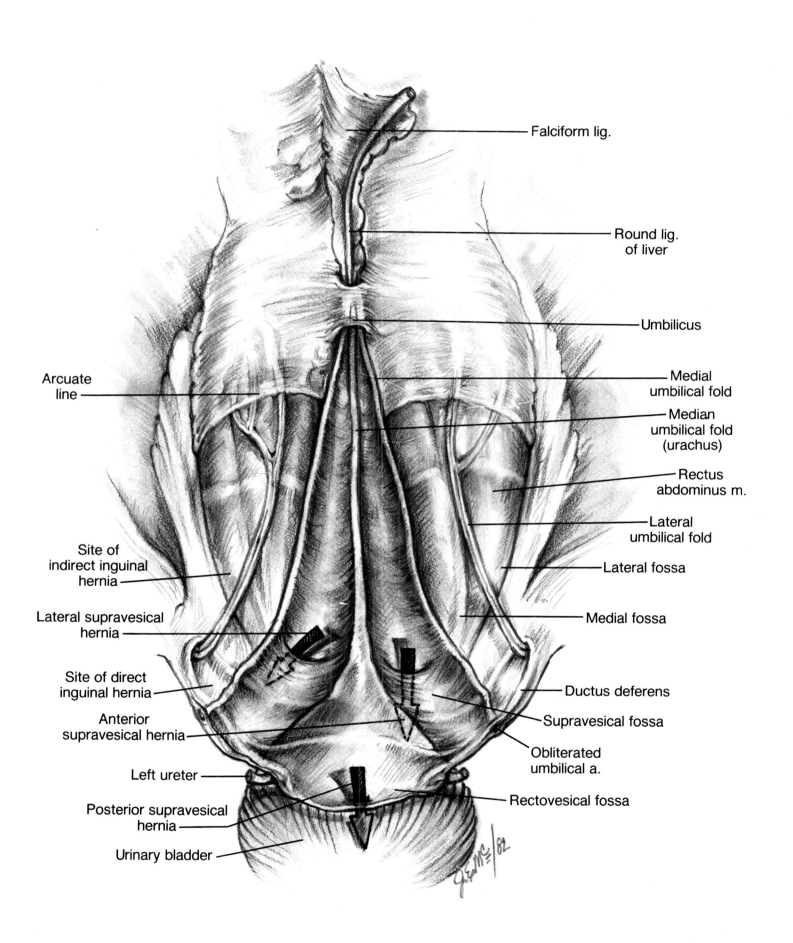

Falciform lig.

Round lig.
of liver

Umbilicus

Medial
umbilical fold

Median
umbilical fold
(urachus)

Rectus
abdominus m.

Lateral
umbilical fold

Lateral fossa

Medial fossa

Ductus deferens

Supravesical fossa

Obliterated
umbilical a.

Rectovesical fossa

Arcuate
line

Site of
indirect inguinal
hernia

Lateral supravesical
hernia

Site of direct
inguinal hernia

Anterior
supravesical hernia

Left ureter

Posterior supravesical
hernia

Urinary bladder

PLATE 14-11
Supravesical Hernia II

If a supravesical hernia does not become a direct or femoral hernia, it may pass into the retropubic space (of Retzius), behind the pubis and in front of the bladder. Such a hernia is said to be an *anterior internal* supravesical hernia.

Another possible pathway is posterior to the bladder and anterior to the rectum in the male, or the uterus in the female. This is a *posterior internal* supravesical hernia.

Remember:

The boundaries of *prevesical* and *paravesical* hernia rings may be described as follows: superior, the upward continuation of the vesical fascia and its fusion with the transversalis fascia and the peritoneum; inferior, fold of vesical fascia and peritoneum; lateral, the lateral umbilical ligament and peritoneum; medial, the medial umbilical ligament and peritoneum. Boundaries of the *retrovesical* hernial ring are superior and anterior, the vesical fascia and peritoneum of the posterior bladder wall; inferior and posterior, the transverse vesical fold.

If enlargement of the ring is necessary, the posterior margins should be incised upward.

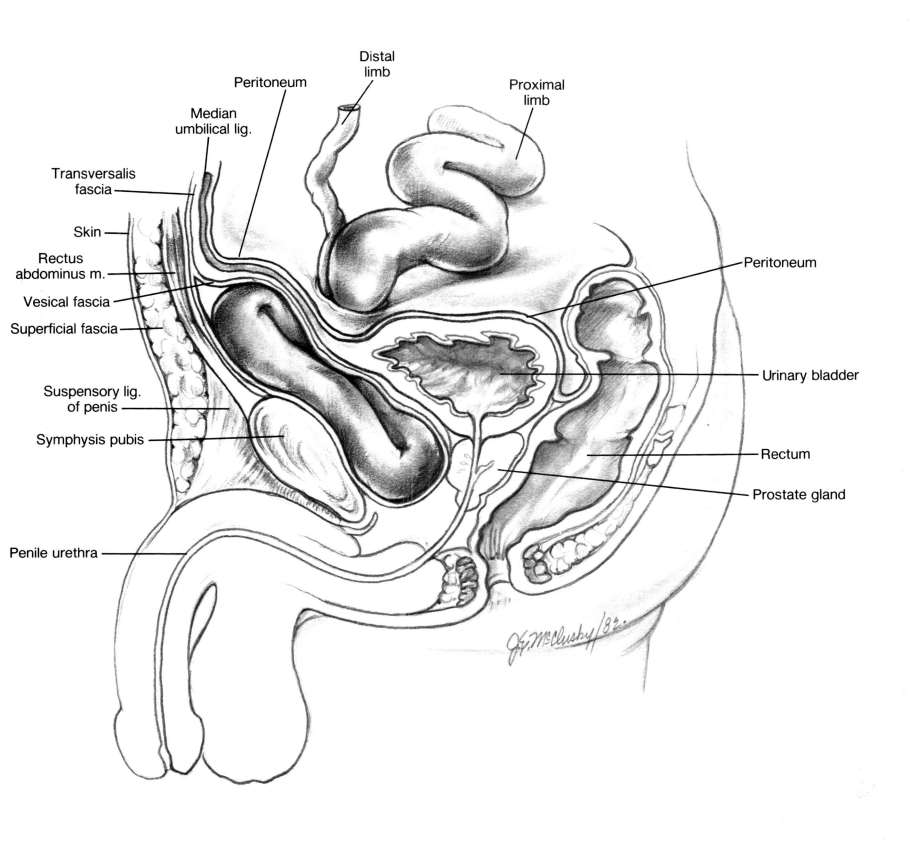

Distal
limb

Peritoneum

Proximal
limb

Median
umbilical lig.

Transversalis
fascia

Skin

Rectus
abdominus m.

Vesical fascia

Superficial fascia

Suspensory lig.
of penis

Symphysis pubis

Penile urethra

Peritoneum

Urinary bladder

Rectum

Prostate gland

PLATE 14-12
Synoptic Table of Groin Hernias

PLATE 14-12
Types of Groin Hernias and Complications of Their Repair

| Type of Hernia | Anatomy | | Complications of Hernia Repair | | |
	Origin	Pathway	Possible Vascular Injury	Possible Organ Injury	Possible Nerve Injury
Indirect Inguinal	Through internal inguinal ring in lateral fossa of anterior abdominal wall	Through external inguinal ring to scrotum	*Hemorrhage from:* Inferior epigastric artery, external iliac artery, vessels of spermatic cord, femoral vein	Ductus deferens Spermatic cord Incarcerated intestinal loop Testicular infarction, swelling, atrophy or necrosis	Iliohypogastric nerve Ilioinguinal nerve Genitofemoral nerve
Direct Inguinal	Through the medial fossa of anterior abdominal wall	Through external inguinal ring to scrotum	*Ischemic from:* Ligation of external iliac artery	Urinary bladder	
Supravesical	Through the supravesical fossa of anterior abdominal wall	*External:* Through external inguinal ring to scrotum *Internal:* Into retropubic space (of Retzius) anteriorly, *or* vesicorectal space posteriorly			
Femoral	Below the inguinal ligament	Through femoral ring and femoral canal to saphenous opening (fossa ovalis)	Aberrant obturator artery Femoral vein		

PLATE 14-13
Obturator Hernia

A. An obturator hernia passes through the obturator canal with the obturator nerve and artery. Superiorly and medially the boundary of the ring is formed by the obturator groove of the superior ramus of the pubic bone, inferiorly by the edge of the obturator membrane, and laterally by the obturator nerve, artery and vein.

The obturator vessels lie lateral to the sac in 50% of patients, and medial, anterior or posterior in the remainder. Because of the relations of the sac to nerves and vessels, the incision should be made at the lower margin of the ring.

B. The sac may follow the anterior division of the obturator nerve, passing between the pectineus and obturator externus muscle.

C. The sac may follow the posterior division of the obturator nerve, passing through the obturator externus muscle.

Remember:

1) The obturator nerve, formed by the second, third and fourth lumbar vertebrae, is found at the medial border of the psoas muscle and lateral to the hypogastric vessels and the ureter. It enters the medial side of the thigh by way of the obturator foramen.

2) Severance of the nerve impairs external rotation and adduction of the thigh. Pressure on the nerve by the hernia produces pain in the medial side of the thigh and knee (Howship-Romberg sign).

3) Injury to both nerves results in serious disability.

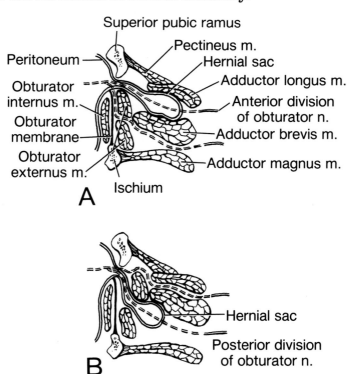

Diagrams of the path of obturator hernias following the anterior or posterior divisions of the obturator nerve.

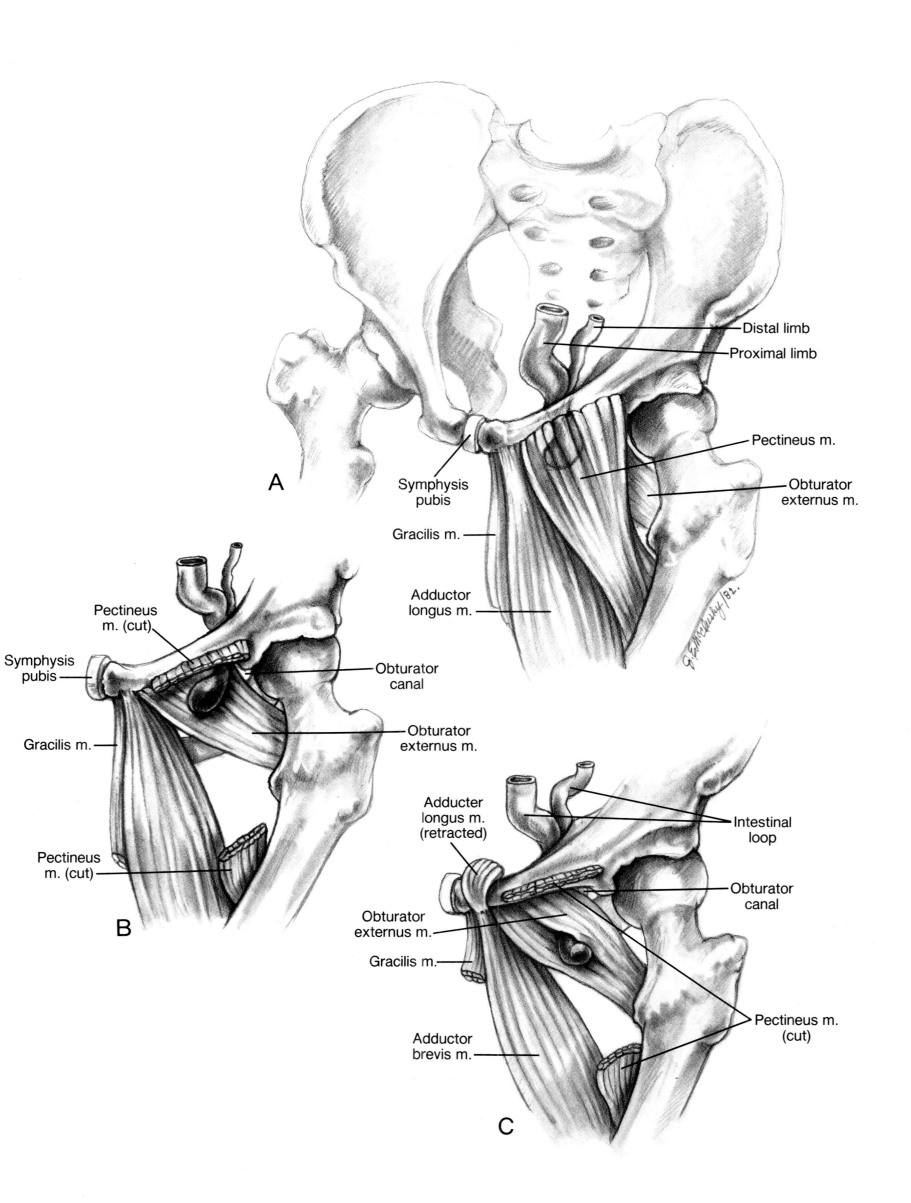

A

Distal limb
Proximal limb

Pectineus m.

Obturator
externus m.

Symphysis
pubis

Gracilis m.

Adductor
longus m.

Pectineus
m. (cut)

Symphysis
pubis

Obturator
canal

Gracilis m.

Obturator
externus m.

Pectineus
m. (cut)

B

Adducter
longus m.
(retracted)

Intestinal
loop

Obturator
canal

Obturator
externus m.

Gracilis m.

Pectineus m.
(cut)

Adductor
brevis m.

C

PLATE 14-14
Sciatic Hernias

1. Suprapiriformis (suprapyramidal) hernia passes through the greater sciatic foramen above the piriformis muscle. Through this foramen pass the piriformis muscle, superior and inferior gluteal nerves and vessels, internal pudendal nerves and vessels, posterior femoral cutaneous nerve, nerves to internal obturator and quadratus femoris muscles and the sciatic nerve. Transection of the piriform muscle by a posterior and inferior incision will relieve an incarcerated hernia.

2. Infrapiriformis (infrapyramidal) hernia passes through the greater sciatic foramen below the muscle. Transection of the muscle will relieve incarceration.

3. Subspinous hernia passes through the lesser sciatic foramen bounded above by the sacrospinous ligament, posteriorly by the sacrotuberous ligament, and anteriorly by the ischium. Reduction without incising the ring is preferred. If reduction is impossible, incise the obturator internus muscle.

Table: The Rings of the Sciatic Hernias

1) Ring of suprapyramidal hernia:

Superior:	anterior sacroiliac ligament
Inferior:	upper border of piriformis muscle
Lateral:	ilium
Medial:	upper part of sacrotuberalis ligament and part of sacrum

2) Ring of subspinous hernia:

Anterior:	ischial tuberosity
Superior:	sacrospinous ligament and ischial spine
Posterior:	sacrotuberous ligament

3) Ring of infrapyramidal hernia

Superior:	lower border of piriformis muscle
Inferior:	sacrospinous ligament
Posterior:	sacrotuberous ligament
Anterior:	ilium

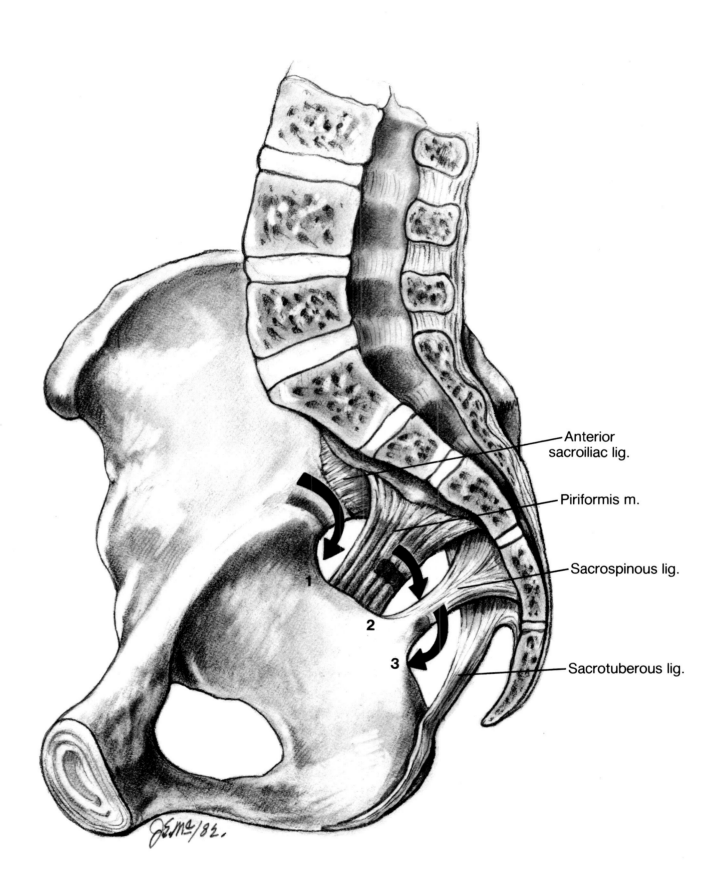

Anterior
sacroiliac lig.

Piriformis m.

Sacrospinous lig.

Sacrotuberous lig.

PLATE 14-15
Perineal Hernia

A perineal hernia may form anterior or posterior to the superficial transverse perineal muscle, through the levator ani muscle or between levator ani and coccygeus.

An anterior hernia protrudes into a triangle formed medially by the bulbocavernosus muscle, laterally by the ischiocavernosus muscle and the transversus perineal muscle posteriorly. It is found only in females and the sac may enter the labium majus (pudendal hernia).

A posterior perineal hernia may pass between component fibers of levator ani muscle or between levator ani and coccygeus muscles. It may emerge halfway between the ischial tuberosity and the anus.

Remember:

Nick the neck to release the incarcerated viscus.

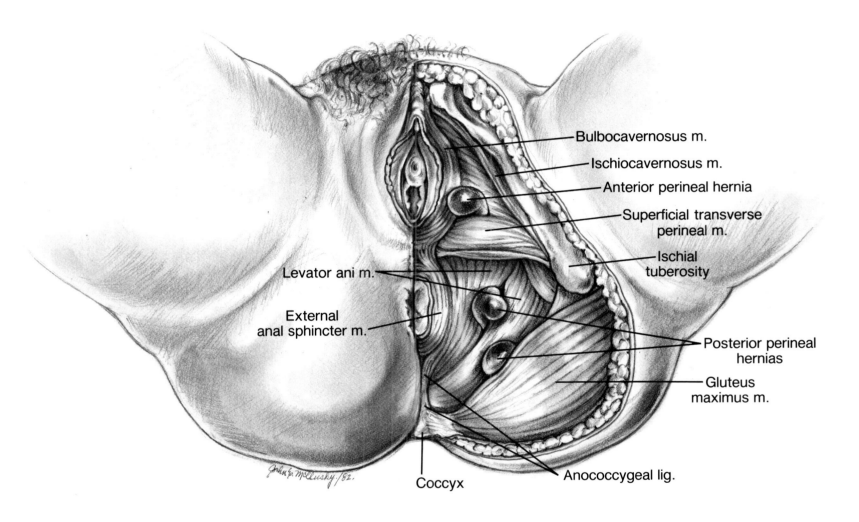

Bulbocavernosus m.

Ischiocavernosus m.

Anterior perineal hernia

Superficial transverse
perineal m.

Ischial
tuberosity

Levator ani m.

External
anal sphincter m.

Posterior perineal
hernias

Gluteus
maximus m.

Coccyx

Anococcygeal lig.

PLATE 14-16
Hernia through the Inferior Lumbar Triangle

This hernia (Petit's hernia) passes through the triangle bounded anteriorly by the posterior border of the external oblique muscle, posteriorly by the anterior border of the latissimus dorsi muscle and inferiorly by the iliac crest. The floor of the triangle is formed by the lumbodorsal fascia and the internal oblique muscle. These structures form the ring of a small hernia. If the hernia is large, the boundaries of the triangle will form the ring. Medial or lateral incision of the lumbodorsal fascia will relieve incarceration.

Hernia may also occur through the superior lumbar triangle (not illustrated). The boundaries are: (1) Anterior (abdominal): posterior border of the internal oblique muscle; (2) Posterior (lumbar): anterior border of the sacrospinalis muscle; (3) Base (costal): serratus posterior inferior muscle and twelfth rib; (4) Floor: transversus abdominis aponeurosis.

If the hernia is small, the transversus abdominis aponeurosis forms the ring; if the hernia is large, the ring is formed by the boundaries of the triangle.

Remember:

1) In hernias through the superior triangle, the ring may be enlarged by incising the lumbodorsal fascia medially or laterally.

2) In hernias through the inferior triangle, the ring should be enlarged by an incision between the 12th rib and the iliac crest.

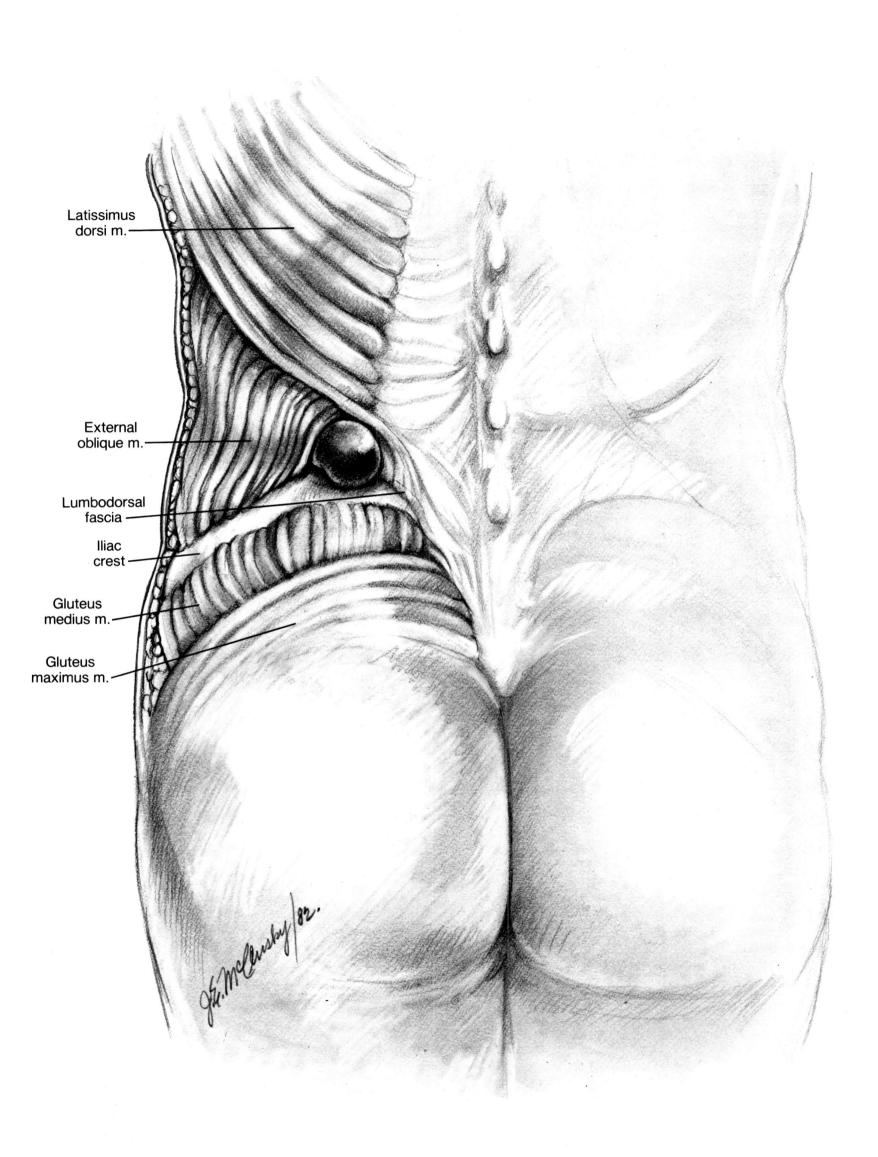

Latissimus
dorsi m.

External
oblique m.

Lumbodorsal
fascia

Iliac
crest

Gluteus
medius m.

Gluteus
maximus m.

PLATE 14-17
Hernias of the Anterior Body Wall

A. The anterior body wall showing sites of hernias.

B. and *inset.* Lateral ventral hernia (Spigelian hernia) occurs in the "semilunar zone" between the muscular fibers and the aponeurosis of the transversus abdominis muscle. Between these, the hernias may occur from above the umbilicus to the symphysis pubis. Most Spigelian hernias are found at the level of the linea semicircularis. The aponeurosis of the internal oblique and transversus abdominis muscles form the hernial ring. If the hernia is above the umbilicus, the defect is formed by a tear in the transversus abdominis muscle and a corresponding defect of the external oblique aponeurosis.

   The sac lies under the aponeurosis of the external oblique muscle which must be incised carefully. The procedures for umbilical herniorrhaphy should be followed.

C. Epigastric hernia (hernia through the linea alba) may occur anywhere from the xiphoid process to the umbilicus. The sac is peritoneum, covered with skin. The linea alba may be incised either upward or downward to release the incarcerated organ.

D. Acquired umbilical hernia in adults is usually through the upper part of the umbilical ring. Fusion of all layers of the abdominal wall forms the ring. The sac is peritoneum covered by skin. The incision should pass around, never over, the hernial sac. The ring should be incised laterally and the incision may extend into the aponeurosis of the rectus muscle if necessary.

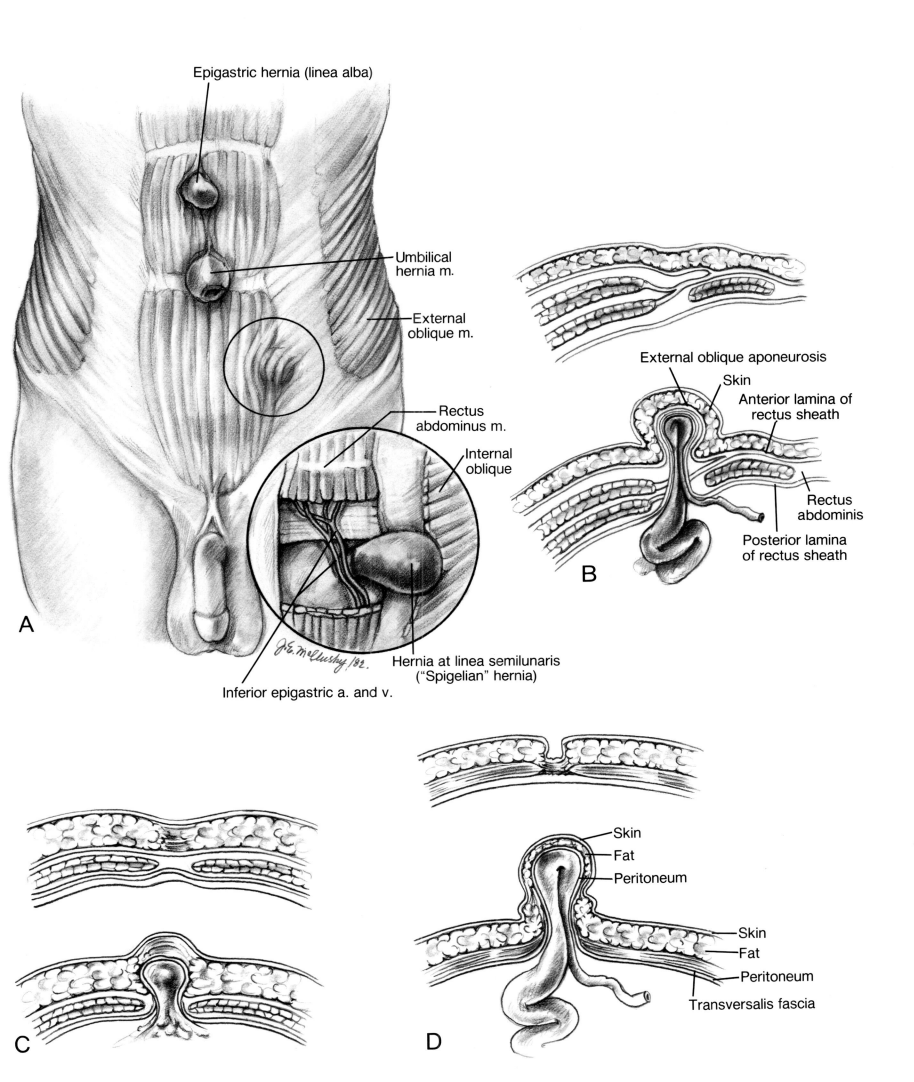

Epigastric hernia (linea alba)

Umbilical
hernia m.

External
oblique m.

Rectus
abdominus m.

Internal
oblique

External oblique aponeurosis

Skin

Anterior lamina of
rectus sheath

Rectus
abdominis

Posterior lamina
of rectus sheath

B

Hernia at linea semilunaris
("Spigelian" hernia)

Inferior epigastric a. and v.

A

J.E. McCleushy /82.

Skin
Fat
Peritoneum

Skin
Fat
Peritoneum
Transversalis fascia

C

D

PLATE 14-18
Gastroschisis and Omphalocele

In both of these conditions the intestines are extra-abdominal at birth. The abdominal cavity is usually too small to accommodate the herniated mass of intestines.

A. Gastroschisis passes through a congenital defect of the abdominal wall to the right or left of the midline. The ring is formed by all of the layers of the abdominal wall and there is no hernial sac. The intestines are usually embedded in a gelatinous matrix. Rarely, the lower edge of the ring must be incised.

B. Section through the abdominal wall at the site of gastroschisis.

C. Omphalocele is a failure of the normal return of the intestines to the abdomen in the third month of gestation. The mass of intestines passes through the umbilical ring in the midline and is covered by a sac of peritoneum. It is not to be confused with the slight bulging of the abdomen between the recti often seen in infants.

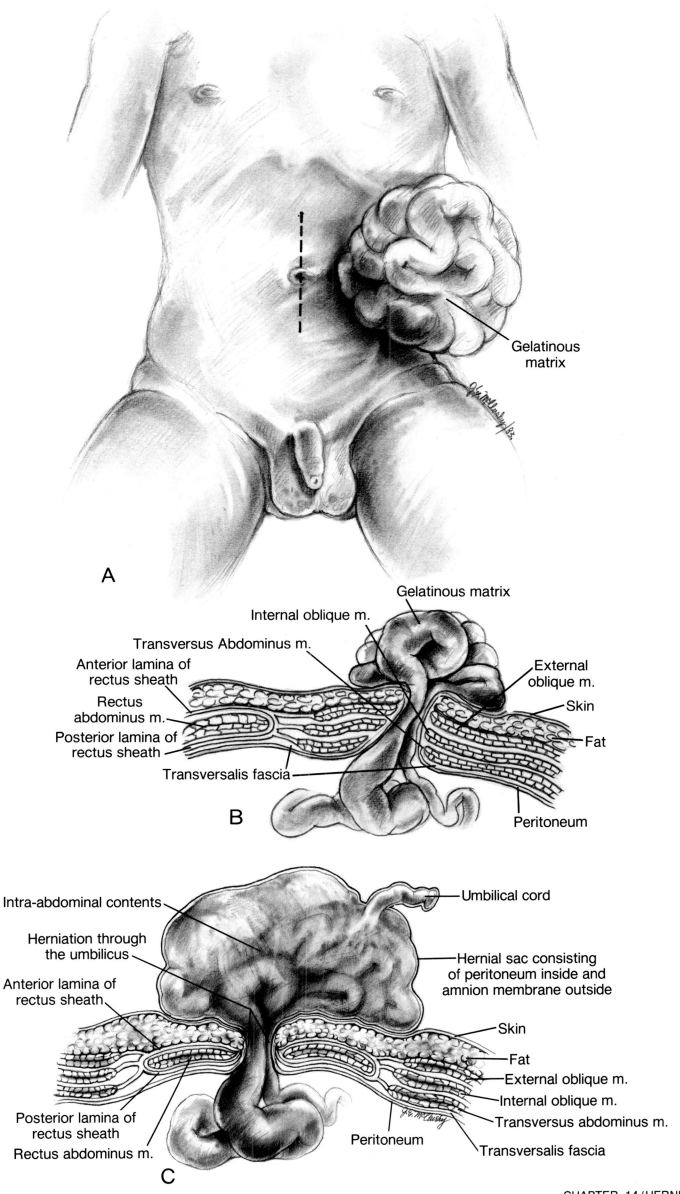

Gelatinous matrix

A

Gelatinous matrix

Internal oblique m.

Transversus Abdominus m.

Anterior lamina of rectus sheath

Rectus abdominus m.

Posterior lamina of rectus sheath

Transversalis fascia

External oblique m.

Skin

Fat

Peritoneum

B

Intra-abdominal contents

Herniation through the umbilicus

Anterior lamina of rectus sheath

Posterior lamina of rectus sheath

Rectus abdominus m.

Umbilical cord

Hernial sac consisting of peritoneum inside and amnion membrane outside

Skin

Fat

External oblique m.

Internal oblique m.

Transversus abdominus m.

Peritoneum

Transversalis fascia

C

PLATE 14-19
Paraduodenal Hernias I

These hernias may occur in a series of inconstant peritoneal fossae with a confusing terminology (see Plate 4–8). "Left" and "right" refer to the direction in which an intestinal loop would pass if it actually herniated into the fossa.

The most frequently encountered hernias are those into the inferior and superior duodenal fossae.

A right paraduodenal fossa and its boundaries are shown in Plate 14–20. The boundaries of the less common left paraduodenal hernial sac are: superiorly, the duodenojejunal flexure; anteriorly, the inferior mesenteric vein; right, the aorta; left, the left kidney.

Table: The Five Most Common Paraduodenal Fossae

Hernial Site	Direction of Hernia	Relative Incidence
1. Intermesocolic fossa (Brösike)	Right	Rare
2. Superior duodenal fossa (Treitz)	Right	50–30%
3. Paraduodenal fossa (Landzert)	Left	2%
4. inferior duodenal fossa (Treitz)	Right	75–50%
5. Mesenterico-parietal fossa (Waldeyer)	Right	1%

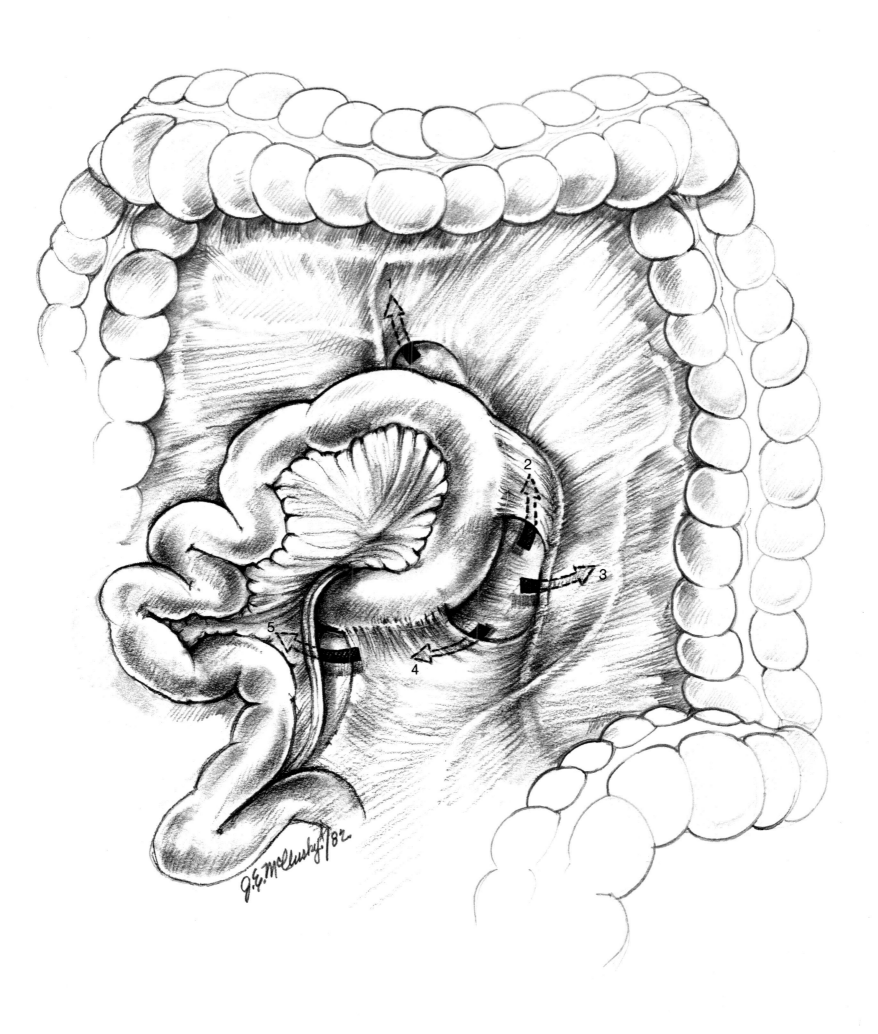

PLATE 14-20
Paraduodenal Hernias II

A right paraduodenal hernia through the mesentericoparietal fossa (of Waldeyer). As the hernia enlarges, its precise origin becomes difficult to determine.

The mouth of the sac lies behind the superior mesenteric artery and vein at the base of the mesentery; the mouth opens to the left; the fundus is directed to the right. The boundaries of the neck are superiorly, the duodenum; anteriorly, the superior mesenteric or ileocolic artery; posteriorly, the lumbar vertebrae.

The incision should be in the lower part of the ring. Decompression before attempting reduction may be necessary.

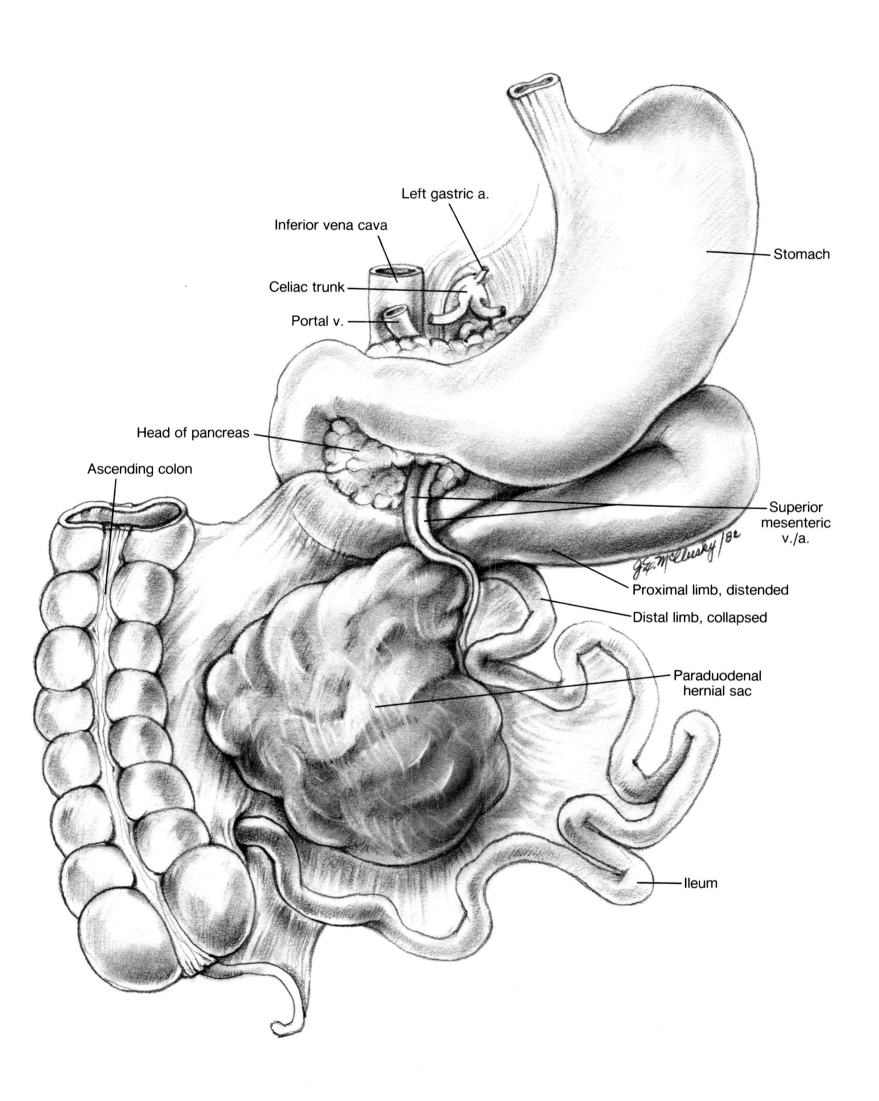

Left gastric a.

Inferior vena cava

Celiac trunk

Portal v.

Head of pancreas

Ascending colon

Stomach

Superior mesenteric v./a.

Proximal limb, distended

Distal limb, collapsed

Paraduodenal hernial sac

Ileum

PLATE 14-21
Hernia through the Sigmoid Mesocolon

As in other transmesenteric hernias, the incarcerated viscus enters a small hole in the mesentery and enlarges it until a large blood vessel limits further expansion and forms at least one free edge. The vessel is usually a branch of the inferior mesenteric artery. There is no hernial sac. The dilated proximal limb of the incarcerated loop should be decompressed and reduced. Do not incise the ring.

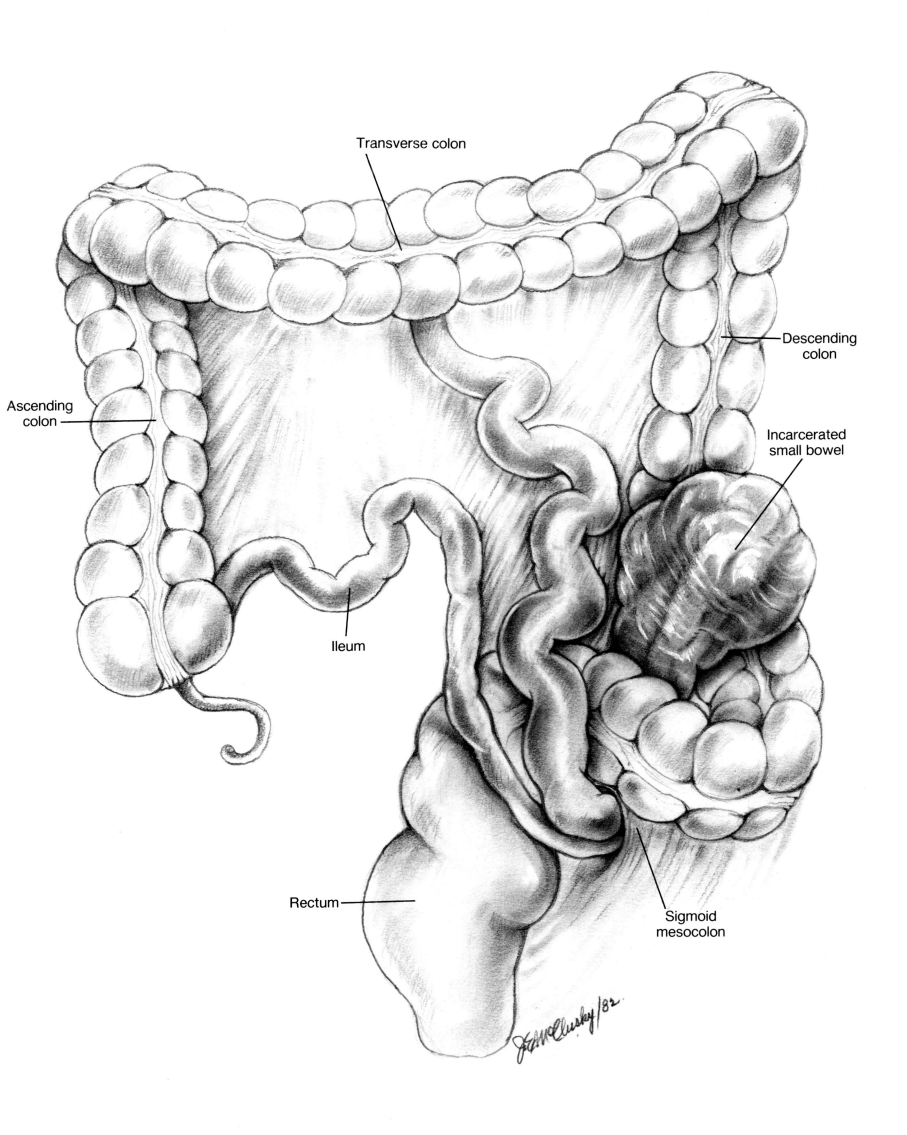

Transverse colon

Descending colon

Ascending colon

Incarcerated small bowel

Ileum

Rectum

Sigmoid mesocolon

PLATE 14-22
Hernia through the Greater Omentum

A large blood vessel will form at least one edge of the hernia ring. Incise the omentum after clamping the vessel.

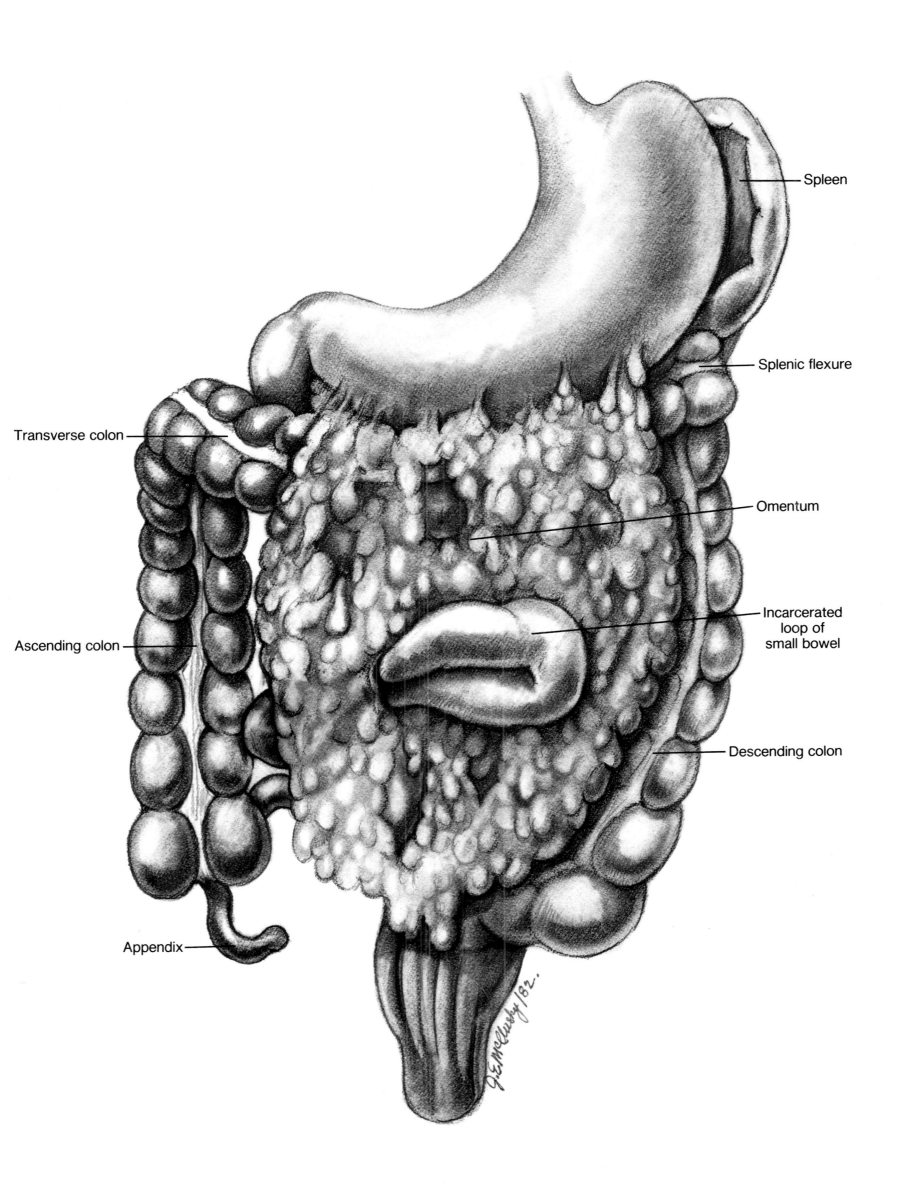

Spleen

Splenic flexure

Omentum

Incarcerated
loop of
small bowel

Descending colon

Transverse colon

Ascending colon

Appendix

PLATE 14-23
Hernia through the Falciform Ligament

This is an extremely rare lesion. It serves to illustrate the fact that any aperture, through any part of the peritoneum, either mesenteric or parietal, is a potential site for herniation.

Remember:

The presence of one hernia does not preclude the presence of another hernia elsewhere in the abdomen or its wall.

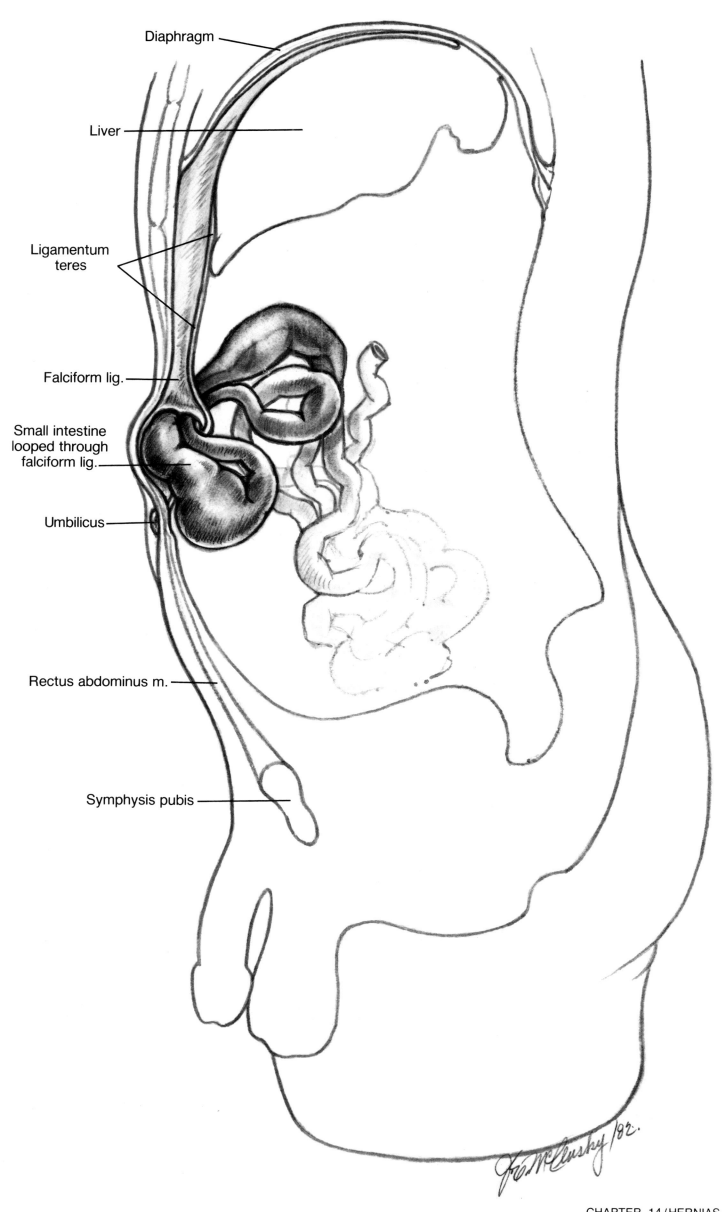

Diaphragm

Liver

Ligamentum
teres

Falciform lig.

Small intestine
looped through
falciform lig.

Umbilicus

Rectus abdominus m.

Symphysis pubis

PLATE 14-24
Hernia through the Epiploic Foramen of Winslow

The neck of the hernia is bounded above by the caudate process of the liver and the inferior layer of the coronary ligament, anteriorly by the hepatoduodenal ligament carrying the portal vein, the hepatic artery and the common bile duct. Posteriorly is the inferior vena cava and inferiorly is the first part of the duodenum and the hepatic artery. Reduction must be by decompression. There is no excuse for dividing the sac.

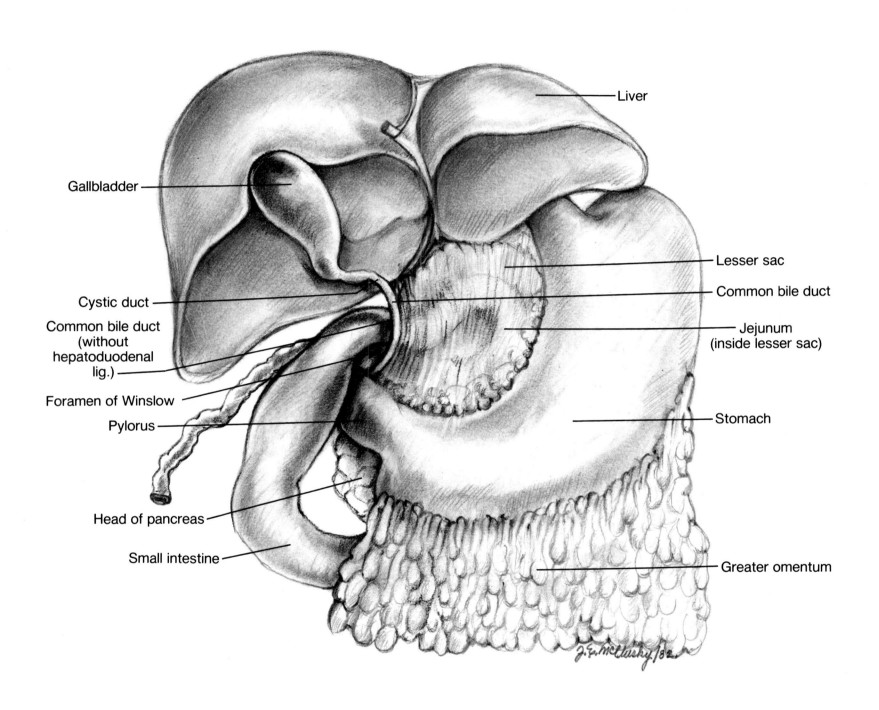

Gallbladder

Cystic duct

Common bile duct
(without
hepatoduodenal
lig.)

Foramen of Winslow

Pylorus

Head of pancreas

Small intestine

Liver

Lesser sac

Common bile duct

Jejunum
(inside lesser sac)

Stomach

Greater omentum

PLATE 14-25
Hernia through the Broad Ligament

This is an extremely rare hernia shown in anterior view. The proper ligament of the ovary bounds the hernial sac superiorly.

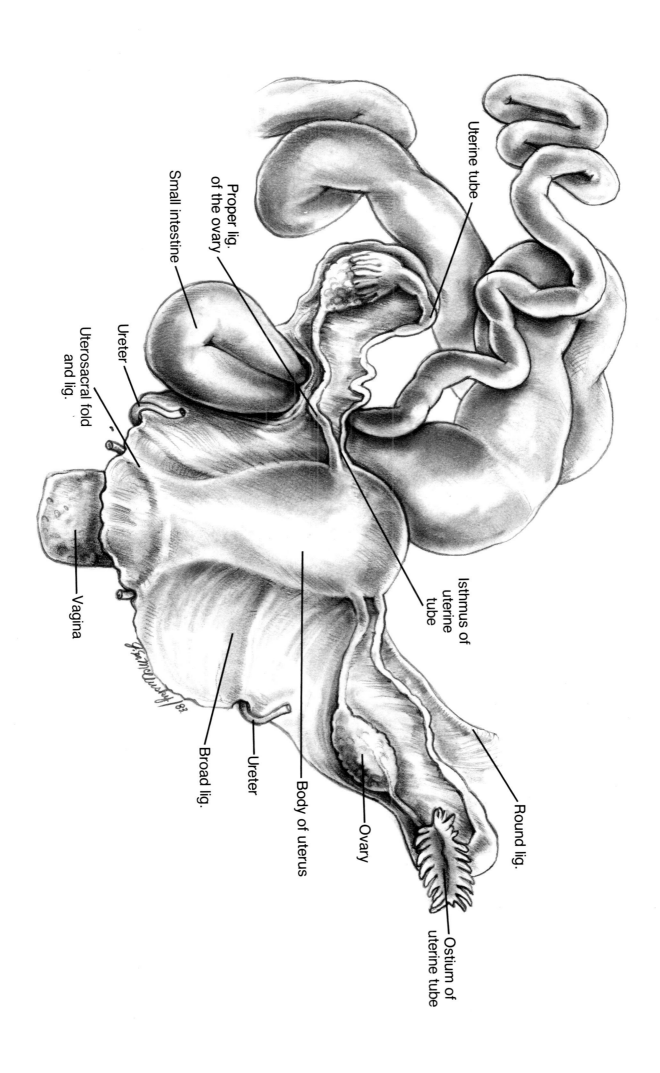

Uterine tube

Proper lig.
of the ovary

Small intestine

Ureter

Uterosacral fold
and lig.

Vagina

Broad lig.

Ureter

Body of uterus

Ovary

Round lig.

Ostium of
uterine tube

Isthmus of
uterine tube

Index

Page numbers in *italics* denote figures; those followed by 't' for 'f' denote tables or footnotes, respectively.